Diabetology: Feature Papers 2022

Diabetology: Feature Papers 2022

Editor

Peter Clifton

MDPI • Basel • Beijing • Wuhan • Barcelona • Belgrade • Manchester • Tokyo • Cluj • Tianjin

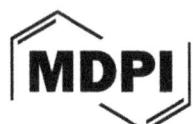

Editor
Peter Clifton
University of South Australia
Australia

Editorial Office
MDPI
St. Alban-Anlage 66
4052 Basel, Switzerland

This is a reprint of articles from the Special Issue published online in the open access journal *Diabetology* (ISSN 2673-4540) (available at: https://www.mdpi.com/si/diabetology/Diabetology_Feature_Papers).

For citation purposes, cite each article independently as indicated on the article page online and as indicated below:

LastName, A.A.; LastName, B.B.; LastName, C.C. Article Title. *Journal Name* **Year**, *Volume Number*, Page Range.

ISBN 978-3-0365-7256-7 (Hbk)
ISBN 978-3-0365-7257-4 (PDF)

© 2023 by the authors. Articles in this book are Open Access and distributed under the Creative Commons Attribution (CC BY) license, which allows users to download, copy and build upon published articles, as long as the author and publisher are properly credited, which ensures maximum dissemination and a wider impact of our publications.

The book as a whole is distributed by MDPI under the terms and conditions of the Creative Commons license CC BY-NC-ND.

Contents

Sally L. Bullock, Telma Menendez, Liz Schwarte, Lisa Craypo, Jennifer T. Mosst, Gabrielle Green, et al.
Transitioning to Telehealth during COVID-19: Experiences and Insights from Diabetes Prevention and Management Program Providers in Los Angeles County
Reprinted from: *Diabetology* **2023**, *4*, 6, doi:10.3390/diabetology4010006 1

Angezwa Siboto, Akinjide Moses Akinnuga, Muhammed Bilaal Ismail, Irvin Noel Booysen, Ntethelelo Hopewell Sibiya, Phikelelani Ngubane and Andile Khathi
Investigating the Protective Effects of a Rhenium (V) Compound with Uracil-Derived Ligands on Liver Damage Associated with Prediabetes in Diet-Induced Prediabetic Rats
Reprinted from: *Diabetology* **2022**, *3*, 40, doi:10.3390/diabetology3040040 17

Dessi P. Zaharieva, Ananta Addala, Priya Prahalad, Brianna Leverenz, Nora Arrizon-Ruiz, Victoria Y. Ding, et al.
An Evaluation of Point-of-Care HbA1c, HbA1c Home Kits, and Glucose Management Indicator: Potential Solutions for Telehealth Glycemic Assessments
Reprinted from: *Diabetology* **2022**, *3*, 37, doi:10.3390/diabetology3030037 33

Sahana Parthasarathy, Natalia Chamorro-Pareja, Amrin Kharawala, Kenneth H Hupart, Joan Curcio, Christina Coyle, et al.
Diabetic Ketoacidosis Was Associated with High Morbidity and Mortality in Hospitalized Patients with COVID-19 in the NYC Public Health System
Reprinted from: *Diabetology* **2022**, *3*, 36, doi:10.3390/diabetology3030036 41

Dimitar Sajkov, Bliegh Mupunga, Jeffrey J. Bowden, Christopher Langton and Nikolai Petrovsky
Narrative Review: Obesity, Type 2 DM and Obstructive Sleep Apnoea—Common Bedfellows
Reprinted from: *Diabetology* **2022**, *3*, 33, doi:10.3390/diabetology3030033 59

Rashid M. Ansari, Mark F. Harris, Hassan Hosseinzadeh and Nicholas Zwar
Implementation of Chronic Care Model for Diabetes Self-Management: A Quantitative Analysis
Reprinted from: *Diabetology* **2022**, *3*, 31, doi:10.3390/diabetology3030031 73

Paul Zimmermann, Felix Aberer, Max L. Eckstein, Sandra Haupt, Maximilian P. Erlmann and Othmar Moser
Verapamil and Its Role in Diabetes
Reprinted from: *Diabetology* **2022**, *3*, 30, doi:10.3390/diabetology3030030 89

Ahmed Abdelhafiz, Shail Bisht, Iva Kovacevic, Daniel Pennells and Alan Sinclair
Insulin in Frail, Older People with Type 2 Diabetes—Low Threshold for Therapy
Reprinted from: *Diabetology* **2022**, *3*, 28, doi:10.3390/diabetology3020028 103

Sandro Gentile, Ersilia Satta, Giuseppina Guarino and Felice Strollo
Lipodystrophies from Insulin Injection: An Update of the Italian Consensus Statement of AMD-OSDI Study Group on Injection Technique
Reprinted from: *Diabetology* **2023**, *4*, 13, doi:10.3390/diabetology4010013 119

Hanako Nakajima, Hiroshi Okada, Akinori Kogure, Takafumi Osaka, Takeshi Tsutsumi, Toru Tanaka, et al.
Multicenter, Open Label, Randomized Controlled Superiority Trial for Availability to Reduce Nocturnal Urination Frequency: Study Protocol for a TOP-STAR Study
Reprinted from: *Diabetology* **2022**, *3*, 48, doi:10.3390/diabetology3040048 129

Felice Strollo, Ersilia Satta and Sandro Gentile
Insulin Injection-Related Skin Lipodystrophies: Blemish or Pathology?
Reprinted from: *Diabetology* **2022**, *3*, 47, doi:10.3390/diabetology3040047 . . . . **143**

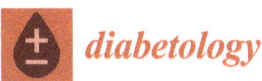

Article

Transitioning to Telehealth during COVID-19: Experiences and Insights from Diabetes Prevention and Management Program Providers in Los Angeles County

Sally L. Bullock [1,*], Telma Menendez [2], Liz Schwarte [3], Lisa Craypo [3], Jennifer T. Mosst [4], Gabrielle Green [2], Noel C. Barragan [2] and Tony Kuo [5,6,7]

1. Department of Public Health, Davidson College, Box 7135, Davidson, NC 28035, USA
2. Division of Chronic Disease and Injury Prevention, Los Angeles County Department of Public Health, 3530 Wilshire Blvd, 8th Floor, Los Angeles, CA 90010, USA
3. Ad. Lucem Consulting, 729 Coventry Rd., Kensington, CA 94707, USA
4. Public Health Consultant, Healthified Consulting Services, Box 671793, Marietta, GA 30006, USA
5. Department of Family Medicine, David Geffen School of Medicine at University of California, Los Angeles (UCLA), 10880 Wilshire Blvd., Suite 1800, Los Angeles, CA 90024, USA
6. Department of Epidemiology, UCLA Fielding School of Public Health, Box 951722, Los Angeles, CA 90095, USA
7. Population Health Program, UCLA Clinical and Translational Science Institute, 10833 Le Conte Ave., BE–144 CHS, Los Angeles, CA 90095, USA
* Correspondence: sabullock@davidson.edu

Abstract: The onset of the COVID-19 pandemic in March 2020 accelerated the efforts of several organizations providing the National Diabetes Prevention Program (National DPP) and the Diabetes Self-Management Education and Support (DSMES) program to rapidly transition from in-person service delivery to program administration via telehealth. Semi-structured interviews were conducted with 35 National DPP and DSMES experts and providers in Los Angeles County to gain a better understanding of the challenges and benefits associated with this transition. Interviews were completed during June to October 2021. Thematic analyses were performed using the Social-Ecological Model as a guiding framework. The analyses revealed several factors that influenced the transition, including at the individual (e.g., technology and health behaviors), interpersonal (e.g., social connections and support), organizational (e.g., provider workload and program enrollment and retention), community (e.g., recruitment), and policy (e.g., government support and reimbursement for telehealth services) levels. Findings suggest that the transition to telehealth was challenging for most National DPP and DSMES providers. However, because of its lower cost, ability to reach long distances virtually, and potential efficiency when employed as part of a hybrid approach, this delivery modality remains viable, offering benefits beyond the traditional program models.

Keywords: key informant interviews; prevention of type 2 diabetes; self-management of type 2 diabetes; National DPP; DSMES; telehealth; provider experiences; COVID-19

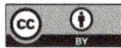

1. Introduction

In the United States, an estimated 34.1 million adults have diabetes, and 88 million have prediabetes [1]. In Los Angeles County, California, approximately 1 in 10 adults has been diagnosed with type 2 diabetes [2]. Individuals with diabetes are at risk for many serious health problems, including heart disease, stroke, chronic kidney failure, amputations of lower limbs, blindness, and premature death [3]. They are also at increased risk for severe disease and death from the coronavirus disease 2019 (COVID-19) [4]; thus, limiting exposure to the virus that causes COVID-19 has been a critical priority for protecting individuals with these conditions throughout the pandemic.

Even before the pandemic, efforts to locally promote diabetes prevention and management have focused on increasing access to and use of the National Diabetes Prevention Program (National DPP) and Diabetes Self-Management Education and Support (DSMES) program services. The National DPP is a year-long lifestyle change program based on the original Diabetes Prevention Program [5–7], which has been shown to reduce the incidence of diabetes in the short term and over time [5,8]. Likewise, DSMES is an evidence-based service model designed for individuals diagnosed with diabetes, with education services that have been shown to improve eating patterns, activity levels, and hemoglobin A1C (HbA1c) levels among program participants [9].

While telehealth is not a novel approach to either program model, the onset of the COVID-19 pandemic in March 2020 accelerated its use by National DPP and DSMES providers across Los Angeles County (LAC) and elsewhere in the United States (U.S.). This rapid transition from in-person service delivery to a virtual format was unprecedented in this regard. Telehealth, by definition and by standard practice, includes the use of telecommunications technologies of various forms to provide healthcare and health education. The modality can involve live videoconferencing, the electronic transmission of health information, and the use of devices to collect and transmit data to providers to assist with clinical decision-making (e.g., remote glucose monitor, remote weight monitoring device) [10].

Prior to the pandemic, both National DPP and DSMES programming were offered in-person, sometimes via telehealth, and through other technology-based modalities [8,11]. Prior studies indicate that programs delivered via telehealth can result in observable improvements to health and behavioral outcomes [11–16]. However, the majority of organizations providing National DPP and DSMES in LAC at the start of the pandemic provided them primarily in-person [17,18]. Nationally, the use of telehealth for these two programs, and for healthcare services more broadly, had been low before the health crisis [19–21]. Reported barriers to telehealth included a lack of technical skills and/or equipment, privacy and security concerns, provider comfort and organizational support of the modality, and a lack of adequate reimbursement for such services [22–24]. The shelter-in-place orders and other efforts to decrease the spread of COVID-19, in a sense, forced providers to come up with innovative solutions to these barriers as they moved from a traditional in-person delivery model to telehealth.

Although pre-pandemic research on telehealth is not sparse in the health services research literature, it has not been conducted for transitions that took place on a very short timeline. For example, little is known about the challenges or the optimal practices that are needed to rapidly switch from primarily in-person sessions to virtual sessions that are facilitated by evolving technology platforms such as Zoom, GoToMeeting, or Doximity. This study explores the experiences and insights of 35 National DPP and DSMES experts and providers in LAC to identify opportunities where integration of telehealth into these 2 program models can help improve the delivery of diabetes prevention and management services, including ways to better increase participation and retention.

2. Methods

2.1. Study Design

A qualitative, key informant study was employed for this project. Thirty-five semi-structured interviews were conducted between June and October 2021. A core project team guided the design, methods, data collection, and analysis of the interview data. The team consisted of staff from Ad Lucem Consulting and the Los Angeles County Department of Public Health (DPH). The DPH's Institutional Review Board reviewed and approved the study protocols and materials.

2.2. Setting

In LAC and at the time of the study, there were approximately 35 organizations that were either accredited by the American Association of Diabetes Care and Education

Specialists (ADCES) or recognized by the American Diabetes Association (ADA) to provide DSMES services [17], and 43 organizations that provided the National DPP [18]. Some of these organizations provided both National DPP and DSMES services. Many that offered the National DPP had applied for and received recognition from the Centers for Disease Control and Prevention (CDC) Diabetes Prevention Recognition Program (DPRP), a program entity that reviews and affirms the effective delivery of DPP services. The organizations providing these services included hospitals and healthcare systems, community-based organizations, Federally Qualified Health Centers (FQHCs), community health centers, pharmacies, universities, and health plans/insurers.

2.3. Participants

Key informant interviews were conducted with experts and providers of National DPP and/or DSMES programs in LAC. The former were not restricted to local experts—they included subject matter experts from across the U.S. For both experts and providers, DPH assisted with recruitment. Some of the expert interviewees were identified through a literature review, and others were identified as "experts" by other interviewees. Experts were primarily selected based on their knowledge of and/or experience with delivering the National DPP and/or the DSMES program. All prospective interviewees were invited via email first, with follow-up phone calls as needed. In total, 56 experts and providers were contacted, and 35 were interviewed (62% response rate).

2.4. Data Collection

Two semi-structured interview guides were developed for the study, one for experts and the other for providers (see Supplementary Materials (S1) for interview guide questions). Both guides include questions about the impact of COVID-19 on National DPP/DSMES program delivery, challenges and optimal practices associated with integrating/implementing telehealth sessions, and policy and systems changes that are likely to be necessary to support and sustain telehealth practices. Experts were asked to assess the value or impacts of telehealth and what the future may look like for National DPP/DSMES that continue telehealth services. Providers were asked questions about the infrastructure and capacity needed to implement telehealth.

All interviewees provided consent prior to being interviewed and did not receive compensation for their participation. Each interview required approximately 45 min to complete, and all interviews were conducted and recorded via videoconferencing software by trained interviewers. Verbatim transcripts were generated, checked for accuracy, and loaded into ATLAS.ti (Version 22.0.6.0, access on 15 December 2022) [25] for sorting and qualitative analysis.

2.5. Qualitative Data Analysis

Interview transcripts were initially coded in ATLAS.ti for themes and subthemes using thematic analysis [26]. A codebook was then developed based on the identified themes. The transcripts were double-coded, and any differences were resolved during team meetings. The lead author coded all the transcripts, and two trained undergraduate research assistants each coded approximately half of the transcripts.

The social-ecological model (SEM) was used as a framework to describe factors that influenced the transition from in-person service delivery to services offered via telehealth. The SEM is a theory-based framework that recognizes the complex interactions between individuals, their social networks, and broader structural factors through five levels: individual, interpersonal, organizational/institutional, community, and policy [27]. The SEM has been used previously to identify factors that impact health and well-being and as the guiding framework for health promotion interventions in the community. This model serves as the organizing framework for themes identified in this study.

3. Results

A total of 35 interviews were conducted with National DPP/DSMES experts and providers. Nine were conducted with experts who represented the following organization types: health management and training ($n = 4$), health professional association ($n = 3$), state public health ($n = 1$), and academia ($n = 1$). Twenty-six were with providers, in particular, with individuals from hospitals/healthcare systems ($n = 8$), community health centers ($n = 7$), private/small businesses ($n = 4$), universities ($n = 3$), Health Resources and Services Administration-funded FQHCs ($n = 3$), and health plans/insurers ($n = 1$). Many of the providers interviewed serve populations with a high burden of diabetes and other chronic diseases.

Two expert interviewees could speak to both National DPP and DSMES delivery, two could speak to just DSMES services, and six could speak to just National DPP programming. Of the experts, two were also DPP providers, and one was delivering both National DPP and DSMES.

Almost all providers were providing in-person sessions prior to the COVID-19 pandemic, and only 2 of the 26 providers were already offering primarily telehealth National DPP and/or DSMES services. Majority of providers switched to providing telehealth services shortly after the start of the pandemic. In most cases, telehealth delivery included videoconferences and/or telephone conference calls with groups or individuals. Experts and providers used different terminology to refer to the virtual delivery of services/programming (e.g., distance learning, telehealth visits, online sessions). For consistency, we use "telehealth sessions" to refer to these services. Table 1 provides an overview of the mode of delivery before and during the pandemic by program type.

Table 1. National Diabetes Prevention Program and Diabetes Self-Management Education and Support program delivery before and after the start of the COVID-19 pandemic among 26 providers that participated in the key informant interviews.

	Program Delivery before the Pandemic		Program Delivery after Start of the Pandemic				
	In-Person Delivery	Telehealth	Continued to Offer Primarily Telehealth	Switched to Telehealth National DPP	Stopped Offering National DPP	Switched to Telehealth DSMES	Stopped Offering DSMES
National DPP ONLY	9	1 *	1	6	3	N/A	N/A
DSMES ONLY	5	0	0	N/A	N/A	5	0
National DPP and DSMES	10	1 *	1	8	2	9	1

* One provider was already offering the National DPP via telehealth, and another provider was offering both the National DPP and DSMES services via telehealth before the pandemic.

3.1. Major Themes

The themes identified during data analysis are described below and in Figure 1 and Table 2 according to the levels of the SEM. It is important to note that some themes included more than one level of influence and were organized according to where they fit best in the conceptual model.

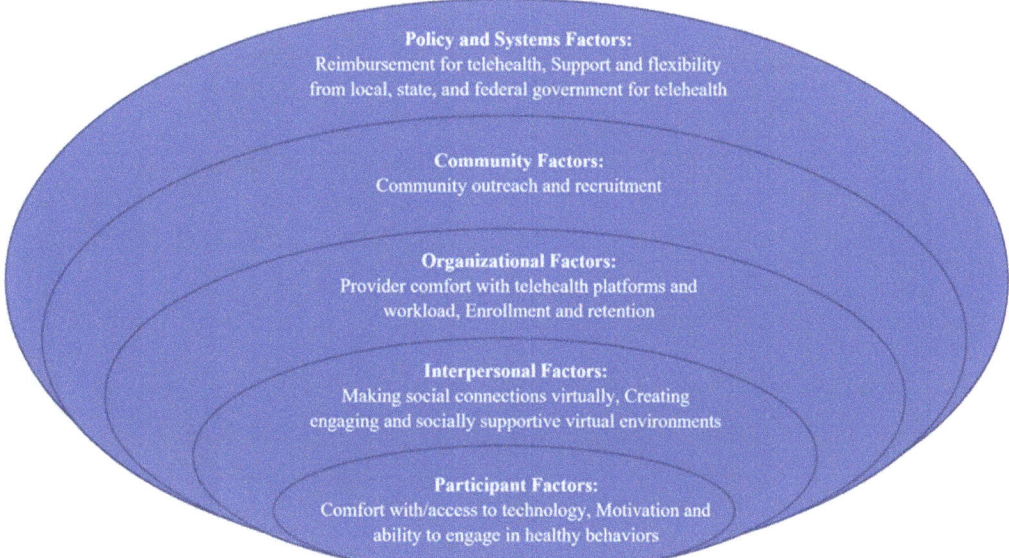

Figure 1. Social-ecological model with factors influencing telehealth delivery of the National Diabetes Prevention Program and Diabetes Self-Management Education and Support program during the COVID-19 pandemic.

Table 2. Themes and representative quotes related to telehealth delivery of the National Diabetes Prevention Program and Diabetes Self-Management Education and Support program during the COVID-19 pandemic by level of the social-ecological model.

Factors	Themes	Representative Quote(s)
Individual Participant Factors: Challenges and optimal practices influencing participants' ability to successfully participate in telehealth National DPP and DSMES		
Access to and comfort with technology	Comfort and access to technology among participants was mixed Tailored and consistent technical assistance helped many participants overcome issues with technology Despite providers' efforts, some participants were not willing or able to engage in telehealth	"We had some groups where 50% of our group didn't have access to a phone ... And then we had other groups that made the switch very easily ... [They had] access to the internet". National DPP Expert and Provider "We created a little handout flyer with like a one pager on the steps on how to connect to the class. And we mailed it to them. We use that and we use phone calls to guide them through it". National DPP and DSMES Provider
Motivation and ability to engage in healthy behaviors	Challenges collecting health data via telehealth made it difficult to determine the impact of the transition on health behaviors Participants' motivation and ability to engage in healthy behaviors and achieve certain health outcomes was mixed Providers helped participants set individualized goals to overcome challenges and provided resources when needed	"They really didn't want to share their weights. Also, we heard several people saying that they don't have access to a weighing scale. So that kind of decreased the number of people reporting weights". National DPP Provider "There was a lot of stress on participants and instead of trying to reach the DPP goal of weight loss, perhaps they would just focus on weight maintenance". National DPP Provider

Table 2. Cont.

Factors	Themes	Representative Quote(s)
Interpersonal Factors: Challenges and optimal practices for facilitating relationships and engagement in a virtual environment		
Creating engaging virtual environments and making social connections virtually	Establishing relationships between participants and between participants and providers was challenging in a virtual environment Modifying materials and delivery of curriculum, using the platform functions, sending group texts, and creating social media groups increased engagement and connection Hybrid approaches (in-person and telehealth) may be useful for establishing relationships and improving telehealth sessions	"They can connect to us. The language, the culture, we live in this community. And that helped us to have a very successful in-person class. But how do I make that connection virtually? It's just not there". National DPP and DSMES Provider "I hate to say that it's kind of like edutainment, so the more colorful and the more interesting your materials are, the more you'll get their attention". National DPP Provider
Organizational Factors: Overcoming provider and organizational barriers to providing telehealth and maintaining enrollment and retention in the programs		
Provider comfort with telehealth platforms	Comfort and familiarity with telehealth platforms and delivery was mixed among providers Training sessions for providers can be helpful for overcoming challenges with platforms and telehealth delivery Contingency plans are needed to deal with technical challenges	"Our Diabetes Prevention Program teams were not on the cutting edge of providing telehealth programming. So, there was a big learning curve for them". National DPP Provider "Your platform might be great and awesome, but the internet might go out ... I always have a dial-in conference line so everyone can get on the phone and talk". National DPP Expert and Provider
Provider workload	Transitioning to telehealth increased the workload of many providers initially but may ultimately save time and allow for program expansion	"You don't have to travel. You don't have to go anywhere. You can run it from your home office ... So those two to three, or even four hours can be used for education ... It can be evolved into providing more classes". National DPP Expert and Provider
Enrollment and retention	Programs experienced an initial drop in enrollment and retention, but many recovered and were able to expand and reach different audiences Telehealth availability increased accessibility of programs to individuals who could not participate in-person	"Now we are able to provide a DPP in summer in Florida or even Hawaii, anywhere they want ... that was a great change that we were able to adapt to be more nationwide rather than just stay in Southern California". National DPP Expert and Provider "Our enrollment actually probably was better, because people didn't have to drive here and try and find a parking space. And it could fit into their time without them really leaving their home". DSMES Provider
Community Factors: Challenges external to organizations resulting from the COVID-19 pandemic		
Community outreach and recruitment	The closure of community recruitment locations due to the pandemic made outreach and recruitment difficult for some providers Providers had to shift recruitment methods	"Recruitment was hard because we couldn't go to places and give our nutrition workshops or hang up flyers". National DPP Provider
Policy and Systems Change Factors: Policy-level barriers and support needed from government agencies for telehealth		
Reimbursement for telehealth and support/flexibility from government agencies for telehealth	Changes to National DPP eligibility requirements and flexibility for maintaining DPRP recognition are needed Adequate and sustained coverage for telehealth is needed from Medicare and Medicaid	"I think once you are recognized, you should be able to go back and forth and do both [in-person and distance learning] if you want to, instead of being pegged into just one track". National DPP Provider "Medicare has to be in-person. And I think for a lot of Medicare participants, being virtual would probably be really good for them because a lot of times they don't have transportation, or they have to be with a caregiver". DSMES Provider "Coverage for services virtually needs to be set in stone ... Now, it's sort of vague, and I don't know how long it's gonna last ... With very clear policies and procedures, and coverage for virtual services, I think in my community, it will increase participation in [DSMES]". DSMES Provider

3.2. Individual Factors

3.2.1. Participant Comfort with and Access to Technology

Interviewees reported a wide range of comfort with and access to technology across and within the populations they work with. While some interviewees described challenges in reaching older populations and lower-income groups because of discomfort with technology and/or limited access to the internet or a computer, others had the opposite experience. One National DPP expert stated:

> "Maybe they are an 89-year-old grandmother who's online all the time and is Queen of the internet . . . or maybe there's someone that is not very familiar with technologies. We saw a big range within our communities."

Participants with less technical knowledge experienced challenges connecting to telehealth platforms and sometimes attended meetings via phone/audio only. In a few cases, participants did not have permanent phones/phone numbers or email accounts. Participants also experienced technical difficulties such as unstable internet connections, dropped calls, or difficulties unmuting to speak. Some participants did have access to technology, but they had a strong preference for in-person learning.

3.2.2. Participant Health Behaviors and Outcomes

The rapid transition to telehealth resulted in challenges in collecting health data from some program participants, so it was difficult for interviewees to determine the full impact of the pandemic on the transition and on telehealth services' delivery as it relates to changes in participant health behaviors and health outcomes.

When program sessions were held in-person, it had been easier for providers to collect participant health data such as weight and HbA1c levels. With the transition to telehealth, providers had to rely on self-reported weight from the participants. Some participants did not want to report their weight or did not have access to a scale at home. Despite lacking complete data on participant weight, some providers mentioned that participants were successful in maintaining their weight, and a minority lost weight. Other interviewees mentioned that participants gained weight. DSMES providers also did not have current data on HbA1c levels because patients were not coming into the office to have laboratory work performed. A few interviewees speculated that participants likely experienced higher HbA1c levels, at least initially. Among those interviewees who had data, they reported similar or better HbA1c levels with telehealth delivery.

Despite the difficulties with collecting health data, a minority of interviewees described how participants improved their eating habits and cooked more after the start of the pandemic due to the large amounts of time they were spending at home. Others mentioned that participants had worse eating habits and described how a few experienced food insecurity and were reliant on food pantries for food, which did not provide enough healthy options. National DPP providers also reported that participants' physical activity levels decreased, and participants had to be highly motivated to exercise during the pandemic. One National DPP provider stated:

> "We saw activity in minutes plunder, and we saw those not so good eating habits go up . . . even though they knew staying healthy and maybe preventing diabetes would hopefully make them weather COVID better."

3.2.3. Meeting Participants Where They Are

To address issues with technology, health behaviors, and health outcomes that resulted from the transition to telehealth and the COVID-19 pandemic, interviewees stressed the need to "meet participants where they are". Technical assistance, health and behavior goals, and resources for participants needed to be tailored to the needs of each participant and/or group. In many cases, providers and participants could work around their initial discomfort with technology and the lack of access to technology, but in other cases, it was too difficult, and some National DPP cohorts ended, or some DSMES participants did not continue receiving services.

Providers described tremendous efforts, especially during the initial transition, to make sure that "everyone's on the same playing field" with technology. These efforts included conducting individual phone meetings with participants, creating simple handouts or guides for connecting to the platform, and following up frequently with participants to make sure they could connect and stay engaged in the program. National DPP providers also hosted "Session Zeroes" before the start of the program to assess participants' readiness to participate and address their technology needs. In addition, providers loaned devices (e.g., tablets, Chromebooks, smartphones) with internet connections to participants without access to the technology.

Tailored assistance for participants was also helpful for overcoming barriers to healthy eating and physical activity habits. Providers helped participants create plans or set goals to work around challenges and provided them with resources when needed. One National DPP and DSMES provider stated:

> "People's lives had to change. People were fearful . . . we would have to tell them these are some exercises you could do at home . . . or these are healthy recipes that you can make with the food that you would get at a food pantry or Food Bank."

3.3. Interpersonal Factors
Social Support and Engagement

Interviewees reported that interpersonal factors such as the relationships between providers and participants were important to the success of DSMES services and to the success that many National DPP cohorts enjoyed. However, interviewees noted that making a "human connection" was "a little harder to do over a virtual connection". One National DPP and DSMES provider stated:

> "The benefit of having an in-person workshop is the social aspect of it. People do feel more connected with each other, and they feel like they have the support of their peers. In the virtual [setting] that was a challenge . . . They're just really not as connected with each other.

Strategies to increase engagement in telehealth sessions and help participants make connections included having round-robin discussions, warm invitations to participate in the conversation, and using breakout rooms and poll functions provided by the telehealth platform. Some providers also mentioned changing the way they delivered content and modifying materials to work for telehealth. One National DPP and DSMES provider mentioned "the more colorful and interesting your materials are, the more you'll get their attention".

Maintaining connections and communication between telehealth sessions was also important for increasing engagement and social cohesion. National DPP providers created group text messages and used social media such as WhatsApp and Facebook to increase communication and connection.

Providers also noted the importance of "knowing your audience and what works for them". Some noted that a hybrid approach with both telehealth and in-person sessions might be good moving forward. One DSMES provider suggested "incorporating face-to-face periodically," as in-person sessions may help establish a relationship with participants and make future telehealth sessions more successful. Despite efforts to engage participants during telehealth sessions, some participants and providers still had a strong preference for in-person sessions.

3.4. Organizational Factors

Providers faced several challenges at the organizational level when transitioning from in-person to telehealth services. Many successfully implemented a range of strategies or optimal practices to overcome these challenges.

3.4.1. Telehealth Platforms and Technical Difficulties

There was a range in comfort levels with the platform (e.g., Zoom, GoToMeeting, Doximity) selected to provide telehealth services. Some providers were very familiar with their platform and had experience delivering telehealth sessions prior to the pandemic, whereas others had very limited or no experience.

Training sessions for providers were implemented at organizations to overcome challenges with platforms and telehealth delivery. Most organizations were also quick to supply providers with the necessary technological equipment (monitors, webcams, etc.) to conduct telehealth sessions. In most cases, providers were able to learn how to use the platform relatively quickly. One National DPP provider stated:

> "We had practice facilitation where I would have them take turns facilitating a class online and then provide feedback. So, there was a lot of training on that for my team."

In other cases, interviewees noted it would have been helpful to have additional training provided by their organization or external experts to increase providers' comfort and effectiveness at delivering telehealth sessions.

Despite providers' quick adjustment to telehealth platforms and the new equipment, a small number of interviewees described remaining challenges with particular platforms that were not fully meeting their needs. Providers also experienced occasional challenges with internet connectivity and noted the need for contingency plans for technical issues or when participants cannot join telehealth sessions.

3.4.2. Provider Workload and Organizational Support

Transitioning to telehealth required providers to spend additional time modifying materials for telehealth delivery, recruiting and retaining participants, and assisting participants. However, interviewees also noted that telehealth delivery of services can be more convenient for providers and save them time or allow them to meet with more cohorts or individuals. One DPP and DSMES provider stated:

> "You can provide a [telehealth] program. It's one hour for the coach. It's not all this travel and set up and talking time that really adds on an additional two hours for every meeting session. So, it's much more streamlined, and that can open the possibilities for delivering the program at hours more populations can attend."

In most cases, providers noted that they felt sufficiently supported by their organizations in the transition to telehealth. A small number of DSMES providers did mention the need for additional organizational support, specifically having enough administrative staff to prepare participants for telehealth sessions and schedule future appointments.

3.4.3. Recruitment and Enrollment

Interviewees reported that programs experienced an initial drop in enrollment because of a pause to program operations and/or recruitment due to the pandemic. Some programs continued to have low enrollment numbers because of recruitment challenges or participant discomfort with telehealth. However, several interviewees noted that telehealth increased access to individuals from a wider geographic area and to those who previously could not commit to a long program and/or had challenges attending in-person. With the enrollment of these additional participants, some programs maintained pre-pandemic numbers, and a few increased their enrollment. For example, one National DPP provider said:

> "Switching to virtual allowed us to reach members that wouldn't normally have the time to attend our in-person workshop. So, these are the working people and maybe the elderly who don't want to drive to a site at night."

Interviewees noted several strategies that could be used to improve outreach and recruitment efforts for telehealth programs. They described the importance of contacting healthcare providers about telehealth services and encouraging them to make referrals, conducting direct marketing to patients through patient portals and newsletters, and marketing through social media. One National DPP and DSMES provider mentioned that regardless of the mode of outreach or recruitment, providers need to tailor the message to fit the needs of the individual participant.

3.4.4. Retention

Interviewees reported two different experiences when it came to the retention of National DPP participants in telehealth programs in comparison to DSMES participants. National DPP providers and experts mentioned that retention rates were mixed across cohorts. Some National DPP providers reported that retention was better with telehealth, especially among well-established cohorts. However, others experienced lower retention rates, especially among participants with a strong preference for in-person sessions or who were not comfortable with technology.

In contrast, many DSMES providers stated that retention stayed the same or improved after transitioning to virtual/distance learning program provision. One DSMES provider commented, "it's about the same as before ... it's not like we saw them for a series of visits. We saw them for the initial and then maybe one follow-up or two. We're still staying about the same".

3.5. Community Factors

Factors external to organizations and occurring in the broader community as a result of the pandemic had an impact on the transition from in-person services to telehealth. The closure of various organizations, churches, senior centers, and other locations was especially challenging for providers that recruited through community outreach efforts. Community outreach often required substantial effort prior to the pandemic and was even more difficult when recruitment locations were closed because of COVID-19. Providers had to conduct other forms of outreach, and some experienced lower enrollments. One National DPP expert stated:

> "In a lot of these communities, the recruitment was very much this high-touch relationship-building with the community where you're going out to health fairs, to congregate meal sites ... Well, senior centers closed, the congregate meal site has become Meals on Wheels, the church is not servicing, senior housing is not letting anyone in, and the assisted living programs are on lockdown."

3.6. Policy and Systems Factors

Interviewees had several suggestions for changes that are needed to support telehealth National DPP and DSMES programs at the local, state, and federal governmental levels.

3.6.1. Local Government

Suggestions for policy and systems changes that could be implemented by the local government or DPH included: assistance with marketing programs to increase enrollment, providing free training and materials for delivering telehealth programs, purchasing technology needed for telehealth and sharing with organizations and program participants, facilitating networking opportunities for providers to share best practices, assisting providers with program compliance, and advocating for policy change at the federal level to increase reimbursement for programs. For example, one National DPP and DSMES provider stated:

> "I think LA County Department of Public Health can continue being an advocate for health plans and vendors that provide the services and really take a role at the federal level to change some of these policies to provide more flexibility for populations covered by Medicare."

3.6.2. State and Federal Government

Interviewees mentioned some general policy changes at the state and federal level that would be helpful for both National DPP and DSMES, such as expanding access to healthcare/insurance and expanding broadband/internet availability. Interviewees also mentioned that insurance companies should cover the technology needed for participants to receive telehealth services. However, in most cases, they suggested program-specific changes.

3.6.3. Policy and Systems Changes Needed for National DPP

Interviewees spoke to the need to increase reimbursement rates for National DPP from Medicaid (Medi-Cal in California) and Medicare, noting that the current reimbursement rates made it difficult for program providers to cover their costs. For example, one National DPP expert stated:

"The reimbursement needs to align, actually align with the high fixed costs of [National DPP] . . . It is very hard to start one of these programs and sustain it over time. You have to be incredibly efficient to be able to do that with Medi-Cal or Medicare DPP reimbursement."

In addition, interviewees mentioned that the process for receiving Medicare reimbursement for National DPP needs to be "less onerous". They noted that few organizations are applying to provide Medicare DPP because of the stringent requirements.

Interviewees also had suggestions for policy and systems changes that need to be made by the CDC, particularly around the Diabetes Prevention Recognition Program (DPRP). Interviewees discussed the need for providing flexibility for maintaining DPRP recognition if organizations were not able to meet program requirements during the pandemic (for example, cohorts that do not achieve required weight loss and activity levels), or if organizations offered the program in a different modality than the one they originally applied for (i.e., offering distance learning versus in-person).

Interviewees also mentioned that National DPP eligibility requirements, the curriculum, and reporting requirements need to be changed or updated. Providers stated that the body mass index (BMI) eligibility requirement for National DPP needs to be removed, as some individuals with lower BMIs may be at risk for diabetes. Providers also recommended the CDC update the National DPP curriculum to meet current nutrition guidelines/science and provide guidance for adapting the curriculum to telehealth. Other providers would like the curriculum to be available in more languages than just English and Spanish. In addition, providers would like the CDC to streamline reporting requirements. One National DPP expert and provider suggested that the CDC should provide a platform for all National DPP programs from which they could provide distance learning, securely enter confidential participant information, and communicate with participants.

3.6.4. Policy and Systems Changes Needed for DSMES

Similar to the National DPP, DSMES experts and providers mentioned the need for adequate and sustained coverage for telehealth programs through Medicare. Interviewees noted that if Medicare continues to cover telehealth and allow a variety of providers to offer telehealth services, other insurers will follow. Interviewees also noted that because of the complexity of Medicare reimbursement, only a small percentage of Medicare beneficiaries utilize the program. For example, a DSMES expert stated:

"[DSMES providers] are afraid to bill [Medicare] because they're afraid they're going to do something wrong. And all they're trying to do is take care of their patients, and they get shut down because they're not sustainable financially."

Other interviewees mentioned that regulations need to be changed to allow providers to be licensed in multiple states, so they can provide services to participants that travel or live in another state.

3.7. Beyond the Pandemic: The Future of Telehealth

When asked about their future plans and whether they would continue to offer National DPP and/or DSMES via telehealth, some providers mentioned that they were excited to go back to all in-person sessions. However, many providers mentioned they were planning to offer both in-person and telehealth programming or some hybrid version. Interviewees noted that telehealth expanded the reach of the program to individuals who could not or would not participate in-person, but in-person was needed for others who either preferred in-person sessions or had technical challenges. One National DPP expert stated:

> "[Telehealth] provides a way in another way into the program. And with 88 million people who have prediabetes, you need as many doors as possible into this program."

After the initial challenges of the rapid transition to telehealth, many providers found that telehealth allowed them to expand their programs to new geographic areas and reduced travel and/or set-up necessary for in-person sessions. Providers noted that continued investment in telehealth modalities and the policy changes mentioned above would be necessary to continue to offer telehealth options.

4. Discussion

Our study analysis shows that several challenges emerged at all levels of the SEM as providers rapidly switched from in-person sessions to telehealth in LAC. Providers implemented several strategies or optimal practices to overcome these challenges and, in many instances, were able to successfully transition to telehealth, retain existing participants, and enroll new participants.

Similar to other studies [23,24], interviewees reported a wide range of comfort with and access to technology among participant populations. Other studies have also found that the elderly, lower-income individuals, and individuals who require translation services may experience greater difficulty in using telehealth services [23,24]. However, in this study, these differences in comfort and access were not always driven by age or income status, as interviewees provided examples of elderly individuals who were very tech-savvy and people with lower incomes who were quickly able to adjust to telehealth.

To overcome technological barriers to engaging in telehealth services, interviewees mentioned that participants needed intense, tailored assistance, at least initially. The extent to which this technical assistance will be necessary in the future, however, is not clear. Overall, participant comfort with and ability to use telehealth likely increased as a result of more frequent use during the pandemic. Studies indicate that interest in telehealth, willingness to use, and use of telehealth increased significantly among U.S. adults throughout the pandemic [28,29], especially among non-Hispanic Black adults and adults with lower education levels [29]. As a result, many new National DPP and DSMES participants may not need as much technical assistance to participate in programs that employ telehealth either exclusively or in a hybrid fashion.

Challenges in collecting participant health data via telehealth made it difficult for interviewees to determine the impact of the pandemic on the transition to telehealth or on individual health behaviors and outcomes. Similar challenges in conducting nutrition assessments and monitoring client health outcomes were also reported by registered dietitian nutritionists that had transitioned to telehealth services during the pandemic [30]. Increasing access to and reimbursement for remote monitoring devices may help overcome data collection challenges associated with telehealth usage [31,32]. Hybrid programming may allow for in-person assessments and data collection while maintaining many of the benefits of services delivered via telehealth.

Challenges with accessing healthy food and safely engaging in physical activity that were exacerbated by the pandemic [33–35] could have resulted in worse health behaviors and outcomes than might normally be seen in programs that utilize telehealth. Studies of telehealth diabetes management programs conducted prior to the pandemic have shown improvements in HbA1c levels and other behavioral and health outcomes [14,15,36]. Additionally, weight loss among individuals with prediabetes that participated in DPP-based programs that used telehealth has been equal to or greater than among those participating in in-person programs [12,13,37–40].

At the interpersonal level, it was challenging to create active, supportive online communities and personal connections among providers and program participants. Other healthcare providers have also had difficulty connecting via telehealth and have called for the development of best practices and training for building rapport [30,41]. There have also been recommendations for additional research to be conducted on strategies and devices that could help increase engagement and social connections to prevention programs that deliver services via telehealth [22].

At the organizational level, providers' comfort and familiarity with telehealth platforms and delivery was mixed, and transitioning to telehealth increased many providers' workloads, at least initially. Similarly, other healthcare providers implementing telehealth services have reported experiencing technical difficulties, a lack of support from administrative staff, and an increased workload [32,42]. Training sessions for providers can help overcome some of these challenges with platforms and telehealth delivery [43,44], and contingency plans are needed to deal with technical barriers. Additional administrative staff may be needed to support programs that rely on telehealth [32,42]. Overall, the number of healthcare providers using telehealth increased significantly during the pandemic [23,30], so provider comfort and familiarity with these virtual platforms have likely increased as well.

Despite the organizational challenges presented by transitioning to telehealth, interviewees noted that delivery via telehealth provided significant opportunities to expand the reach of the National DPP and DSMES programs, especially for individuals from various geographic areas, including rural communities, and for individuals who cannot or will not, otherwise, participate in in-person services. Telehealth delivery has been effective at reaching individuals who live in areas where transportation and access to in-person services can be limited [37–39,42,45]. As a modality, telehealth allows services to continue without disruption during travel or relocation [39]. Many telehealth participants are highly satisfied with these services because of the time savings, convenience, and reduction in travel time associated with using telehealth [24,46].

4.1. Limitations

This study has limitations. First, interviews were not conducted with program participants themselves, so the perspectives of individuals involved in the transition to telehealth were based on the impressions of experts and providers and not directly on the perspectives of participants. Since most providers interviewed were able to switch from in-person to telehealth services during the pandemic, additional perspectives may be needed from providers who were not successful in making this switch to complete a full story of this process. However, some of the experts who were interviewed could speak to the experiences of providers who were not able to transition to telehealth. The interviewees were also selected because of their positions as National DPP and/or DSMES experts and providers, and we did not collect demographic information from them. It is possible that responses to interview questions could have been influenced by demographic variables. Finally, while we did interview experts familiar with programs and services in other states and localities, majority of the interviewees were based in LAC. As a result, findings from this study may not be generalizable to other jurisdictions and areas across the U.S.

4.2. Implications for Policy and Practice

While interviewees made policy and systems change recommendations across different levels of government, the most critical changes identified were at the federal level. Specifically, interviewees mentioned the need for more flexible program requirements and adequate reimbursement of the telehealth services being delivered. Although great strides have been made in response to the COVID-19 pandemic, the rapid transition to telehealth for many of these programs remains a temporary change. Reimbursement policies for telehealth delivery instituted by Medicare, Medicaid, and private health insurers during the health crisis will likely need to continue to sustain these gains made in service delivery. In addition, these policies will need to be adjusted to allow for greater coverage and payment of services provided via telehealth, at the equivalent level as in-person sessions [47,48]. There have been calls for the Centers for Medicare and Medicaid Services, as well as for health plans, to make these changes permanent and expand telehealth delivery options to increase coverage of chronic disease, dietary counseling, and remote support services that are needed to better manage chronic conditions [42,49,50]. To further increase access to and the convenience of telehealth services, policy changes may also be needed to allow providers to be licensed in multiple states and/or practice in a different state than their patients are receiving treatment. Policymakers can also improve upon the incentives used for providing more comprehensive services via telehealth. More research may be needed to study these policy options and to provide evidence of telehealth effectiveness for this type of coverage expansion, especially for Medicare and Medicaid populations across the nation.

5. Conclusions

The COVID-19 pandemic provided a rare opportunity for increasing access to and use of telehealth services for National DPP and DSMES programs. Despite the challenges of implementing telehealth under the difficult circumstances created by the health crisis, many providers appreciated the benefits of telehealth for participants and for their organizations. Additional program flexibility and adequate reimbursement will be key to these programs continuing to offer telehealth services.

Supplementary Materials: The following are available online at https://www.mdpi.com/article/10.3390/diabetology4010006/s1, File S1: Interview Guides.

Author Contributions: Conceptualization, T.K., N.C.B., T.M., J.T.M., G.G., L.S. and L.C.; methodology, L.S. and L.C.; formal analysis, S.L.B.; investigation, S.L.B.; data curation, S.L.B.; writing—original draft preparation, S.L.B.; writing—review and editing, all authors; visualization, S.L.B.; supervision, T.K. and N.C.B.; project administration, T.M. and J.T.M.; funding acquisition, T.K. and N.C.B. All authors have read and agreed to the published version of the manuscript.

Funding: This project was supported in part by a cooperative agreement from the Centers for Disease Control and Prevention (CDC, U58DP006619).

Institutional Review Board Statement: The project was considered exempt from full review by the Los Angeles County Department of Public Health Institutional Review Board, as it was originally conducted for program fidelity/improvement purposes.

Informed Consent Statement: Each interviewee verbally consented to participate in the project prior to each interview.

Data Availability Statement: Data can be made available upon request if the request is appropriate and feasible.

Acknowledgments: The authors thank the Los Angeles County Diabetes Coalition for its partnership and efforts in helping to recruit and facilitate the key informant interviews with the various National Diabetes Prevention Program and Diabetes Self-Management Education and Support program experts and providers. The authors would also like to thank Caroline Wachino and Lizabella Nadelson for their assistance with the analysis. The decision to develop and publish this study's results was that of the authors and was not influenced by the funder nor any of the affiliated institutions. The contents presented do not represent the positions or views of the organizations or agencies mentioned in the text.

Conflicts of Interest: The authors declare no conflict of interest.

References

1. The Centers for Disease Control and Prevention. The National Diabetes Statistics Report. Available online: https://www.cdc.gov/diabetes/pdfs/data/statistics/national-diabetes-statistics-report.pdf (accessed on 23 September 2021).
2. Los Angeles County Department of Public Health. Key Indicators of Health by Service Planning Area. Available online: http://publichealth.lacounty.gov/ha/docs/2015LACHS/KeyIndicator/PH-KIH_2017-sec%20UPDATED.pdf (accessed on 9 December 2021).
3. Centers for Disease Control and Prevention. Diabetes Report Card 2019. Available online: https://www.cdc.gov/diabetes/pdfs/library/Diabetes-Report-Card-2019-508.pdf (accessed on 6 December 2021).
4. Sacks, L.J.; Pham, C.T.; Fleming, N.; Neoh, S.L.; Ekinci, E.I. Considerations for people with diabetes during the Coronavirus Disease (COVID-19) pandemic. *Diabetes Res. Clin. Pract.* **2020**, *166*, 108296. [CrossRef] [PubMed]

5. Diabetes Prevention Program Research Group. Reduction in the incidence of type 2 diabetes with lifestyle intervention or metformin. *N. Engl. J. Med.* **2002**, *346*, 393–403. [CrossRef] [PubMed]
6. Albright, A.L.; Gregg, E.W. Preventing type 2 diabetes in communities across the U.S.: The National Diabetes Prevention Program. *Am. J. Prev. Med.* **2013**, *44*, S346–S351. [CrossRef] [PubMed]
7. United States Congress. H.R.4124–Diabetes Prevention Act of 2009. Available online: https://www.congress.gov/bill/111th-congress/house-bill/4124 (accessed on 5 August 2021).
8. Diabetes Prevention Program Research Group. Long-term effects of lifestyle intervention or metformin on diabetes development and microvascular complications over 15-year follow-up: The Diabetes Prevention Program Outcomes Study. *Lancet Diabetes Endocrinol* **2015**, *3*, 866–875. [CrossRef]
9. Chrvala, C.A.; Sherr, D.; Lipman, R.D. Diabetes self-management education for adults with type 2 diabetes mellitus: A systematic review of the effect on glycemic control. *Patient Educ. Couns.* **2016**, *99*, 926–943. [CrossRef]
10. National Consortium of Telehealth Resource Centers. A Framework for Defining Telehealth. Available online: https://cchp.nyc3.digitaloceanspaces.com/2021/04/Telehealth-Definintion-Framework-for-TRCs_0.pdf (accessed on 26 October 2021).
11. Powers, M.A.; Bardsley, J.K.; Cypress, M.; Funnell, M.M.; Harms, D.; Hess-Fischl, A.; Hooks, B.; Isaacs, D.; Mandel, E.D.; Maryniuk, M.D.; et al. Diabetes self-management education and support in adults with type 2 diabetes: A consensus report of the American Diabetes Association, the Association of Diabetes Care & Education Specialists, the Academy of Nutrition and Dietetics, the American Academy of Family Physicians, the American Academy of PAs, the American Association of Nurse Practitioners, and the American Pharmacists Association. *Diabetes Care* **2020**, *43*, 1636–1649. [CrossRef]
12. Joiner, K.L.; Nam, S.; Whittemore, R. Lifestyle interventions based on the diabetes prevention program delivered via eHealth: A systematic review and meta-analysis. *Prev. Med.* **2017**, *100*, 194–207. [CrossRef]
13. Grock, S.; Ku, J.H.; Kim, J.; Moin, T. A review of technology-assisted interventions for diabetes prevention. *Curr. Diab. Rep.* **2017**, *17*, 107. [CrossRef]
14. Appuswamy, A.V.; Desimone, M.E. Managing diabetes in hard to reach populations: A review of telehealth interventions. *Curr. Diab. Rep.* **2020**, *20*, 28. [CrossRef]
15. McDaniel, C.C.; Kavookjian, J.; Whitley, H.P. Telehealth delivery of motivational interviewing for diabetes management: A systematic review of randomized controlled trials. *Patient Educ. Couns.* **2021**, *105*, 805–820. [CrossRef]
16. Robson, N.; Hosseinzadeh, H. Impact of telehealth care among adults living with type 2 diabetes in primary care: A systematic review and meta-analysis of randomised controlled trials. *Int. J. Environ. Res. Public Health* **2021**, *18*, 12171. [CrossRef] [PubMed]
17. Los Angeles County Public Health Department. Find a Diabetes Self–Management Education and Support Program Near You. Available online: http://publichealth.lacounty.gov/phcommon/public/dsmesearch.cfm (accessed on 9 December 2021).
18. Los Angeles County Public Health Department. Find a National Diabetes Prevention Program. Available online: http://publichealth.lacounty.gov/phcommon/public/nationaldpp.cfm (accessed on 9 December 2021).
19. Modi, P.K.; Kaufman, S.R.; Portney, D.S.; Ryan, A.M.; Hollenbeck, B.K.; Ellimoottil, C. Telemedicine utilization by providers in accountable care organizations. *Mhealth* **2019**, *5*, 10. [CrossRef] [PubMed]
20. Crossen, S.; Raymond, J.; Neinstein, A. Top 10 tips for successfully implementing a diabetes telehealth program. *Diabetes Technol. Ther.* **2020**, *22*, 920–928. [CrossRef]
21. Harvey, J.B.; Valenta, S.; Simpson, K.; Lyles, M.; McElligott, J. Utilization of outpatient telehealth services in parity and nonparity states 2010–2015. *Telemed J. E Health* **2019**, *25*, 132–136. [CrossRef] [PubMed]
22. O'Connor, S.; Hanlon, P.; O'Donnell, C.A.; Garcia, S.; Glanville, J.; Mair, F.S. Understanding factors affecting patient and public engagement and recruitment to digital health interventions: A systematic review of qualitative studies. *BMC Med. Inform. Decis. Mak.* **2016**, *16*, 120. [CrossRef] [PubMed]
23. Phimphasone-Brady, P.; Chiao, J.; Karamsetti, L.; Sieja, A.; Johnson, R.; Macke, L.; Lum, H.; Lee, R.; Farro, S.; Loeb, D.; et al. Clinician and staff perspectives on potential disparities introduced by the rapid implementation of telehealth services during COVID-19: A mixed-methods analysis. *Transl. Behav. Med.* **2021**, *11*, 1339–1347. [CrossRef]
24. Almathami, H.K.Y.; Win, K.T.; Vlahu-Gjorgievska, E. Barriers and facilitators that influence telemedicine-based, real-time, online consultation at patients' homes: Systematic literature review. *J. Med. Internet Res.* **2020**, *22*, e16407. [CrossRef]
25. ATLAS.ti Scientific Software Development GmbH. *ATLAS.ti 22 Windows*, Version 22.0.6.0. 2022.
26. Braun, V.; Clarke, V. Using thematic analysis in psychology. *Qual. Res. Psychol.* **2006**, *3*, 77–101. [CrossRef]
27. McLeroy, K.R.; Bibeau, D.; Steckler, A.; Glanz, K. An ecological perspective on health promotion programs. *Health Educ. Q* **1988**, *15*, 351–377. [CrossRef]
28. Hong, Y.R.; Lawrence, J.; Williams, D., Jr.; Mainous, I.A. Population-level interest and telehealth capacity of US hospitals in response to COVID-19: Cross-sectional analysis of google search and national hospital survey data. *JMIR Public Health Surveill* **2020**, *6*, e18961. [CrossRef]
29. Fischer, S.H.; Predmore, Z.; Roth, E.; Uscher-Pines, L.; Baird, M.; Breslau, J. Use of and willingness to use video telehealth through the COVID-19 pandemic. *Health Aff.* **2022**, *41*, 1645–1651. [CrossRef] [PubMed]
30. Rozga, M.; Handu, D.; Kelley, K.; Jimenez, E.Y.; Martin, H.; Schofield, M.; Steiber, A. Telehealth during the COVID-19 pandemic: A cross-sectional survey of registered dietitian nutritionists. *J. Acad. Nutr. Diet.* **2021**, *121*, 2524–2535. [CrossRef] [PubMed]
31. Kirley, K.; Sachdev, N. Digital health-supported lifestyle change programs to prevent type 2 diabetes. *Diabetes Spectr.* **2018**, *31*, 303–309. [CrossRef] [PubMed]

32. Odom, J.; Beauchamp, C.; Fiocchi, C.; Eicken, M.; Stancil, M.; Turner, J.; Bruch, J. Rapid innovation in diabetes care during Covid-19. *ADCES Pract.* **2020**, *8*, 28–32. [CrossRef]
33. Ansari, R.M.; Harris, M.F.; Hosseinzadeh, H.; Zwar, N. Experiences of diabetes self-management: A focus group study among the middle-aged population of rural pakistan with type 2 diabetes. *Diabetology* **2022**, *3*, 17–29. [CrossRef]
34. Naja, F.; Hamadeh, R. Nutrition amid the COVID-19 pandemic: A multi-level framework for action. *Eur. J. Clin. Nutr.* **2020**, *74*, 1117–1121. [CrossRef]
35. Mattioli, A.V.; Sciomer, S.; Cocchi, C.; Maffei, S.; Gallina, S. Quarantine during COVID-19 outbreak: Changes in diet and physical activity increase the risk of cardiovascular disease. *Nutr. Metab. Cardiovasc. Dis.* **2020**, *30*, 1409–1417. [CrossRef]
36. Davis, T.C.; Hoover, K.W.; Keller, S.; Replogle, W.H. Mississippi diabetes telehealth network: A collaborative approach to chronic care management. *Telemed. J. E Health* **2020**, *26*, 184–189. [CrossRef]
37. Vadheim, L.M.; McPherson, C.; Kassner, D.R.; Vanderwood, K.K.; Hall, T.O.; Butcher, M.K.; Helgerson, S.D.; Harwell, T.S. Adapted diabetes prevention program lifestyle intervention can be effectively delivered through telehealth. *Diabetes Educ.* **2010**, *36*, 651–656. [CrossRef]
38. Vadheim, L.M.; Patch, K.; Brokaw, S.M.; Carpenedo, D.; Butcher, M.K.; Helgerson, S.D.; Harwell, T.S. Telehealth delivery of the diabetes prevention program to rural communities. *Transl. Behav. Med.* **2017**, *7*, 286–291. [CrossRef]
39. Taetzsch, A.; Gilhooly, C.H.; Bukhari, A.; Das, S.K.; Martin, E.; Hatch, A.M.; Silver, R.E.; Montain, S.J.; Roberts, S.B. Development of a videoconference-adapted version of the community diabetes prevention program, and comparison of weight loss with in-person program delivery. *Mil. Med.* **2019**, *184*, 647–652. [CrossRef]
40. Tate, D.F.; Jackvony, E.H.; Wing, R.R. Effects of Internet behavioral counseling on weight loss in adults at risk for type 2 diabetes: A randomized trial. *JAMA Am. Med. Assoc.* **2003**, *289*, 1833–1836. [CrossRef] [PubMed]
41. Schwartz, D.; DeMasi, M. The importance of teaching virtual rapport-building skills in telehealth curricula. *Acad. Med.* **2021**, *96*, 1231–1232. [CrossRef] [PubMed]
42. Knotowicz, H.; Haas, A.; Coe, S.; Furuta, G.T.; Mehta, P. Opportunities for innovation and improved care using telehealth for nutritional interventions. *Gastroenterology* **2019**, *157*, 594–597. [CrossRef]
43. Thomas, E.E.; Haydon, H.M.; Mehrotra, A.; Caffery, L.J.; Snoswell, C.L.; Banbury, A.; Smith, A.C. Building on the momentum: Sustaining telehealth beyond COVID-19. *J. Telemed. Telecare* **2022**, *28*, 301–308. [CrossRef] [PubMed]
44. Smith, A.C.; Thomas, E.; Snoswell, C.L.; Haydon, H.; Mehrotra, A.; Clemensen, J.; Caffery, L.J. Telehealth for global emergencies: Implications for coronavirus disease 2019 (COVID-19). *J. Telemed. Telecare* **2020**, *26*, 309–313. [CrossRef] [PubMed]
45. Ariel-Donges, A.H.; Gordon, E.L.; Dixon, B.N.; Eastman, A.J.; Bauman, V.; Ross, K.M.; Perri, M.G. Rural/urban disparities in access to the National Diabetes Prevention Program. *Transl. Behav. Med.* **2020**, *10*, 1554–1558. [CrossRef] [PubMed]
46. Gruß, I.; Mayhew, M.; Firemark, A.; Fitzpatrick, S.L. Participants' perspectives on perceived usefulness of digital and in-person diabetes prevention programs: A qualitative study to inform decisions related to program participation. *Obes. Sci. Pract.* **2022**, *8*, 176–184. [CrossRef]
47. The Center for Connected Health Policy. COVID-19 Telehealth Coverage Policies. Available online: https://www.cchpca.org/resources/covid-19-telehealth-coverage-policies/ (accessed on 19 October 2021).
48. Centers for Medicare & Medicaid Services. President Trump Expands Telehealth Benefits for Medicare Beneficiaries During COVID-19 Outbreak. Available online: https://www.cms.gov/newsroom/press-releases/president-trump-expands-telehealth-benefits-medicare-beneficiaries-during-covid-19-outbreak (accessed on 5 October 2021).
49. Anthony Jnr, B. Implications of telehealth and digital care solutions during COVID-19 pandemic: A qualitative literature review. *Inform. Health Soc. Care* **2021**, *46*, 68–83. [CrossRef]
50. Hoffman, D.A. Increasing access to care: Telehealth during COVID-19. *J. Law Biosc.* **2020**, *7*, lsaa049. [CrossRef] [PubMed]

Disclaimer/Publisher's Note: The statements, opinions and data contained in all publications are solely those of the individual author(s) and contributor(s) and not of MDPI and/or the editor(s). MDPI and/or the editor(s) disclaim responsibility for any injury to people or property resulting from any ideas, methods, instructions or products referred to in the content.

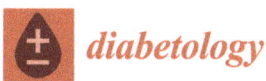

Article

Investigating the Protective Effects of a Rhenium (V) Compound with Uracil-Derived Ligands on Liver Damage Associated with Prediabetes in Diet-Induced Prediabetic Rats

Angezwa Siboto [1,*], Akinjide Moses Akinnuga [1], Muhammed Bilaal Ismail [2], Irvin Noel Booysen [2], Ntethelelo Hopewell Sibiya [3], Phikelelani Ngubane [1] and Andile Khathi [1]

[1] School of Laboratory Medicine and Medical Sciences, College of Health Sciences, University of KwaZulu-Natal, Durban 4000, South Africa
[2] School of Chemistry and Physics, College of Agriculture, Engineering Sciences, University of KwaZulu-Natal, Pietermaritzburg 3209, South Africa
[3] Pharmacology Division, Rhodes University, Grahamstown 6140, South Africa
* Correspondence: 212518628@stu.ukzn.ac.za

Abstract: Non-alcoholic fatty liver disease (NAFLD) is associated with prediabetes and can be treated by using a combination of metformin and dietary modification. However, people often fail to adhere to dietary modifications and become more dependent on pharmaceutical intervention, and this affects the effectiveness of the drug. In this study, we investigated the effects of rhenium (V) compound with uracil-derived ligands on liver health in diet-induced prediabetic rats in both the presence and absence of dietary modification. Prediabetic male Sprague Dawley rats were treated with the rhenium (V) compound for 12 weeks in both the presence and absence of dietary modification while monitoring fasting blood glucose levels. Antioxidant enzyme activity, inflammation markers and liver enzymes were measured together with liver glycogen and plasma triglycerides after sacrificing. The administration of rhenium (V) compound to prediabetic rats in both the presence and absence of dietary modification resulted in reduced concentrations of fasting blood glucose and triglycerides. There was also reduced liver glycogen, oxidative stress and liver enzymes while increasing antioxidant enzymes. Altogether, the rhenium (V) compound ameliorated liver injury and prevented hepatotoxicity.

Keywords: prediabetes; liver enzymes; rhenium (V) compound; triglycerides; NAFLD; fructose

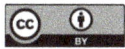

1. Introduction

Non-alcoholic fatty liver disease (NAFLD) has recently become the most frequent chronic liver disease that occurs across all age groups due to the growing prevalence of obesity and prediabetes [1,2]. NAFLD is strongly associated with insulin resistance, dyslipidemia and hypertriglyceridemia. Diets that are high in carbohydrates and saturated fats have been shown to predispose individuals to developing both prediabetes and NAFLD [3,4]. Additionally, fizzy drinks that are high in fructose activate lipogenesis in the hepatocytes, resulting in a fatty liver [5–7]. Prediabetes is linked with moderate levels of insulin resistance and has been shown to play a primary role in the pathogenesis of NAFLD [8,9]. Liver dysfunction is associated with hepatic insulin resistance and an increase in hepatic glycogen production, whereas liver injury is shown by abnormal liver enzymes such as alanine transaminase (ALT), aspartate transaminase (AST) and lactic dehydrogenase [10,11]. These may be due to alternations in the permeability of the cell membrane and damage in the liver tissue [5,12].

The treatment of NAFLD involves a combination of dietary modification to enhance weight loss, along with the use of different insulin-sensitizing agents such as metformin [13–16]. However, studies have shown that patients become more dependent on the pharmaceutical interventions while neglecting the lifestyle modification, resulting in a reduction in the efficacy of metformin [17,18]. Therefore, there exists a need for novel pharmacological compounds that can work in both the presence and absence of lifestyle modifications. Transition metals have been used to try and manage diabetes and other metabolic conditions, but they have been shown to disrupt lipid and protein metabolism as well as induce oxidative stress in the liver [5]. However, recent studies from our laboratory have shown that the incorporation of organic ligands to the transition metals results in reduced cellular toxicity [19,20]. We have previously shown that our novel rhenium (V) compound with uracil-derived ligands improves glucose homeostasis in high-fat–high-carbohydrate diet-induced prediabetic animals in both the absence and presence of dietary modifications [20,21]. In this study, we sought to further investigate the effects of the rhenium (V) compound on selected liver function markers in diet-induced prediabetic rats.

2. Methods and Materials

2.1. Animals

Thirty-six (36) male Sprague Dawley rats (150–180 g) obtained from Biomedical Research Unit, University of KwaZulu-Natal (UKZN), were kept under standard environmental conditions, i.e., constant humidity (55 ± 5%), temperature (22 ± 2 °C), 12 h day:12 h night cycle. The animals were acclimatized for 2 weeks with free access to a standard rat chow (Meadow Feeds, South Africa) and water ad libitum before being fed on the experimental high-fat–high-carbohydrate (HFHC) diet (AVI Products (Pty) Ltd., Waterfall, South Africa) to induce prediabetes. The HFHC diet consists of carbohydrates (55% kcal/g), fats (30% kcal/g) and proteins (15% kcal/g), as described in our previous study [3,20]. All the experimental designs and procedures were carried out according to the ethics and guidelines of the Animal Research Ethics Committee (AREC, ethical clearance code: AREC/039/018M) of the UKZN, Durban, South Africa.

2.1.1. Induction of Prediabetes on Male Sprague Dawley Rats

Sprague Dawley rats (n = 6 per group) were divided into groups based on the diet they received: a standard rat chow with normal drinking water (ND + H_2O), high-fat–high-carbohydrate diet with drinking water supplemented with fructose (HFHC + fructose). Prediabetes induction took 20 weeks using a previously established protocol [3,22]. Rats with fasting blood levels that were higher than 5.6 mmol/L were considered prediabetic and grouped further for pharmacological studies [23,24]. The treatment commenced on the subsequent day, and this was considered as day 1 of treatment.

2.1.2. Study Design for Experiments

In this study, rats were randomly divided into 6 groups of 6 animals in each (30 prediabetic persisting, 6 normal). Group 1: normal healthy control rats received vehicle (NC); Group 2: prediabetic control rats continued with HFHC diet and received vehicle (PD); Group 3: prediabetic treated rats switched to the STD diet and received metformin (MET + DI); Group 4: prediabetic treated rats continued with HFHC diet received metformin (MET + HFHC); Group 5: prediabetic rats switched to the STD diet and received rhenium (V) compound (Re + DI); Group 6: prediabetic treated rats continued with diet received rhenium (V) compound (Re + HFHC). See Figure 1.

2.1.3. Treatment of Prediabetic Animals

After 20 weeks of inducing prediabetes, the treatment period started and lasted an additional 12 weeks. During the treatment period, the animals were treated once every third day at 9:00 a.m., where metformin (500 mg/kg) was given through oral dosing to the MET + HFHC and MET + DI, while rhenium (V) compound (15 mg/kg) was given via subcutaneous injection to the Re + HFHC and Re + DI groups. Parameters including fasting blood glucose (FBG) concentration, food intake and body weights were monitored every 4 weeks during the treatment period. See Figure 1.

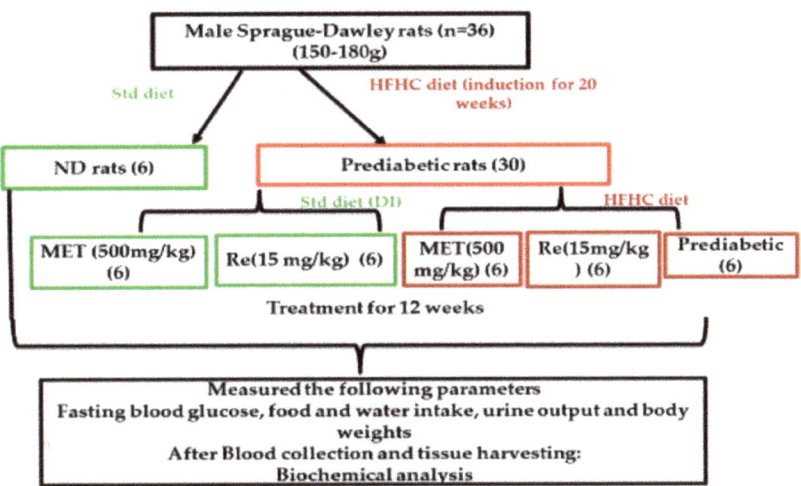

Figure 1. The experimental protocol for the study.

2.1.4. Blood Collection and Tissue Harvesting

For blood collection, all animals were anesthetized with Isofor (100 mg/kg) (Safeline Pharmaceuticals (Pty) Ltd., Roodeport, South Africa) via a gas anesthetic chamber (Biomedical Resource Unit, UKZN, Durban, South Africa) for 3 min in line with the guidelines for use of anesthesia. While the rats were unconscious, blood was collected by cardiac puncture into individual pre-cooled heparinized containers. The blood was then centrifuged (Eppendorf centrifuge 5403, Germany) at 4 °C, 503× g for 15 min. Plasma was collected and stored at −80 °C in a Bio Ultra freezer (Snijers Scientific, Holland, Netherlands) until ready for biochemical analysis. Thereafter, liver tissue was removed, weighed and rinsed with cold normal saline solution and snap frozen in liquid nitrogen before storage in a BioUltra freezer (Snijers Scientific, Tilburg, Netherlands) at −80 °C until biochemical analysis.

2.1.5. Relative Liver Weight

The relative liver weights of all the animals in each experimental group were determined from the percentage of the ratio of liver weight to the body weight using the formula below:

$$\text{Relative liver weight} = \frac{\text{liver weight}}{\text{body weight}} \times 100\% \qquad (1)$$

2.2. Biochemical Analysis

2.2.1. Quantification of Hepatic Glycogen, Plasma Triglycerides, TNF α and Liver Function Enzymes

Glycogen concentration analysis was performed in liver tissues. The glycogen assay was conducted using a well-established laboratory protocol [20].

Triglycerides (TGs) were measured using a colorimetric assay kit (catalog No: E-BC-K238; Manufacturer: Elabscience), single reagent, GPO-PAP method. Briefly, 50 mg of liver tissue was homogenized on 0.9% saline in a ratio of 9:1. The tissue was homogenized on ice for 2 min, and then the sample was centrifuged at 1000× g for 5–10 min. After centrifugation, the aqueous phase extraction was used in the assay. The protein quantification was conducted using Bradford assay. The assay was carried out according to the manufacturer's instructions. Furthermore, for TNF α measurements, 50 mg of liver tissue was homogenized, and the concentration was determined using an ELISA kit following the manufacturer's instructions (catalog no.: E-EL-R2856; manufacturer: Elabscience). Liver AST and ALT concentrations were measured using the Catalyst One Chemistry Analyzer (IDEXX Laboratories, Westbrook, ME, USA).

2.2.2. Antioxidant Activity Profile

Antioxidant activity in the liver was measured on selected antioxidant markers. Glutathione peroxidase (GPx) (catalog no.: E-EL-R2491; manufacturer: Elabscience) and superoxide dismutase (SOD) (catalog no.: E-EL-R1424; manufacturer: Elabscience) concentrations were determined using assay kits as per manufacturer's instructions.

2.3. Statistical Analysis

All data are expressed as means ± SD. Statistical comparisons were performed with GraphPad InStat Software (version 5.00, GraphPad Software, Inc., San Diego, CA, USA) using two-way analysis of variance (ANOVA) followed by Tukey–Kramer multiple comparison test. A value of $p < 0.05$ was considered statistically significant.

3. Results

3.1. Fasting Blood Glucose Concentration

Figure 2 shows fasting blood glucose concentrations in the normal control (NC), prediabetic control (PD), metformin and diet intervention (MET + DI), metformin and high fat–high carbohydrate (MET + HFHC), rhenium (V) compound and diet intervention (Re + DI) and rhenium (V) compound and high fat–high carbohydrate (Re + HFHC) groups after 12 weeks of treatment. By comparison with the NC, there was a significant increase in fasting blood glucose concentration in the PD group ($p < 0.05$, Figure 2). The administration of the rhenium (V) compound in both the HFHC and diet intervention groups resulted in significant reduction in fasting blood glucose concentration by comparison to PD ($p < 0.05$, Figure 1). A similar observation was shown by the MET + DI treated group as compared to the PD group (see Figure 2).

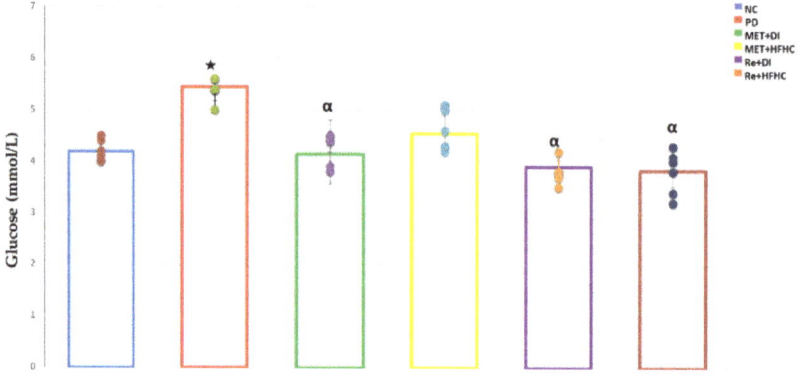

Figure 2. Fasting blood glucose in NC, PD, MET + DI, MET + HFHC, Re + DI and Re + HFHC at 12 weeks of treatment. Values are presented as means ± SD ($n = 6$). ★ $p < 0.05$ by comparison with NC, α $p < 0.05$ by comparison with PD, MET + DI, MET + HFHC, Re + DI and Re + HFHC.

3.2. Liver Glycogen Concentration

Figure 3 shows liver glycogen levels in the normal control (NC), prediabetic control (PD), metformin and diet intervention (MET + DI), metformin and high fat–high carbohydrate (MET + HFHC), rhenium (V) compound and diet intervention (Re + DI) and rhenium (V) compound and high fat–high carbohydrate (Re + HFHC) groups after 12 weeks of treatment. By comparison with the NC group, the PD group showed a significant increase in liver glycogen concentration ($p < 0.05$) (Figure 3). The administration of rhenium (V) compound in both diet intervention and high fat–high carbohydrate groups resulted in a significant decrease of liver glycogen concentration when compared with the PD group ($p < 0.05$). A similar effect was observed with the MET + DI treated group when compared with the PD group ($p < 0.05$) (see Figure 3).

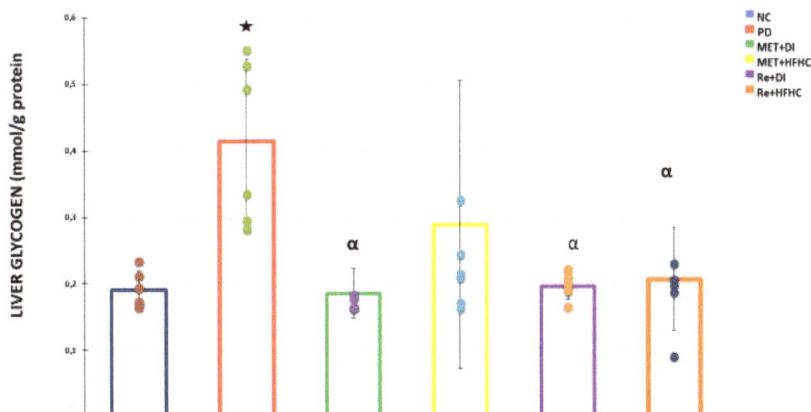

Figure 3. Liver glycogen concentration in NC, PD, MET + DI, MET + HFHC, Re + DI and Re + HFHC after 12 weeks of treatment. Values are presented as means ± SD and individual data points ($n = 6$). ★ $p < 0.05$ by comparison with NC, α $p < 0.05$ by comparison with PD, MET + DI, MET + HFHC, Re + DI and Re + HFHC.

3.3. Liver Triglycerides (TGs) Concentration

Figure 4 shows liver triglyceride concentration in the normal control (NC), prediabetic control (PD), metformin and diet intervention (MET + DI), metformin and high fat–high carbohydrate (MET + HFHC), rhenium (V) compound and diet intervention (Re + DI) and rhenium (V) compound and high fat–high carbohydrate (Re + HFHC) groups after 12 weeks of treatment. By comparison with the NC group, the PD group showed a significant increase in liver triglycerides concentration ($p < 0.05$) (Figure 4). The administration of rhenium (V) compound in both diet intervention and high fat–high carbohydrate groups resulted in a significant decrease of liver triglycerides concentration when compared with the PD group ($p < 0.05$). A similar effect was observed with the MET + DI treated group when compared with the PD group ($p < 0.05$) (see Figure 4).

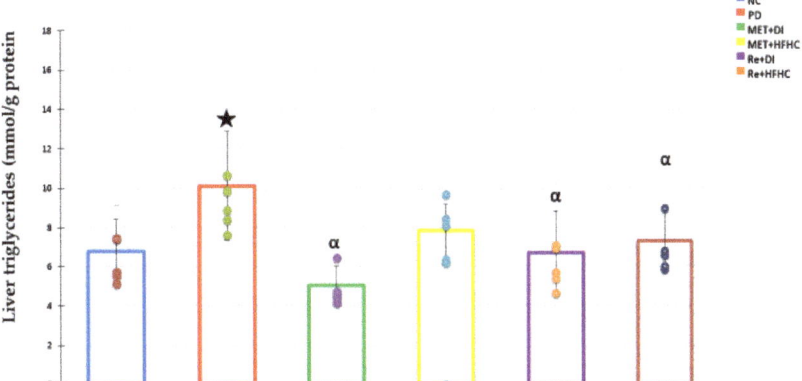

Figure 4. Liver triglycerides concentration in NC, PD, MET + DI, MET + HFHC, Re + DI and Re + HFHC after 12 weeks of treatment. Values are presented as means ± SD and individual data points ($n = 6$). ★ $p < 0.05$ by comparison with NC, α $p < 0.05$ by comparison with PC, MET + DI, MET + HFHC, Re + DI and Re + HFHC.

3.4. Relative Liver Weight

Figure 5 shows relative liver weight in the normal control (NC), prediabetic control (PD), metformin and diet intervention (MET + DI), metformin and high fat–high carbohydrate (MET + HFHC), rhenium (V) compound and diet intervention (Re + DI) and rhenium (V) compound and high fat–high carbohydrate (Re + HFHC) groups after 12 weeks of treatment. In comparison with the NC group, the PD group showed a significant increase in relative liver weight ($p < 0.05$) (Figure 5). The administration of rhenium (V) compound in both diet intervention and high fat–high carbohydrate groups resulted in a significant decrease of relative liver weight when compared with the PD group ($p < 0.05$). A similar effect was observed with the MET + DI treated group when compared with the PD group ($p < 0.05$) (see Figure 5).

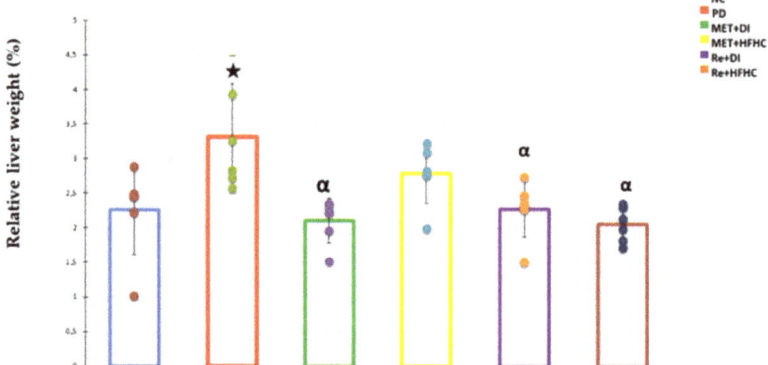

Figure 5. Relative liver weight in normal control (NC), prediabetic control (PD), metformin and diet intervention (MET + DI), metformin and high fat–high carbohydrate (MET + HFHC), rhenium (V) compound and diet intervention (Re + DI) and rhenium (V) compound and high fat–high carbohydrate (Re + HFHC) groups after 12 weeks of treatment. Values are presented as means ± SD and individual data points ($n = 6$). ★ $p < 0.05$ by comparison with NC, α $p < 0.05$ by comparison with PD, MET + DI, MET + HFHC, Re + DI and Re + HFHC.

3.5. Liver Antioxidant Activity

Figure 6 shows antioxidant SOD activity in the normal control (NC), prediabetic control (PD), metformin and diet intervention (MET + DI), metformin and high fat–high carbohydrate (MET + HFHC), rhenium (V) compound and diet intervention (Re + DI) and rhenium (V) compound and high fat–high carbohydrate (Re + HFHC) groups after 12 weeks of treatment. In comparison with the NC group, the PD group showed a significant decrease in SOD activity ($p < 0.05$) (Figure 6). The administration of rhenium (V) compound in both diet intervention and high fat–high carbohydrate groups resulted in a significant increase of SOD activity when compared with the PD group ($p < 0.05$). A similar effect was observed with the MET + DI treated group when compared with the PD group ($p < 0.05$) (see Figure 6).

Figure 6 shows antioxidant GPx activity in the normal control (NC), prediabetic control (PD), metformin and diet intervention (MET + DI), metformin and high fat–high carbohydrate (MET + HFHC), rhenium (V) compound and diet intervention (Re + DI) and rhenium (V) compound and high fat–high carbohydrate (Re + HFHC) groups after 12 weeks of treatment. In comparison with the NC group, the PD group showed a significant decrease in GPx activity ($p < 0.05$) (Figure 7). The administration of rhenium (V) compound in both diet intervention and high fat–high carbohydrate groups resulted in a significant increase of GPx activity when compared with the PD group ($p < 0.05$). A similar effect was observed with the MET + DI treated group when compared with the PD group ($p < 0.05$) (see Figure 7).

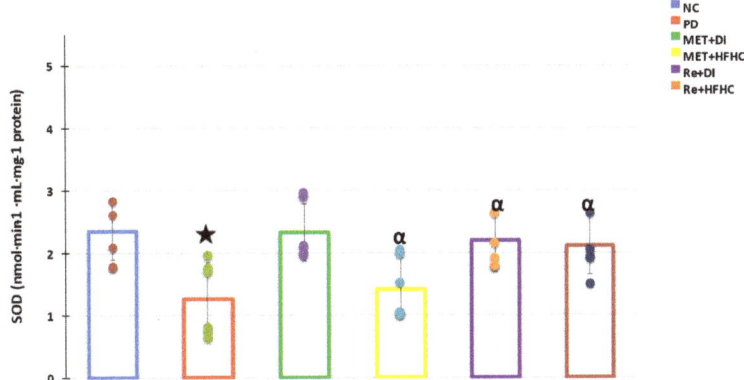

Figure 6. SOD activity in normal control (NC), prediabetic control (PD), metformin and diet intervention (MET + DI), metformin and high fat–high carbohydrate (MET + HFHC), rhenium (V) compound and diet intervention (Re + DI) and rhenium (V) compound and high fat–high carbohydrate (Re + HFHC) groups after 12 weeks of treatment. Values are presented as means ± SD and individual data points ($n = 6$). ★ $p < 0.05$ by comparison with NC, α $p < 0.05$ by comparison with PD, MET + DI, MET + HFHC, Re + DI and Re + HFHC.

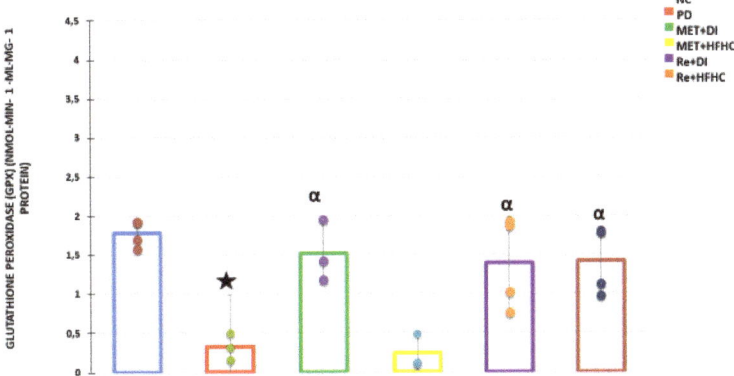

Figure 7. GPx activity in normal control (NC), prediabetic control (PD), metformin and diet intervention (MET + DI), metformin and high fat–high carbohydrate (MET + HFHC), rhenium (V) compound and diet intervention (Re + DI) and rhenium (V) compound and high fat–high carbohydrate (Re + HFHC) groups after 12 weeks of treatment. Values are presented as means ± SD and individual data points ($n = 6$). ★ $p < 0.05$ by comparison with NC, α $p < 0.05$ by comparison with PD, MET + DI, MET + HFHC, Re + DI and Re + HFHC.

3.6. Liver TNF α Concentration

Figure 8 shows TNF α concentrations in the normal control (NC), prediabetic control (PD), metformin and diet intervention (MET + DI), metformin and high fat–high carbohydrate (MET + HFHC), rhenium (V) compound and diet intervention (Re + DI) and rhenium (V) compound and high fat–high carbohydrate (Re + HFHC) groups after 12 weeks of treatment. In comparison with the NC group, the PD group showed a significant increase in TNF α concentration ($p < 0.05$) (Figure 8). The administration of rhenium (V) compound in both diet intervention and high fat–high carbohydrate groups resulted in a significant decrease of TNF α concentration when compared with the PD group ($p < 0.05$). A similar effect was observed with the MET + DI treated group when compared with the PD group ($p < 0.05$) (see Figure 8).

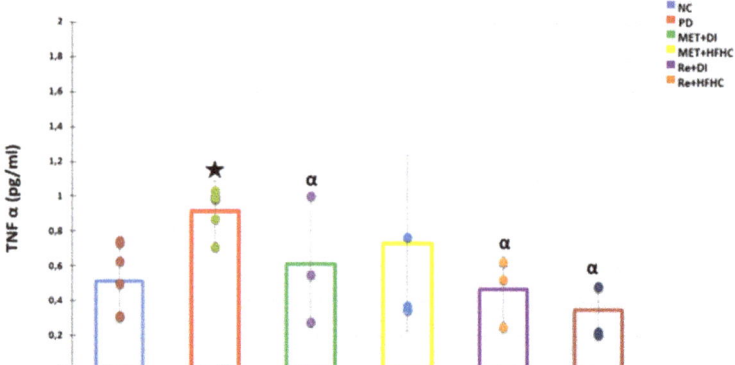

Figure 8. TNF α concentration in normal control (NC), prediabetic control (PD), metformin and diet intervention (MET + DI), metformin and high fat–high carbohydrate (MET + HFHC), rhenium (V) compound and diet intervention (Re + DI) and rhenium (V) compound and high fat–high carbohydrate (Re + HFHC) groups after 12 weeks of treatment. Values are presented as means ± SD and individual data points (n = 6). ★ p < 0.05 by comparison with NC, α p < 0.05 by comparison with PC, MET + DI, MET + HFHC, Re + DI and Re + HFHC.

3.7. Plasma ALT Concentration

Figure 9 shows plasma ALT concentration in the normal control (NC), prediabetic control (PD), metformin and diet intervention (MET + DI), metformin and high fat–high carbohydrate (MET + HFHC), rhenium (V) compound and diet intervention (Re + DI) and rhenium (V) compound and high fat–high carbohydrate (Re + HFHC) after 12 weeks of treatment. In comparison with the NC group, the PD group showed a significant increase in plasma ALT concentration (p < 0.05) (Figure 9). The administration of rhenium (V) compound in both diet intervention and high fat–high carbohydrate groups resulted in a significant decrease of plasma ALT concentration when compared with the PD group (p < 0.05). A similar effect was observed with the MET + DI treated group when compared with the PD group (p < 0.05) (see Figure 9).

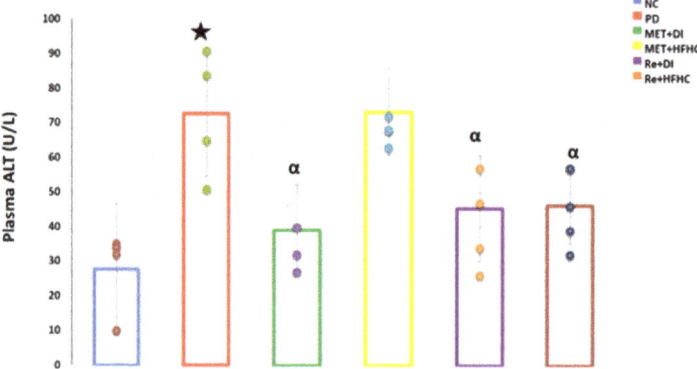

Figure 9. Plasma ALT concentration in normal control (NC), prediabetic control (PD), metformin and diet intervention (MET + DI), metformin and high fat–high carbohydrate (MET + HFHC), rhenium (V) compound and diet intervention (Re + DI) and rhenium (V) compound and high fat–high carbohydrate (Re + HFHC) groups after 12 weeks of treatment. Values are presented as means ± SD and individual data points (n = 6). ★ p < 0.05 by comparison with NC, α p < 0.05 by comparison with PC, MET + DI, MET + HFHC, Re + DI and Re + HFHC.

3.8. Plasma AST Concentration

Figure 10 shows plasma AST concentration in the normal control (NC), prediabetic control (PD), metformin and diet intervention (MET + DI), metformin and high fat–high carbohydrate (MET + HFHC), rhenium (V) compound and diet intervention (Re + DI) and rhenium (V) compound and high fat–high carbohydrate (Re + HFHC) groups after 12 weeks of treatment. In comparison with the NC group, the PD group showed a significant increase in plasma AST concentration ($p < 0.05$) (Figure 10). The administration of rhenium (V) compound in both diet intervention and high fat–high carbohydrate groups resulted in a significant decrease of plasma AST concentration when compared with the PD group ($p < 0.05$). A similar effect was observed with the MET + DI treated group when compared with the PD group ($p < 0.05$) (see Figure 10).

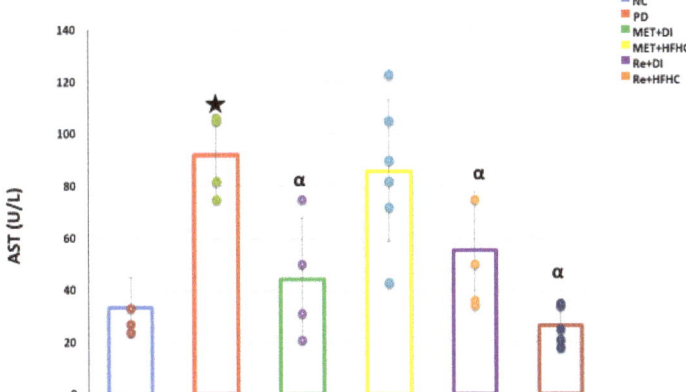

Figure 10. Plasma AST concentration in normal control (NC), prediabetic control (PD), metformin and diet intervention (MET + DI), metformin and high fat–high carbohydrate (MET + HFHC), rhenium (V) compound and diet intervention (Re + DI) and rhenium (V) compound and high fat–high carbohydrate (Re + HFHC) groups after 12 weeks of treatment. Values are presented as means ± SD and individual data points ($n = 6$). ⋆ $p < 0.05$ by comparison with NC, α $p < 0.05$ by comparison with PD, MET + DI, MET + HFHC, Re + DI and Re + HFHC.

4. Discussion

There is growing evidence that associates prediabetes with disorders that were previously thought to co-exist with type 2 diabetes [25,26]. These disorders include impaired glucose homeostasis, dyslipidemia, NAFLD and cardiovascular disease [27,28]. The development of NAFLD is strongly linked with chronic consumption of high calorie diets and is considered the most frequent liver disease in developing countries [28]. Prediabetes is associated with insulin resistance, which can increase peripheral lipolysis, triglyceride synthesis and hepatic uptake of free fatty acids, which ultimately leads to NAFLD [27,29]. Studies have revealed that individuals with prediabetes and NAFLD have a higher risk of progressing to T2DM [27].

Studies have shown that anti-diabetic drugs can be used to manage NAFLD and to prevent it from developing into non-alcoholic steatohepatitis (NASH) [12,30]. Metformin has been used to treat NAFLD, as it is known to increase insulin action and reduce plasma glucose levels [31]. However, metformin has been shown to reach optimal efficacy when combined with lifestyle modifications that increase physical activity and lower caloric intake [30,32]. However, studies on patients show that there is an over-reliance on pharmacological interventions leading to a neglect on the lifestyle modification that results in reduced efficacy of the drugs [33]. Therefore, there is a great need for drugs which could perhaps assist those individuals who struggle with lifestyle modification [15,18].

There is a growing interest in using transition metal compounds to treat complications associated with metabolic disorders due to their high biological activity [9,34]. Our novel transition metal compound, rhenium (V) compound with uracil-derived ligands, has been previously shown to have anti-diabetic and anti-oxidant effects [20]. However, the effects of this metal-based compound on prediabetes induced NAFLD are yet to be investigated. In this study, we sought to further investigate the effects of this rhenium (V) compound on selected liver function markers in diet-induced prediabetic rats.

To maintain an individual's health, processes such as glucose homeostasis are tightly regulated to meet the energy needs for important organs. The liver plays an important role in the maintenance of glucose homeostasis by being involved many pathways of glucose metabolism including glycogenesis, glycogenolysis, glycolysis and gluconeogenesis [6,35]. During fasting conditions, the liver has a vital role in producing glucose through gluconeogenesis as a fuel for other tissues, such as the brain, red blood cells and muscles [35]. The main function of insulin is to inhibit glycogenolysis and gluconeogenesis in the hepatocytes [33]. However, in the prediabetic state, there is increased energy demand due to insulin resistance in some tissues, while there is also dysregulation of metabolic pathways such as gluconeogenesis [36,37]. Gluconeogenesis is increased in the liver due to peripheral insulin resistance [38]. Insulin-resistant muscle and other tissues require energy; therefore, signals are sent to the liver to produce glucose [39,40]. Gluconeogenesis is activated, resulting in glucose production from the liver to the plasma, while hepatic steatosis leads to increased hepatic gluconeogenesis [41,42]. Indeed, the untreated prediabetic group in this study showed high fasting plasma glucose levels. This could be due to unregulated gluconeogenesis and energy demand from insulin-resistant peripheral tissues [32,43]. Furthermore, the treated groups with rhenium (V) compound were shown to have reduced plasma glucose in both the presence and absence of dietary intervention. The rhenium (V) compound has been previously shown to restore peripheral insulin sensitivity through increased GLUT 4 expression, thus ameliorating insulin sensitivity and improving glycemic control [37]. Another transition metal with an organic ligand such as the dioxidovanadium complex (V) for this compound was shown to lower plasma glucose by increasing glucose transport and insulin-receptor tyrosine-kinase activity in NAFLD [44].

The hepatocytes play a vital role in regulating carbohydrate metabolism [45]. The storage of glycogen in the liver during feeding conditions provides a storage form of glucose that can be used during fasting periods. Normally, stored glycogen is critical for maintaining glucose homeostasis in individuals during an overnight fasting period [11,45]. However, in the prediabetic state, the liver has to store glucose due to insulin resistance in other tissues such as muscle and adipose tissues [11]. GLUT 2 transports glucose independently of insulin, and this results in a higher rate of hepatic glycogenesis occurring due to the shunting of glucose during the prediabetic state [46]. In this study, the untreated prediabetic group was shown to have high hepatic glycogen concentration. This could be due to high glucose uptake through GLUT 2. Further observations show that the treated groups with the rhenium (V) compound in both the presence and absence of dietary intervention had reduced glycogen concentration. A possible reason for the observed reduction in glycogen levels in the rhenium (V) compound treated group may be because this compound has been shown to improve insulin sensitivity by increasing the expression of GLUT4 in the skeletal muscle and fat tissue, as shown in a study conducted by Siboto, A. et al., 2020 [20]. This reduction in the amount of glucose being shunted to the liver could result in reduced storage of hepatic glycogen [34]. Other studies on transition metals on NAFLD treatment showed that metal complexes including ruthenium and vanadium reduce hepatic glycogen concentration by channeling excess glucose to be metabolized in skeletal muscle and adipose tissue [19,44]. Glucose from excess dietary carbohydrates goes through glycolysis in hepatocytes and is later converted into fatty acids to be esterified into triglycerides (TGs), which are eventually secreted via very low-density lipoproteins [45].

In NAFLD patients with insulin resistance, the increased lipolysis in adipose tissue causes enhanced liver glucose synthesis, which further activates de novo lipogenesis, resulting in hepatic fat deposition [12,38]. Enhanced de novo lipogenesis and reduced fatty acid oxidation had been reported in patients with insulin resistance and contribute to a critical biochemical pathway for the pathogenesis of NAFLD [47,48].

Consumption of diets high in fructose also results in the activation of the de novo lipogenesis pathway. PPARγ-coactivator-1β (PGC-1β), which acts as a co-activator of SREBP1c, can be stimulated by fructose. Moreover, fructose inhibits hepatic fatty acid β-oxidation, which mainly occurs by inhibiting the transcriptional activities of PPARα [7,49]. Thus, the shift towards lipogenesis over fatty acid oxidation contributes to hepatic steatosis. In a hyper-insulinemic state, insulin continues to drive lipogenesis via the SREBP1 pathway in addition to failing to suppress gluconeogenesis, contributing to exacerbating hepatic steatosis. Due to hyperinsulinemia and hyperglycemia, SREBP-1c is activated resulting in high storage of TGs observed in the untreated prediabetic group. However, the administration of the rhenium (V) compound in both the presence and absence of diet intervention resulted in reduced hepatic TGs storage on the treated prediabetic rats. This may be because the rhenium (V) compound facilitated weight loss through suppressing the secretion of ghrelin and reducing food intake. The food consumption results are on a glucose homeostasis paper by Siboto, A. et al., 2020 [20].

Due to a decrease in hepatic TGs concentration in the treated groups, we can also speculate that the rhenium (V) compound may decrease free fatty deposition to the liver by divergence of the substrates to other tissues for metabolism, increased β oxidation of fat or increased triglyceride disposal via very low-density lipoprotein (VLDL) exportation from the liver. Other metals such a dioxidovanadium lowered plasma TGs in diabetic rats via improving insulin sensitivity in adipose tissue and skeletal muscle [44]. Literature research on metal complexes such as ruthenium (ii) complex facilitated weight loss in prediabetic rat resulting in less fatty acid deposition in the liver [19].

The administration of rhenium (V) compound in both the presence and the absence of diet intervention on treated prediabetic rats resulted in both reduction of hepatic glycogen concentration and hepatic TGs storage. This positive effect caused by the administration of the rhenium (V) compound resulted in reduced liver weight as compared to the untreated prediabetic group. Several studies suggest that increased liver weights in prediabetes and NAFLD are associated with increased hepatic lipid accumulation [33]. Furthermore, this may imply that the rhenium (V) compound manages NAFLD delaying from becoming NASH. Relative liver weights results may also be a reflection of triacylglycerol and liver weights due to hepatic very-low-density lipoprotein–triglyceride (VLDL-TG) secretion rates. Studies have shown that liver weight is directly related to hepatic VLDL-TG secretion, independently of body weight. Therefore, since there is reduction of liver TGs in the prediabetic treated group, the liver weight is also reduced. We speculate that with improved insulin sensitivity on the adipose tissue, fat molecules are metabolized, resulting in enhanced HDL reducing the risk of hepatic steatosis associated with insulin resistance.

Oxidative stress is balanced by a number of antioxidant enzymes [50]. Antioxidant enzymes are ROS scavenging agents to protect the cells against oxidative stress under physiological conditions [4]. Uncontrolled oxidative stress can result in liver injury [51]. Increased oxidative stress is independently associated with NAFLD [50]. NAFLD is characterized by insulin resistance, which results in elevated concentrations of free fatty acids, providing substrates for triglyceride formation and subsequent progression of the disease in the liver [51]. It is suggested that increased accumulation of liver triglycerides leads to increased oxidative stress in the hepatocytes [52,53]. NAFLD is also associated with mitochondrial dysfunction, and an increase of mitochondrial β-oxidation activity, due to a lipid overload, may induce an impairment of electron transport chain, resulting in electron leakage and increased ROS [54]. Oxidative stress causes hepatocellular damage through many different mechanisms, including lipid peroxidation, that can directly stimulate cell necrosis and activation of apoptosis [41,55]. Oxidation stress can directly lead to the synthesis of reactive oxygen species (ROS) that are usually removed by antioxidant pathways; however, in the prediabetic state, antioxidant activity is reduced. Indeed, this is also observed in the untreated prediabetic group. The administration of the rhenium (V) compound in both the presence and the absence of diet intervention in the prediabetic rats showed reduced lipid peroxidation and improved antioxidant activity in both SOD and GPx. We speculate that since the rhenium (V) compound reduces fat deposition in the liver, this prevents mitochondrial dysfunction. Therefore, the rhenium (V) compound can prevent liver injury that can be caused by oxidative stress. Vanadium and ruthenium complexes have also been shown to prevent oxidative stress through enhanced glycemic control [19,21,44].

Inflammation, oxidative stress and insulin resistance are involved in NAFLD. The progression of NAFLD to NASH is identified through increased inflammation. NASH patients with increased serum TNF-a concentrations also show higher levels of interleukin (IL)-6 [54]. The administration of the rhenium (V) compound in both the presence and the absence of diet intervention was showed to reduce oxidative stress and improve antioxidant activity, reducing liver injury. The rhenium (V) compound has been shown to have anti-inflammatory properties by reducing plasma TNF α in the treated prediabetic group, protecting progressive liver damage.

Liver enzymes, AST and ALT, are used as clinical biomarkers to identify the degree of hepatocyte damage occurring in the liver [45]. The reason the liver enzyme levels better reflect the presence of injury is that these enzymes are components of hepatocytes that are released into circulation upon hepatocyte damage [45]. Literature trends have variably shown that high AST and ALT occur in blood due to necrosis of the hepatocyte during liver damage [33,55]. Metals are strongly known to be toxic on the liver [39]. The rhenium (V) compound was administered via subcutaneous injection in order for the drug to bypass liver metabolism and be absorbed in the bloodstream. This allows the drug to avoid first-pass metabolism in the liver, as the rhenium complex is known to be relatively harmless. The literature has shown that metal complexes are often associated with increased plasma AST and ALT levels, suggesting liver toxicity [33,55]. However, the rhenium (V) compound is synthesized with uracil-derived ligands that increase bioactivity and uracil-derived ligands. This has been shown to have the capability of coordination through a variety of donor atoms [56]. These uracil-derived ligands make the rhenium (V) compound have reduced cellular toxicity [56,57].

Liver enzymes such as AST and ALT are released into the bloodstream whenever hepatocytes are damaged, and this has been reported to occur during prediabetes [55]. The untreated prediabetic group had a high level of liver AST and ALT [27]. This observation of increased liver enzymes in the plasma suggested that liver cells are damaged through oxidative stress and increased hepatic lipogenesis or glycogenesis. However, administration of the rhenium (V) compound in prediabetic rats resulted in a decreased concentration of liver enzymes. This can be a result that is observed in this study. The rhenium (V) compound seems to improve hepatic health via its antioxidant, antilipidemic and anti-inflammatory effects. Studies have shown that metal-based compounds such as ruthenium (II) compounds ameliorated liver disarrangement and prevented hepatotoxicity [19,58].

5. Conclusions

The administration of the rhenium compound is associated with an improved liver health as evidenced by decreased liver triglyceride, glycogen and fasting blood glucose concentrations. Additionally, the observations suggest that this compound may attenuate liver injury associated with prediabetes, as evidenced by the reduction of oxidative stress, liver function marker enzymes and inflammatory markers in the liver. Given the beneficial effects of the rhenium (V) compound presented in this study, further investigations are warranted to fully assess the therapeutic value of rhenium (V) administration during prediabetes.

Author Contributions: Conceptualization, A.S., A.K. and A.M.A.; methodology, A.S., M.B.I. and A.M.A.; software, A.S.; validation, A.S., A.K. and N.H.S.; formal analysis, A.S. and A.K.; investigation, A.S.; resources, A.K., P.N. and I.N.B.; data curation, A.S.; writing—original draft preparation, A.S.; writing—review and editing, I.N.B., A.K., N.H.S. and P.N.; visualization, A.S.; supervision, N.H.S. and A.K.; project administration A.K.; funding acquisition, A.K. All authors have read and agreed to the published version of the manuscript.

Funding: National Research Foundation (NRF) (grant 106041) and University of KwaZulu Natal College of Health Science funding.

Institutional Review Board Statement: The animal study protocol was approved by the Institutional Animal Research Ethics Committee of University of KwaZulu-Natal UKZN (protocol code AREC/00003221/2021 (previous AREC reference number: AREC/039/018M) and date of approval: 23 June 2022).

Informed Consent Statement: Not applicable.

Data Availability Statement: The data presented in this study are available on request from the corresponding author.

Acknowledgments: The authors acknowledge the personnel at the UKZN Biomedical Resource Unit for their technical assistance.

Conflicts of Interest: The authors declare no conflict of interest.

References

1. Stefan, N.; Häring, H.-U.; Cusi, K. Non-alcoholic fatty liver disease: Causes, diagnosis, cardiometabolic consequences, and treatment strategies. *Lancet Diabetes Endocrinol.* **2018**, *7*, 313–324. [CrossRef]
2. Cusi, K.; Sanyal, A.J.; Zhang, S.; Hartman, M.L.; Bue-Valleskey, J.M.; Hoogwerf, B.J.; Haupt, A. Non-alcoholic fatty liver disease (NAFLD) prevalence and its metabolic associations in patients with type 1 diabetes and type 2 diabetes. *Diabetes Obes. Metab.* **2017**, *19*, 1630–1634. [CrossRef] [PubMed]
3. Khathi, A.; Luvuno, M.; Mabandla, M. Voluntary Ingestion of a High-Fat High-Carbohydrate Diet: A Model for Prediabetes. Master's Thesis, University of KwaZulu-Natal, KwaZulu-Natal, South Africa, 2017. [CrossRef]
4. Maghsoudi, Z.; Ghiasvand, R.; Salehi-Abargouei, A. Empirically derived dietary patterns and incident type 2 diabetes mellitus: A systematic review and meta-analysis on prospective observational studies. *Public Health Nutr.* **2015**, *19*, 230–241. [CrossRef] [PubMed]
5. Kalender, S.; Apaydin, F.G.; Baş, H.; Kalender, Y. Protective effects of sodium selenite on lead nitrate-induced hepatotoxicity in diabetic and non-diabetic rats. *Environ. Toxicol. Pharmacol.* **2015**, *40*, 568–574. [CrossRef]
6. Jensen, T.; Abdelmalek, M.F.; Sullivan, S.; Nadeau, K.J.; Green, M.; Roncal, C.; Nakagawa, T.; Kuwabara, M.; Sato, Y.; Kang, D.-H.; et al. Fructose and sugar: A major mediator of non-alcoholic fatty liver disease. *J. Hepatol.* **2018**, *68*, 1063–1075. [CrossRef]
7. Ter Horst, K.W.; Serlie, M.J.J.N. Fructose consumption, lipogenesis, and non-alcoholic fatty liver disease. *Nutrients* **2017**, *9*, 981. [CrossRef]
8. Newton, K.P.; Hou, J.; Crimmins, N.A.; LaVine, J.E.; Barlow, S.E.; Xanthakos, S.A.; Africa, J.; Behling, C.; Donithan, M.; Clark, J.M.; et al. Prevalence of Prediabetes and Type 2 Diabetes in Children With Nonalcoholic Fatty Liver Disease. *JAMA Pediatr.* **2016**, *170*, e161971. [CrossRef]
9. Ortiz-Lopez, C.; Lomonaco, R.; Orsak, B.; Finch, J.; Chang, Z.; Kochunov, V.G.; Hardies, J.; Cusi, K. Prevalence of Prediabetes and Diabetes and Metabolic Profile of Patients With Nonalcoholic Fatty Liver Disease (NAFLD). *Diabetes Care* **2012**, *35*, 873–878. [CrossRef]
10. Sanyal, D.; Mukherjee, P.; Raychaudhuri, M.; Ghosh, S.; Mukherjee, S.; Chowdhury, S. Profile of liver enzymes in non-alcoholic fatty liver disease in patients with impaired glucose tolerance and newly detected untreated type 2 diabetes. *Indian J. Endocrinol. Metab.* **2015**, *19*, 597–601. [CrossRef]
11. Neuschwander-Tetri, B.A.J.B. Non-alcoholic fatty liver disease. *BMC medicine.* **2017**, *15*, 45. [CrossRef]
12. Bhatt, H.B.; Smith, R.J. Fatty liver disease in diabetes mellitus. *Hepatobiliary Surg. Nutr.* **2015**, *4*, 101–108. [CrossRef]
13. Shurrab, N.T.; Arafa, E.-S.A. Metformin: A review of its therapeutic efficacy and adverse effects. *Obes. Med.* **2020**, *17*, 100186. [CrossRef]
14. Gupta, A.; Behl, T.; Sachdeva, M. Key milestones in the diabetes research: A comprehensive update. *Obes. Med.* **2020**, *17*, 100183. [CrossRef]
15. El-Kader, S.M.A.; El-Den Ashmawy, E.M.S. Non-alcoholic fatty liver disease: The diagnosis and management. *World J. Hepatol* **2015**, *7*, 846. [CrossRef]
16. Leite, N.C. Non-alcoholic fatty liver disease and diabetes: From physiopathological interplay to diagnosis and treatment. *World J. Gastroenterol.* **2014**, *20*, 8377–8392. [CrossRef]

17. Malin, S.K.; Gerber, R.; Chipkin, S.R.; Braun, B. Independent and Combined Effects of Exercise Training and Metformin on Insulin Sensitivity in Individuals with Prediabetes. *Diabetes Care* **2011**, *35*, 131–136. [CrossRef]
18. Roberts, S.; Barry, E.; Craig, D.; Airoldi, M.; Bevan, G.; Greenhalgh, T. Preventing type 2 diabetes: Systematic review of studies of cost-effectiveness of lifestyle programmes and metformin, with and without screening, for pre-diabetes. *BMJ Open* **2017**, *7*, e017184. [CrossRef]
19. Mabuza, L.P.; Gamede, M.W.; Maikoo, S.; Booysen, I.N.; Nguban, P.S.; Khathi, A. Hepatoprotective Effects of a Ruthenium(II) Schiff Base Complex in Rats with Diet-Induced Prediabetes. *Curr. Ther. Res.* **2019**, *91*, 66–72. [CrossRef]
20. Siboto, A.; Akinnuga, A.M.; Khumalo, B.N.; Ismail, M.B.; Booysen, I.N.; Sibiya, N.H.; Ngubane, P.S.; Khathi, A. The effects of a [3+1] oxo-free rhenium (V) compound with uracil-derived ligands on selected parameters of glucose homeostasis in diet-induced pre-diabetic rats. *Obes. Med.* **2020**, *19*, 100258. [CrossRef]
21. Mabuza, L.P.; Gamede, M.W.; Maikoo, S.; Booysen, I.N.; Ngubane, P.S.; Khathi, A. Effects of a Ruthenium Schiff Base Complex on Glucose Homeostasis in Diet-Induced Pre-Diabetic Rats. *Molecules* **2018**, *23*, 1721. [CrossRef]
22. Luvuno, M.; Mbongwa, H.; Khathi, A. Development of a novel prediabetes animal model using a high fat high carbohydrate diet: Implications for type 2 diabetes. *PLoS ONE* **2017**, *13*, 8–14.
23. Wallace, T.M.; Levy, J.C.; Matthews, D.R. Use and Abuse of HOMA Modeling. *Diabetes Care* **2004**, *27*, 1487–1495. [CrossRef]
24. Heikes, K.E.; Eddy, D.M.; Arondekar, B.; Schlessinger, L. Diabetes Risk Calculator: A simple tool for detecting undiagnosed diabetes and pre-diabetes. *Diabetes Care* **2008**, *31*, 1040–1045. [CrossRef]
25. Ngubane, P.S.; Masola, B.; Musabayane, C.T. The Effects of *Syzygium aromaticum*-Derived Oleanolic Acid on Glycogenic Enzymes in Streptozotocin-Induced Diabetic Rats. *Ren. Fail.* **2011**, *33*, 434–439. [CrossRef]
26. Mkhwanazi, B.N.; Serumula, M.R.; Myburg, R.B.; Van Heerden, F.R.; Musabayane, C.T. Antioxidant effects of maslinic acid in livers, hearts and kidneys of streptozotocin-induced diabetic rats: Effects on kidney function. *Ren. Fail.* **2013**, *36*, 419–431. [CrossRef]
27. Buysschaert, M.; Medina, J.L.; Bergman, M.; Shah, A.; Lonier, J. Prediabetes and associated disorders. *Endocrine* **2014**, *48*, 371–393. [CrossRef]
28. Bungau, S.; Behl, T.; Tit, D.M.; Banica, F.; Bratu, O.G.; Diaconu, C.C.; Nistor-Cseppento, C.D.; Bustea, C.; Aron, R.A.C.; Vesa, C.M. Interactions between leptin and insulin resistance in patients with prediabetes, with and without NAFLD. *Exp. Ther. Med.* **2020**, *20*, 1. [CrossRef]
29. Rajput, R.; Ahlawat, P. Prevalence and predictors of non-alcoholic fatty liver disease in prediabetes. *Diabetes Metab. Syndr.* **2019**, *13*, 2957–2960. [CrossRef]
30. Targher, G.; Corey, K.E.; Byrne, C.D.; Roden, M. The complex link between NAFLD and type 2 diabetes mellitus—Mechanisms and treatments. *Nat. Rev. Gastroenterol. Hepatol.* **2021**, *18*, 599–612. [CrossRef]
31. Portillo-Sanchez, P.; Cusi, K. Treatment of Nonalcoholic Fatty Liver Disease (NAFLD) in patients with Type 2 Diabetes Mellitus. *Clin. Diabetes Endocrinol.* **2016**, *2*, 9. [CrossRef]
32. Gaggini, M.; Morelli, M.; Buzzigoli, E.; DeFronzo, R.A.; Bugianesi, E.; Gastaldelli, A. Non-Alcoholic Fatty Liver Disease (NAFLD) and Its Connection with Insulin Resistance, Dyslipidemia, Atherosclerosis and Coronary Heart Disease. *Nutrients* **2013**, *5*, 1544–1560. [CrossRef] [PubMed]
33. Adiels, M.; Taskinen, M.-R.; Borén, J.J.C. Fatty liver, insulin resistance, and dyslipidemia. *Curr. Diabetes Rep.* **2008**, *8*, 60–64. [CrossRef] [PubMed]
34. Chang, L.; Chiang, S.-H.; Saltiel, A.R. Insulin Signaling and the Regulation of Glucose Transport. *Mol. Med.* **2004**, *10*, 65–71. [CrossRef] [PubMed]
35. Sharabi, K.; Tavares, C.D.; Rines, A.K.; Puigserver, P. Molecular pathophysiology of hepatic glucose production. *Mol. Asp. Med.* **2015**, *46*, 21–33. [CrossRef]
36. Katsiki, N.; Mikhailidis, D.P.; Mantzoros, C.S. Non-alcoholic fatty liver disease and dyslipidemia: An update. *Metabolism* **2016**, *65*, 1109–1123. [CrossRef]
37. Sunny, N.E.; Parks, E.J.; Browning, J.D.; Burgess, S.C. Excessive Hepatic Mitochondrial TCA Cycle and Gluconeogenesis in Humans with Nonalcoholic Fatty Liver Disease. *Cell Metab.* **2011**, *14*, 804–810. [CrossRef]
38. Chao, H.-W.; Chao, S.-W.; Lin, H.; Ku, H.-C.; Cheng, C.-F. Homeostasis of Glucose and Lipid in Non-Alcoholic Fatty Liver Disease. *Int. J. Mol. Sci.* **2019**, *20*, 298. [CrossRef]
39. Watterworth, B.; Wright, T.B. *Diabetic Peripheral Neuropathy, in Pain*; Springer: Berlin/Heidelberg, Germany, 2019; pp. 911–913. [CrossRef]
40. Bernardes, N.; Ayyappan, P.; De Angelis, K.; Bagchi, A.; Akolkar, G.; Dias, D.D.S.; Belló-Klein, A.; Singal, P.K. Excessive consumption of fructose causes cardiometabolic dysfunctions through oxidative stress and inflammation. *Can. J. Physiol. Pharmacol.* **2017**, *95*, 1078–1090. [CrossRef]
41. Rowell, R.J.; Anstee, Q.M.J.C. An overview of the genetics, mechanisms and management of NAFLD and ALD. *Clin. Med.* **2015**, *15* (Suppl. S6), s77–s82. [CrossRef]
42. Abdul-Ghani, M.A.; DeFronzo, R.A. Pathophysiology of prediabetes. *Curr. Diabetes Rep.* **2009**, *9*, 193–199. [CrossRef]
43. Samuel, V.T.; Shulman, G.I.J.T.J. The pathogenesis of insulin resistance: Integrating signaling pathways and substrate flux. *J. Clin. Investig.* **2016**, *126*, 12–22. [CrossRef]

44. Sibiya, S.; Msibi, B.; Khathi, A.; Sibiya, N.; Booysen, I.; Ngubane, P. The effect of dioxidovanadium complex (V) on hepatic function in streptozotocin-induced diabetic rats. *Can. J. Physiol. Pharmacol.* **2019**, *97*, 1169–1175. [CrossRef]
45. Kalra, A.; Yetiskul, E.; Wehrle, C.J.; Tuma, F. Physiology, Liver. In *StatPearls*; StatPearls Publishing: Treasure Island, FL, USA, 2022.
46. Akehi, Y.; Yanase, T.; Motonaga, R.; Umakoshi, H.; Tsuiki, M.; Takeda, Y.; Yoneda, T.; Kurihara, I.; Itoh, H.; Katabami, T.; et al. High Prevalence of Diabetes in Patients With Primary Aldosteronism (PA) Associated With Subclinical Hypercortisolism and Prediabetes More Prevalent in Bilateral Than Unilateral PA: A Large, Multicenter Cohort Study in Japan. *Diabetes Care* **2019**, *42*, 938–945. [CrossRef]
47. Goodpaster, B.H.; DeLany, J.P.; Otto, A.D.; Kuller, L.; Vockley, J.; South-Paul, J.E.; Thomas, S.B.; Brown, J.; McTigue, K.; Hames, K.C.; et al. Effects of diet and physical activity interventions on weight loss and cardiometabolic risk factors in severely obese adults: A randomized trial. *JAMA* **2010**, *304*, 1795–1802. [CrossRef]
48. Manne, V.; Handa, P.; Kowdley, K.V. Pathophysiology of Nonalcoholic Fatty Liver Disease/Nonalcoholic Steatohepatitis. *Clin. Liver Dis.* **2018**, *22*, 23–37. [CrossRef]
49. Sodum, N.; Kumar, G.; Bojja, S.L.; Kumar, N.; Rao, C.M. Epigenetics in NAFLD/NASH: Targets and therapy. *Pharmacol. Res.* **2021**, *167*, 105484. [CrossRef]
50. Narasimhan, S.; Gokulakrishnan, K.; Sampathkumar, R.; Farooq, S.; Ravikumar, R.; Mohan, V.; Balasubramanyam, M. Oxidative stress is independently associated with non-alcoholic fatty liver disease (NAFLD) in subjects with and without type 2 diabetes. *Clin. Biochem.* **2010**, *43*, 815–821. [CrossRef]
51. Asmat, U.; Abad, K.; Ismail, K. Diabetes mellitus and oxidative stress—A concise review. *Saudi Pharm. J.* **2015**, *24*, 547–553. [CrossRef]
52. Arroyave-Ospina, J.C.; Wu, Z.; Geng, Y.; Moshage, H. Role of Oxidative Stress in the Pathogenesis of Non-Alcoholic Fatty Liver Disease: Implications for Prevention and Therapy. *Antioxidants* **2021**, *10*, 174. [CrossRef]
53. Videla, L.A.; Rodrigo, R.; Araya, J.; Poniachik, J. Insulin resistance and oxidative stress interdependency in non-alcoholic fatty liver disease. *Trends Mol. Med.* **2006**, *12*, 555–558. [CrossRef]
54. Masarone, M.; Rosato, V.; Dallio, M.; Gravina, A.G.; Aglitti, A.; Loguercio, C.; Federico, A.; Persico, M. Role of oxidative stress in pathophysiology of nonalcoholic fatty liver disease. *Oxidative Med. Cell. Longev.* **2018**, *2018*, 9547613. [CrossRef]
55. Clark, J.M.; Brancati, F.L.; Diehl, A.M.J.G. Nonalcoholic fatty liver disease. *N. Engl. J. Med.* **2002**, *122*, 1649–1657. [CrossRef]
56. Ismail, M.B.; Booysen, I.N. Complexes of the fac-[Re(CO)3]+ and [ReO]3+ Moieties with Aromatic, Multidentate, NDonor Ligands. *Ther. Drug Monit.* **2013**, *357*, 1499–1516.
57. Ismail, M.B.; Booysen, I.N.; Akerman, M. DNA interaction studies of rhenium compounds with Schiff base chelates encompassing biologically relevant moieties. *Nucleosides Nucleotides Nucleic Acids* **2019**, *38*, 950–971. [CrossRef]
58. Ismail, M.B.; Booysen, I.N.; Akerman, M.P. Rhenium(I) complexes with aliphatic Schiff bases appended to bio-active moieties. *Inorg. Chem. Commun.* **2017**, *78*, 78–81. [CrossRef]

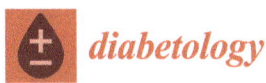

Article

An Evaluation of Point-of-Care HbA1c, HbA1c Home Kits, and Glucose Management Indicator: Potential Solutions for Telehealth Glycemic Assessments

Dessi P. Zaharieva [1,*], Ananta Addala [1], Priya Prahalad [1,2], Brianna Leverenz [1], Nora Arrizon-Ruiz [1], Victoria Y. Ding [3], Manisha Desai [3], Amy B. Karger [4] and David M. Maahs [1,2]

[1] Division of Endocrinology, Department of Pediatrics, School of Medicine, Stanford University, Stanford, CA 94304, USA
[2] Stanford Diabetes Research Center, Stanford, CA 94304, USA
[3] Quantitative Sciences Unit, Division of Biomedical Informatics Research, Stanford University, Stanford, CA 94305, USA
[4] Department of Laboratory Medicine and Pathology, School of Medicine, University of Minnesota, Minneapolis, MN 55455, USA
* Correspondence: dessi@stanford.edu; Tel.: +1-(628)-238-9420; Fax: +1-(650)-475-8375

Abstract: During the COVID-19 pandemic, fewer in-person clinic visits resulted in fewer point-of-care (POC) HbA1c measurements. In this sub-study, we assessed the performance of alternative glycemic measures that can be obtained remotely, such as HbA1c home kits and Glucose Management Indicator (GMI) values from Dexcom Clarity. Home kit HbA1c (n = 99), GMI, (n = 88), and POC HbA1c (n = 32) were collected from youth with T1D (age 9.7 ± 4.6 years). Bland–Altman analyses and Lin's concordance correlation coefficient (ρ_c) were used to characterize the agreement between paired HbA1c measures. Both the HbA1c home kit and GMI showed a slight positive bias (mean difference 0.18% and 0.34%, respectively) and strong concordance with POC HbA1c (ρ_c = 0.982 [0.965, 0.991] and 0.823 [0.686, 0.904], respectively). GMI showed a slight positive bias (mean difference 0.28%) and fair concordance (ρ_c = 0.750 [0.658, 0.820]) to the HbA1c home kit. In conclusion, the strong concordance of GMI and home kits to POC A1c measures suggest their utility in telehealth visits assessments. Although these are not candidates for replacement, these measures can facilitate telehealth visits, particularly in the context of other POC HbA1c measurements from an individual.

Keywords: type 1 diabetes; pediatrics; HbA1c; telemedicine; continuous glucose monitoring

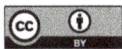

Citation: Zaharieva, D.P.; Addala, A.; Prahalad, P.; Leverenz, B.; Arrizon-Ruiz, N.; Ding, V.Y.; Desai, M.; Karger, A.B.; Maahs, D.M. An Evaluation of Point-of-Care HbA1c, HbA1c Home Kits, and Glucose Management Indicator: Potential Solutions for Telehealth Glycemic Assessments. *Diabetology* 2022, 3, 494–501. https://doi.org/10.3390/diabetology3030037

Academic Editor: Jie Hu

Received: 27 June 2022
Accepted: 31 August 2022
Published: 13 September 2022

Publisher's Note: MDPI stays neutral with regard to jurisdictional claims in published maps and institutional affiliations.

Copyright: © 2022 by the authors. Licensee MDPI, Basel, Switzerland. This article is an open access article distributed under the terms and conditions of the Creative Commons Attribution (CC BY) license (https:// creativecommons.org/licenses/by/ 4.0/).

1. Introduction

For individuals with type 1 diabetes (T1D), hemoglobin A1c (HbA1c), self-monitoring of blood glucose (SMBG), and continuous glucose monitoring (CGM) are common metrics used to assess glycemic management. HbA1c has long been considered the gold standard in glucose monitoring [1]. Although HbA1c remains an important measure of glucose values over time and overall diabetes management, various conditions can impact the accuracy of HbA1c measures, including hemoglobinopathies, chronic kidney disease, or iron-deficiency anemia [1]. In routine clinical care, point-of-care (POC) HbA1c measurements using fingerstick samples with National Glycohemoglobin Standardization Program (NGSP) certification offer healthcare providers a method for real-time assessment of glycemic control [2].

With the increasing use of CGM technology [3], various CGM-derived estimations of HbA1c have evolved over the years. The term "estimated A1c" has also been replaced with terms such as Glucose Management Indicator (GMI) to reduce confusion if laboratory HbA1c and estimated A1c differ. CGM-derived glucose metrics offer promising, real-time, and effective data to better manage T1D [4] by focusing on the glucose time-in-range (i.e., time spent between 70–180 mg/dL).

CGM-derived metrics have become particularly relevant during the COVID-19 pandemic, where fewer in-person clinic visits resulted in fewer POC HbA1c measurements. Therefore, as reported by Beck and colleagues [5], there is an increased need for alternate methods to assess HbA1c, including academic laboratories' fingerstick capillary blood collection kits suitable for home use (HbA1c home kit) and CGM-derived GMI [6]. This work aimed to assess the accuracy and concordance between POC HbA1c, HbA1c home kit, and GMI in pediatric patients with T1D within the 4T Study when the COVID-19 pandemic required creative solutions to monitor glucose control. We report these findings as they may expand options for evaluating diabetes care.

2. Materials & Methods

This sub-study was part of the larger 4T Study, which aims to initiate CGM (Dexcom G6; Dexcom, San Diego, CA, USA) shortly after T1D diagnosis, approved by the Stanford University Institutional Review Board (clinicaltrials.gov: NCT03968055 and NCT04336969) [7–16]. Inclusion criteria for the 4T Study included all youth within one month of the T1D diagnosis seen in the Stanford Lucile Packard Children's Hospital ages six months to 21. A formal diagnosis of T1D included at least one positive autoantibody. The exclusion criteria for the 4T Study included a diabetes diagnosis other than T1D, diagnosis greater than one month before the initial study visit, individuals to obtain diabetes care at another clinic, individuals who do not consent to CGM use, and individuals greater than 21 years of age.

HbA1c measurements were collected from 71 youth with T1D (age 9.7 ± 4.6 years, 41% female, and 48% Non-Hispanic White, Table 1). Of the 71 unique participants, 23 (32.4%) contributed more than one HbA1c home kit measurement (University of Minnesota's Advanced Research and Diagnostic Laboratory [ARDL]) for a total of 99 HbA1c values for which there were GMI (n = 88) and concurrent POC HbA1c (n = 32; DCA Vantage® Analyzer, Siemens, Germany) to evaluate these three methods for measuring glycemic control. The ARDL HbA1c measurements were performed on the Tosoh G8 HPLC system in variant mode (Tosoh Bioscience, Inc., South San Francisco, CA, USA). Although there are a variety of methods for computing a HbA1c value from CGM data [17–19], we chose GMI in this study because all of the participants enrolled in the 4T Study were started on a Dexcom G6 CGM system, and we were able to determine GMI readily using Dexcom Clarity reports.

The HbA1c home kit and POC HbA1c (n = 32) measurements were collected on the same day in the clinic with the guidance of the study staff. The HbA1c home kit and GMI (n = 88) and POC A1c and GMI (n = 27) were also collected on the same day. The HbA1c home kit included an alcohol wipe, gauze, a single-use lancing device, a capillary tube, a Bio-Rad hemoglobin capillary collection vial with ethylenediaminetetraacetic acid (EDTA) and potassium cyanide; a cardboard stand to hold the collection vial, written instructions, a blood collection form, a biohazard bag, a gel pack for freezing, an absorbent pad, and a cardboard shipping box with a pre-paid return label. The HbA1c home kits were collected, packaged according to instructions, and mailed via United States Postal Service (USPS) as first-class mail to the ARDL at the University of Minnesota for analysis.

The POC vs. GMI only had 27 paired samples (versus 32 for POC vs. the home kit) due to missing GMI data in five participants. Similarly, for the home kit vs. GMI, there were 88 paired samples (of the 99 total home kits) due to the 11 participants missing GMI data. Overall, there were fewer matched comparisons available for the POC HbA1c because fewer families attended in-clinic visits during the COVID-19 pandemic. GMI values were captured on the same day the home kit and POC HbA1c were collected, and we used a 90-day retrospective GMI measurement period via Dexcom Clarity reports.

Table 1. Participant Demographics. Note: N = 71 unique participants (25 contributed more than one measurement).

Demographics	Mean ± SD Median [IQR]
Age, years	9.7 ± 4.6 10 [6–14]
Sex	
Male	29 (41%)
Female	42 (59%)
Race/Ethnicity	
Non-Hispanic White	34 (48%)
Non-Hispanic Black	0 (0%)
Hispanic	7 (10%)
Asian/Pacific Islander	10 (14%)
Other	2 (3%)
Unknown	18 (25%)
Body Mass Index (BMI)	18.6 ± 6.1 17 [15–21]
Insurance Type	
Private	55 (77%)
Public	16 (23%)
HbA1c at Diagnosis (%)	12.5 ± 2.2
HbA1c Home Kit (%)	6.9 ± 1.2
Months Since Diagnosis	8.6 ± 5.1 8 [4–12]

3. Statistical Analysis

Matched pairs were used for Bland–Altman analyses and Lin's concordance correlation coefficient (ρ_c) to evaluate the agreement among glycemic control measures. Paired measures include the following: POC vs. home kit = 32 paired; POC vs. GMI = 27 paired; and home kit vs. GMI = 88 paired samples. Bias was defined as the difference between the alternative glycemic control measure and the reference POC A1c as presented for each measure. When comparing home kits' A1c and GMI, the home kit was used as the reference measure since the standard of care POC HbA1c was not available for these matched pairs. All matched HbA1c measurements were collected on the same day, and 90-day GMI data were captured using the CGM mean glucose value from Dexcom Clarity. To confirm that the observed differences fell within the equivalence bounds (i.e., between −0.5 and 0.5%), a TOST analysis for equivalency was conducted using paired t-tests.

4. Results

The median CGM wear time to evaluate GMI was 98.9% (IQR 86.7, 100%). In relation to POC HbA1c (Figure 1), both HbA1c home kit (panel (A)) and GMI (panel (B)) showed a slight positive bias (mean difference 0.18% and 0.34%, respectively). The HbA1c home kit and GMI showed strong concordance with POC HbA1c (ρ_c = 0.982 [0.965, 0.991] and 0.823 [0.686, 0.904], respectively). The GMI (panel (C)) also showed a slight positive bias (mean difference 0.28%) and fair concordance (ρ_c = 0.750 [0.658, 0.820]) with the HbA1c home kit.

In addition, the percentage of the paired HbA1c values that deviated by a clinically meaningful amount (>0.5%) was 0% (POC versus home kit, 0/32), 44% (POC versus GMI, 12/27), and 27% (home kit versus GMI, 24/88); Figure 2. For each pairwise comparison, we tested the composite null hypotheses H0$_1$: $\Delta \leq -0.5$ and H0$_2$: $\Delta \geq 0.5$. Upon rejection at the 0.05 alpha level, we concluded that the observed differences fall within the predefined equivalence bounds of −0.5 and 0.5%.

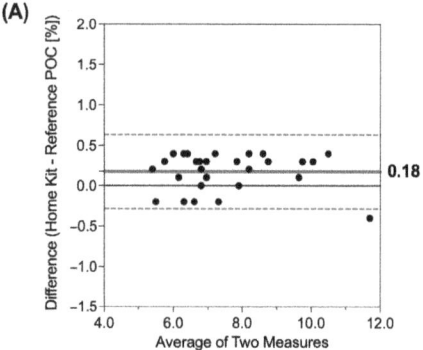
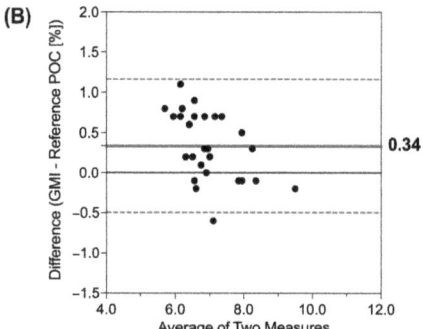
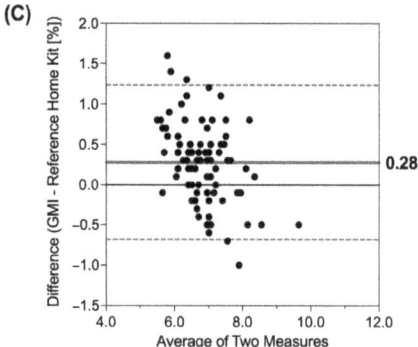

Figure 1. Bland–Altman comparison of the HbA1c home kit, GMI, and POC HbA1c measurements. The solid line (blue) represents the mean difference between comparator and reference, and the dashed lines (red) represent the 95% limits of agreement. In (**A**), the HbA1c home kit is the comparator, and POC HbA1c is the reference. In (**B**), GMI is the comparator, and POC HbA1c is the reference. In (**C**), GMI is the comparator, and HbA1c home kit is the reference. GMI = Glucose Management Indicator; POC = point-of-care HbA1c.

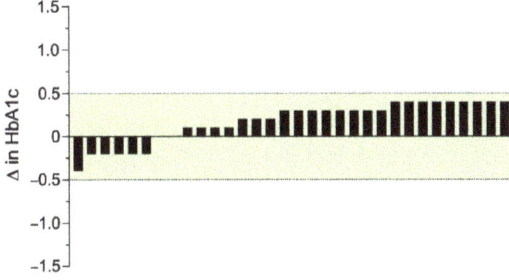

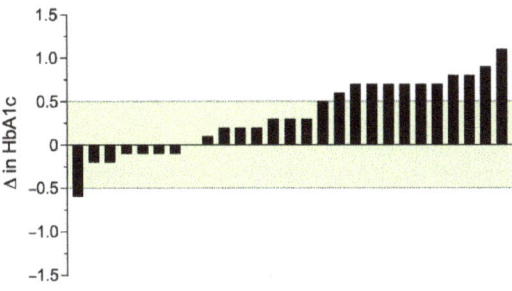

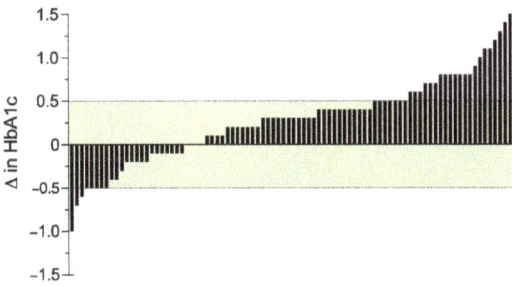

Figure 2. Paired HbA1c values are as follows: (**A**) POC versus Home Kit A1c, (**B**) POC versus GMI, and (**C**) home kit versus GMI. The green shaded area denotes HbA1c values that did not deviate by a clinically meaningful amount (>0.5%).

The Bland–Altman analyses revealed that 30 and 90 days of GMI data showed slightly less bias than using 14-day GMI data (mean difference of 0.34% for both 30 and 90 days of the GMI data versus 0.38% for 14-day GMI data, respectively).

5. Discussion

In this sub-study, we assessed the accuracy and concordance between POC HbA1c, HbA1c home kit, and Glucose Management Indicator (GMI) values in pediatric patients with type 1 diabetes. The COVID-19 pandemic has led to changes and rapid adoption of diabetes care delivery in a telehealth model. Even with more openings, patients and families often choose telehealth for convenience [9]. Therefore, implementation and accessibility to HbA1c home kits will allow for regular glycemia and patient-centered care monitoring. This sub-study demonstrates that the HbA1c home kit and GMI show a strong concordance with the standard of care POC HbA1c, and these data support the use of the ARDL home HbA1c kits within the 4T study [7–16], as well as verified home HbA1c kits as an option for clinical care for telehealth diabetes care. Beck et al. [5] recently reported similar findings with two capillary blood collection kits (one of which was the ARDL HbA1c home kit described here) and venous HbA1c. They show compelling evidence that HbA1c measurements from these two capillary blood collection kits can be used interchangeably with venous HbA1c. In our analysis, we extend these findings and demonstrate the added utility of GMI in youth wearing CGM technology.

There are limitations in this sub-study worth noting. We used the Dexcom G6 CGM system in the present study, so these conclusions may not be generalizable across different types of CGM systems. In addition, our POC reference device used in this analysis was the DCA Vantage analyzer based on latex immunoagglutination inhibition, a commonly used POC A1c measurement system. Different POC HbA1c instruments may work by different methodologies (e.g., boronate affinity chromatography); therefore, we also note the lack of generalizability of these conclusions across other HbA1c POC systems that were not tested. Similarly, in this sub-study, we obtained a relatively small number of matched pairs (specifically for POC measurements due to the COVID-19 pandemic). This may warrant a more robust analysis to confirm the current findings.

The use of telehealth-specific options for A1c measures (i.e., GMI and home kit) has its own unique set of pros and cons. In our analysis, the A1c home kit outperformed GMI in concordance. However, the A1c home kit also requires additional collection kit instructions for patients, the possibility of user error in sample collection, and challenges around timely shipment and analysis of samples. GMI calculations do not correct glycation rates, and studies have shown that similar methods may yield more accurate A1c estimations [17–19]. Therefore, future studies might consider different methods for calculating HbA1c from CGM tracings that may correct the rate of glycation and, in turn, the lifetime of red blood cells. The convenience of GMI is that it does not require additional testing or associated costs like the A1c home kit and is obtainable from the CGM device already in use.

6. Conclusions

In conclusion, these data demonstrate that the HbA1c home kit and GMI show strong concordance with POC HbA1c. The use of GMI data in this analysis is not intended to replace future POC or venous blood samples for HbA1c. However, using GMI may be particularly helpful for families and individuals that may not have access to POC HbA1c or the HbA1c home kit and to facilitate telehealth visits. CGM data also provide additional information on hypoglycemia and glucose variability [20]. Overall, the HbA1c home kit and GMI may be potential solutions to glycemic assessment during the COVID-19 pandemic and for future telehealth visits.

Author Contributions: D.P.Z. wrote and edited the technical report. D.P.Z. performed statistical analyses that were reviewed and approved by V.Y.D. and M.D. All authors (D.P.Z., V.Y.D., A.A., P.P., B.L., N.A.-R., A.B.K., D.M.M. and M.D.) contributed to the revisions and approved the submitted letter. All authors have read and agreed to the published version of the manuscript.

Funding: Funding was provided in part by the NIDDK (R18 DK122422), Stanford Diabetes Research Center (P30DK116074), Leona M. and Harry B. Helmsley Charitable Trust (G-2002-04251), Lucile Packard Children's Hospital Auxiliaries, and ISPAD-JDRF Research Fellowship.

Institutional Review Board Statement: The study was conducted in accordance with the Declaration of Helsinki and approved by the Institutional Review Board of Stanford University (protocol code clinicaltrials.gov: NCT03968055 and NCT04336969 on 30 May 2019, and 7 April 2020, approval).

Informed Consent Statement: Informed consent was obtained from all individuals involved in the study.

Data Availability Statement: Data is contained within the article.

Acknowledgments: We would like to thank the other members of the 4T Study Group for their help with this project. Study team members include: Julie Hooper, Ana Cortes, Erica Pang, Carolyn Herrera, Rachel Tam, Dom Mitchell,, Liz Heckard, Andrea Bonilla Ospina, Franziska Bishop, Natalie Pageler, Jeannine Leverenz, Piper Sagan, Anjoli Martinez-Singh, Barry Conrad, Annette Chmielewski, Julie Senaldi, Rebecca Gardner, Kim Clash, Erin Hodgson, Diana Naranjo, Molly Tanenbaum, Johannes Ferstad, Ryan Pi, Michael Gao, Annie Chang, Ransalu Senanayake, Anastasiya Vitko, Simrat Ghuman, Esli Osmanlliu, Emily Fox, Carlos Guestrin, Alex Wang, and Juan Langlois.

Conflicts of Interest: D.P.Z. has received speaker's honoraria from Medtronic Diabetes, Ascensia Diabetes, and Insulet Canada; and research support from the Helmsley Charitable Trust and ISPAD-JDRF Research Fellowship. She is also on the Dexcom Advisory board. A.B.K. has served as an external consultant for Roche Diagnostics and received research funding from Siemens Healthcare Diagnostics and Kyowa Kirin Pharmaceutical Development. A.B.K. has also received speaker honoraria from the National Kidney Foundation and the American Kidney Fund. All funding is unrelated to this manuscript. D.M.M. has had research support from the National Kidney Foundation, Juvenile Diabetes Research Foundation, NSF, and the Helmsley Charitable Trust and his institution has had research support from Medtronic, Dexcom, Insulet, Bigfoot Biomedical, Tandem, and Roche. D.M.M. has consulted for Abbott, Aditxt, the Helmsley Charitable Trust, Lifescan, Mannkind, Sanofi, Novo Nordisk, Eli Lilly, Medtronic, Insulet, Dompe, and Biospex. The remaining authors have no conflicts of interest.

References

1. American Diabetes Association. 6. Glycemic Targets: Standards of Medical Care in Diabetes—2021. *Diabetes Care* **2021**, *44* (Suppl. S1), S73–S84. [CrossRef] [PubMed]
2. Whitley, H.P.; Yong, E.V.; Rasinen, C. Selecting an A1C Point-of-Care Instrument. *Diabetes Spectr.* **2015**, *28*, 201–208. [CrossRef] [PubMed]
3. Battelino, T.; Danne, T.; Bergenstal, R.M.; Amiel, S.A.; Beck, R.; Biester, T.; Bosi, E.; Buckingham, B.A.; Cefalu, W.T.; Close, K.L.; et al. Clinical Targets for Continuous Glucose Monitoring Data Interpretation: Recommendations from the International Consensus on Time in Range. *Diabetes Care* **2019**, *42*, 1593–1603. [CrossRef] [PubMed]
4. American Diabetes Association Professional Practice Committee. 6. Glycemic Targets: Standards of Medical Care in Diabetes—2022. *Diabetes Care* **2022**, *45* (Suppl. S1), S83–S96. [CrossRef] [PubMed]
5. Beck, R.W.; Bocchino, L.E.; Lum, J.W.; Kollman, C.; Barnes-Lomen, V.; Sulik, M.; Haller, M.J.; Bode, B.; Cernich, J.T.; Killeen, A.A.; et al. An Evaluation of Two Capillary Sample Collection Kits for Laboratory Measurement of HbA1c. *Diabetes Technol. Ther.* **2021**, *23*, 537–545. [CrossRef] [PubMed]
6. Bergenstal, R.M.; Beck, R.W.; Close, K.L.; Grunberger, G.; Sacks, D.B.; Kowalski, A.; Brown, A.S.; Heinemann, L.; Aleppo, G.; Ryan, D.B.; et al. Glucose Management Indicator (GMI): A New Term for Estimating A1C From Continuous Glucose Monitoring. *Diabetes Care* **2018**, *41*, 2275–2280. [CrossRef] [PubMed]
7. Prahalad, P.; Zaharieva, D.P.; Addala, A.; New, C.; Scheinker, D.; Desai, M.; Hood, K.K.; Maahs, D.M. Improving Clinical Outcomes in Newly Diagnosed Pediatric Type 1 Diabetes: Teamwork, Targets, Technology, and Tight Control—The 4T Study. *Front. Endocrinol.* **2020**, *11*, 360. [CrossRef] [PubMed]
8. Prahalad, P.; Ding, V.Y.; Zaharieva, D.P.; Addala, A.; Johari, R.; Scheinker, D.; Desai, M.; Hood, K.; Maahs, D.M. Teamwork, Targets, Technology, and Tight Control in Newly Diagnosed Type 1 Diabetes: Pilot 4T Study. *J. Clin. Endocrinol. Metab.* **2021**, *107*, 998–1008. [CrossRef] [PubMed]
9. Tanenbaum, M.; Zaharieva, D.P.; Addala, A.; Hooper, J.; Leverenz, B.; Cortes, A.; Arrizon-Ruiz, N.; Pang, E.; Bishop, F.; Maahs, D. Initiating CGM over telehealth is well accepted by parents of newly diagnosed youth with T1D. *Diabetes Technol. Ther.* **2022**, *24* (Suppl. 1), A157.
10. Ferstad, J.O.; Vallon, J.J.; Jun, D.; Gu, A.; Vitko, A.; Morales, D.P.; Leverenz, J.; Lee, M.Y.; Leverenz, B.; Vasilakis, C.; et al. Population-level management of type 1 diabetes via continuous glucose monitoring and algorithm-enabled patient prioritization: Precision health meets population health. *Pediatr. Diabetes* **2021**, *22*, 982–991. [CrossRef] [PubMed]
11. Scheinker, D.; Gu, A.; Grossman, J.; Ward, A.; Ayerdi, O.; Miller, D.; Leverenz, J.; Hood, K.; Lee, M.Y.; Maahs, D.M.; et al. Algorithm-Enabled, Personalized Glucose Management for Type 1 Diabetes at the Population Scale: Prospective Evaluation in Clinical Practice. *JMIR Diabetes* **2022**, *7*, e27284. [CrossRef] [PubMed]
12. Prahalad, P.; Addala, A.; Scheinker, D.; Hood, K.K.; Maahs, D.M. CGM Initiation Soon After Type 1 Diabetes Diagnosis Results in Sustained CGM Use and Wear Time. *Diabetes Care* **2019**, *43*, e3–e4. [CrossRef] [PubMed]
13. Addala, A.; Zaharieva, D.P.; Gu, A.J.; Prahalad, P.; Scheinker, D.; Buckingham, B.; Hood, K.K.; Maahs, D.M. Clinically serious hypoglycemia is rare and not associated with time-in-range in youth with newly diagnosed type 1 diabetes. *JCEM* **2021**, *106*, 3239–3247. [CrossRef] [PubMed]
14. Grossman, J.; Ward, A.; Crandell, J.L.; Prahalad, P.; Maahs, D.M.; Scheinker, D. Improved individual and population-level HbA1c estimation using CGM data and patient characteristics. *J. Diabetes Its Complicat.* **2021**, *35*, 107950. [CrossRef]

15. Zaharieva, D.P.; Bishop, F.; Maahs, D.M. Advancements and Future Directions in the Teamwork, Targets, Technology, and Tight Control—The 4T Study: Improving Clinical Outcomes in Newly Diagnosed Pediatric Type 1 Diabetes. *Curr. Opin. Pediatr.* **2022**, *34*, 423–429. [CrossRef] [PubMed]
16. Tanenbaum, M.L.; Zaharieva, D.P.; Addala, A.; Ngo, J.; Prahalad, P.; Leverenz, B.; New, C.; Maahs, D.M.; Hood, K.K. 'I was ready for it at the beginning': Parent experiences with early introduction of continuous glucose monitoring following their child's Type 1 diabetes diagnosis. *Diabet. Med.* **2021**, *38*, e14567. [CrossRef]
17. Xu, Y.; Grimsmann, J.M.; Karges, B.; Hofer, S.E.; Danne, T.; Holl, R.W.; Ajjan, R.A.; Dunn, T.C. Personal Glycation Factors and Calculated Hemoglobin A1c for Diabetes Management: Real-World Data from the Diabetes Prospective Follow-up (DPV) Registry. *Diabetes Technol. Ther.* **2021**, *23*, 452–459. [CrossRef]
18. Chrzanowski, J.; Michalak, A.; Łosiewicz, M.A.; Kuśmierczyk, M.H.; Mianowska, M.B.; Szadkowska, M.A.; Fendler, W. Improved Estimation of Glycated Hemoglobin from Continuous Glucose Monitoring and Past Glycated Hemoglobin Data. *Diabetes Technol. Ther.* **2021**, *23*, 293–305. [CrossRef] [PubMed]
19. Fabris, C.; Heinemann, L.; Beck, R.; Cobelli, C.; Kovatchev, B. Estimation of Hemoglobin A1c from Continuous Glucose Monitoring Data in Individuals with Type 1 Diabetes: Is Time In Range All We Need? *Diabetes Technol. Ther.* **2020**, *22*, 501–508. [CrossRef] [PubMed]
20. Danne, T.; Nimri, R.; Battelino, T.; Bergenstal, R.M.; Close, K.L.; DeVries, J.H.; Garg, S.; Heinemann, L.; Hirsch, I.; Amiel, S.A.; et al. International Consensus on Use of Continuous Glucose Monitoring. *Diabetes Care* **2017**, *40*, 1631–1640. [CrossRef] [PubMed]

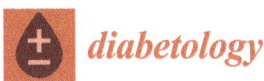

Article

Diabetic Ketoacidosis Was Associated with High Morbidity and Mortality in Hospitalized Patients with COVID-19 in the NYC Public Health System

Sahana Parthasarathy [1,2], Natalia Chamorro-Pareja [1,2], Amrin Kharawala [1,2], Kenneth H Hupart [1,3,4], Joan Curcio [1,5,6], Christina Coyle [1,2], Daniel Buchnea [1,7], Dimitris Karamanis [8], Robert Faillace [1,2], Leonidas Palaiodimos [1,2] and Preeti Kishore [1,2,*]

1. NYC Health + Hospitals, New York, NY, USA
2. Jacobi Medical Center, Albert Einstein College of Medicine, Bronx, NY 10461, USA
3. Coney Island Hospital, Brooklyn, NY 11235, USA
4. Albert Einstein College of Medicine, Yeshiva University, New York, NY 10461, USA
5. Elmhurst Hospital Center, Queens, NY 11373, USA
6. Mount Sinai School of Medicine/Icahn School of Medicine, New York, NY 10029, USA
7. Kings County Hospital Center, Brooklyn, NY 11203, USA
8. Department of Health Informatics, Rutgers School of Health Professions, Newark, NJ 07107, USA
* Correspondence: preeti.kishore@nychhc.org

Abstract: Background: COVID-19 has been associated with a higher risk of death in patients with diabetes mellitus (DM). However, there is a dearth of data regarding the effects of diabetic ketoacidosis (DKA) in these patients. We explored the in-hospital outcomes of patients who presented with COVID-19 and DKA. Methods: A propensity score-matched observational retrospective cohort study was conducted in hospitalized patients with COVID-19 in the public healthcare system of New York City from 1 March 2020 to 31 October 2020. Patients were matched, and a subgroup analysis of patients with DKA and COVID-19 and patients without COVID-19 was conducted. Results: 13,333 (16.0%) patients with COVID-19 and 70,005 (84.0%) without COVID-19 were included in the analysis. The in-hospital mortality rate was seven-fold in patients with DKA and COVID-19 compared to patients with COVID-19 and without DKA (80 (36.5%) vs. 11 (5.4%), $p < 0.001$). Patients with COVID-19 and DKA had a two-fold higher likelihood for in-hospital death (OR: 1.95; 95% CI: 1.41–2.70; $p < 0.001$) after adjusting for multiple variables. Conclusions: DKA was associated with significantly higher in-hospital mortality in hospitalized patients with COVID-19.

Keywords: coronavirus disease 2019; COVID-19; severe acute respiratory syndrome coronavirus 2; SARS-CoV-2; diabetes; diabetic ketoacidosis; DKA; hyperglycemia; mortality; innate immunity; cytokine storm; angiotensin-converting enzyme 2; pancreatic β-cell damage

1. Introduction

New-onset diabetes and severe metabolic complications such as diabetic ketoacidosis (DKA) and hyperosmolar hyperglycemic state (HHS) have been observed in patients infected with severe acute respiratory syndrome coronavirus 2 (SARS-CoV2) [1], the virus that causes Coronavirus disease 2019 (COVID-19). Initially, DKA was more commonly associated with patients with type 1 diabetes mellitus (T1DM) as compared to type 2 diabetes mellitus (T2DM). However, some studies have shown that patients with T2DM can present with DKA, but they are usually older, require more insulin, and tend to have a longer course of stay [2,3]. Interestingly, patients with COVID-19 have presented with DKA without a previously known diagnosis of DM [4,5]. Since the beginning of the pandemic, there have been reports of worse outcomes and increased mortality in patients with DKA and COVID-19 [6,7]. It has been proposed that the higher mortality in these patients can be attributed to advanced age, the higher severity of COVID-19, and the use of steroids [8,9]. COVID infection resulted in an increased incidence of DKA in patients with T2DM. These patients required a longer ICU stay and were found to have worse mortality [10]. We previously reported significantly higher mortality in patients with COVID-19 that presented with DKA compared to the previously known mortality rate of DKA [11]. In this study, we compared the in-hospital outcomes of patients with DKA prior to the start of the COVID-19 pandemic in our hospital system to the mortality of patients that presented with DKA in the setting of COVID-19 during the first phase of the pandemic in 2020.

2. Materials and Methods

2.1. Study Design and Patient Population

This was a propensity score-matched observational cohort study performed at the eleven acute care hospitals of the New York City Health + Hospitals (NYC H + H) system. The study group included patients ≥18 years of age who presented to the emergency room and were admitted to any inpatient service, including intensive care units (ICU), with laboratory-confirmed COVID-19 from 1 March 2020 to 31 October 2020. The control group included patients that were admitted from 1 July 2019 to 31 December 2019, before the pandemic was declared and prior to the first diagnosed case of COVID-19 in the USA. These populations were matched, and a subgroup analysis of patients with COVID-19 and DKA and patients with DKA but without COVID-19 was performed. DKA was defined as blood glucose > 250 mg/dL, pH < 7.3, a bicarbonate level of <18 mEq/L, an elevated anion gap, and positive ketones in blood or urine [12]. Laboratory-confirmed COVID-19 was defined as a SARS-CoV-2 positive result in the real-time reverse transcriptase-polymerase chain reaction (RT-PCR) analysis of nasopharyngeal or nasal swab samples (Bio Reference Laboratories, Elmwood Park, NJ, USA). We excluded patients that had the following criteria: patients that were discharged from the emergency department, patients without laboratory-confirmed COVID-19, and patients who were still hospitalized at the time of data collection. The study was approved by the Biomedical Research Alliance of New York Institutional Review Board with a waiver of informed consent (IRB #20-12-318-373). The data were fully de-identified and anonymized before they were accessed, and IRB waived the requirement for informed consent.

2.2. Data Sources

The study data were obtained from electronic health records via appropriate diagnostic codes (Epic systems, Verona, WI, USA). The dataset was reviewed by two independent investigators for missing data and completeness. The extracted data included baseline demographic variables (age, sex, race), clinical characteristics (body mass index (BMI), history of tobacco use, hypertension, hyperlipidemia, asthma, coronary artery disease (CAD), heart failure, stroke/transient ischemic attack (TIA), chronic kidney disease (CKD), end-stage renal disease (ESRD)), medication list (including insulin, biguanides, dipeptidyl peptidase- 4 (DPP-4) inhibitors, glucagon like peptide-1 (GLP-1) agonists, sulfonylureas, insulin, angiotensin-converting enzyme (ACE) inhibitors, and statins), laboratory data (hemoglobin A1C, C-reactive protein (CRP), lactate dehydrogenase (LDH), Ferritin, D-Dimer, creatinine, aspartate aminotransferase (AST), alanine aminotransferase (ALT)), and outcomes including invasive mechanical ventilation, admission to the intensive care unit (ICU), the need for renal replacement therapy (RRT), and death from all causes. The data were processed and analyzed without any personal identifiers to maintain patient confidentiality, as per the Health Insurance Portability and Accountability Act (HIPAA).

2.3. Exposure of Interest and Outcomes

The primary outcome was the in-hospital mortality in patients with COVID-19 and DKA. The secondary outcomes were length of stay (LOS), invasive mechanical ventilation, admission to the ICU, and need for RRT.

2.4. Statistical Analysis

Propensity score matching was conducted to create comparable groups controlling for imbalances of covariates [13] [Supplemental Material Figures S1 and S2]. The propensity score was estimated using a logistic regression model and is the subject-specific probability of being infected with COVID-19, in which the following covariates were used: age, sex, BMI, race, DKA, comorbidities (history of diabetes mellitus, hypertension, hyperlipidemia, Chronic obstructive pulmonary disease (COPD), asthma, CAD, heart failure, stroke TIA, ESRD, CKD), and medications (biguanides, DPP4 inhibitors, SGLT2 inhibitors, GLP-1 agonists, insulin, ACE inhibitors, sulfonylureas, and statins). A nearest-neighbor matching without replacement was performed using a caliper of 0.2, which has been found to be optimal [14,15].

A stepwise logistic regression model identified the baseline variables associated with in-hospital mortality, invasive mechanical ventilation/intubation [Tables S1–S3] admission to ICU [Tables S4–S6], and the need for RRT [Tables S7–S9] in three different data panels: (a) matched groups (COVID-19 and control), (b) COVID-19 group, and (c) DKA group. Univariate analysis was performed, and four multivariate models with different definitions of our variable of interest are presented for robustness: model 1: age, sex, and BMI; model 2: age, sex, BMI, and all comorbidities; model 3: age, sex, BMI, all comorbidities, and diabetes medications; model 4: age, sex, BMI, all comorbidities, diabetes medications, and all medications used during inpatient status. Additional variables are included in the multivariable models 1–4 for every different panel, specifically: for panel (a), models 1–4 also include positive COVID-19 status and the presence of DKA; for panel (b), models 1–4 also include the presence of DKA; and for panel (c), models 1–4 also include positive COVID-19 status.

T-tests compared continuous variables, while Chi-Square tests compared discrete variables. Continuous data are presented as median values with the interquartile range (IQR) specified, and categorical data are presented as absolute and relative frequencies. A *p*-value < 0.05 was considered statistically significant.

3. Results

3.1. Descriptive Analyses

3.1.1. Baseline Characteristics

A flowchart of the analysis is presented in Figure 1. In total, 83,338 patients were included in our analysis. A total of 13,333 (16.0%) were patients with COVID-19, and 70,005 (84.0%) were patients without COVID-19. The propensity score matching between the COVID-19 and control groups yielded a cohort of 22,694 patients (COVID-19 group: 11,347 and control group: 11,347). In the COVID-19 group, 58.8% were men, the median age was 62 (IQR 49–74) years, and the median BMI was 28.1 (24.4–32.8) kg/m^2. From the non-COVID-19 group, 57.8% were men, the median age was 62 (IQR 48–75) years, and the median BMI was 27.9 (23.8–33.3) kg/m^2. The matching in DKA patients yielded a cohort of 422 patients (DKA/COVID-19 group: 219 and control group: 203). In the DKA/COVID-19 group, 63.5% were men, the median age was 56 (69–41) years, and the median BMI was 25.7 (22.6–30.2) kg/m^2. In the DKA/non-COVID-19 group, 67.0% were men, the median age was 50 (38–63) years, and the median BMI was 26.1 (22.4–30.8) kg/m^2. Detailed baseline characteristics are included in Table 1.

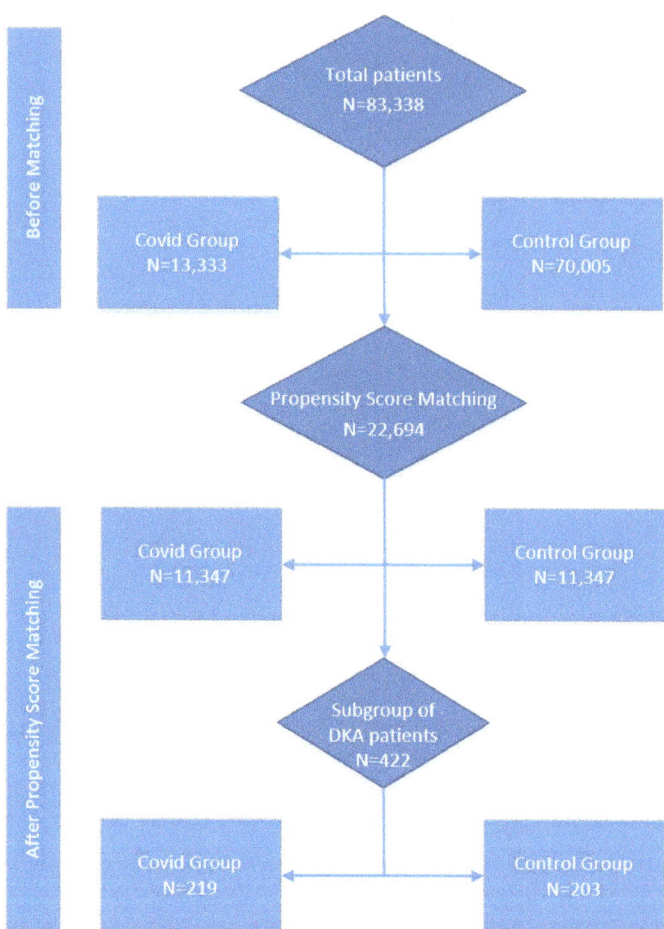

Figure 1. Flowchart of the analysis.

Table 1. Baseline characteristics.

	COVID-19 and Control Group				DKA/COVID-19 vs. DKA/Non-COVID-19			
	Total (N = 22,694)	COVID-19 Group (N = 11,347)	Control Group (N = 11,347)	p-Value	Total (N = 422)	COVID-19 Group (N = 219)	Control Group (N = 203)	p-Value
Male sex—no. (%)	13,224 (52.2)	6672 (58.8)	6552 (57.7)	0.106	275 (65.1)	139 (63.4)	136 (67.0)	0.448
Age—years—Median (IQR)	62 (48–74)	62 (49–74)	62 (48–75)	0.233	53 (40–66)	56 (41–69)	50 (38–63)	0.004
BMI—kg/m^2—Median (IQR)	27.9 (24.1–33.1)	28.1 (24.4–32.8)	27.9 (23.8–33.3)	0.063	25.8 (22.5–30.4)	25.7 (22.6–30.2)	26.1 (22.4–30.8)	0.429
Race/Ethnicity—no. (%)								
Asian	1395 (6.21)	643 (5.7)	752 (6.7)	<0.001	16 (3.8)	9 (4.1)	7 (3.5)	0.255
Black	7264 (32.3)	3577 (31.8)	3687 (32.8)		153 (36.7)	74 (34.1)	79 (45.2)	
White	3003 (13.3)	1174 (10.4)	1829 (16.3)		40 (9.6)	17 (7.8)	23 (11.5)	
Other/Latino	10,791 (48.0)	5846 (52.0)	4945 (44.1)		207 (49.7)	117 (53.9)	90 (45.2)	
Coexisting disorder—no. (%)								
Diabetic Ketoacidosis	422 (1.8)	219 (1.9)	203 (1.7)	0.432	422 (100)	219 (100)	203 (100)	-
History of DM	9951 (43.8)	4938 (43.5)	5013 (44.1)	0.316	422 (100)	219 (100)	203 (100)	-

Table 1. Cont.

		COVID-19 and Control Group				DKA/COVID-19 vs. DKA/Non-COVID-19		
	Total (N = 22,694)	COVID-19 Group (N = 11,347)	Control Group (N = 11,347)	p-Value	Total (N = 422)	COVID-19 Group (N = 219)	Control Group (N = 203)	p-Value
Type 1 Diabetes	139 (0.6)	61 (0.5)	78 (0.6)	0.148	93 (22.0)	44 (20.0)	49 (24.1)	0.316
HTN	5127 (22.5)	2532 (22.3)	2595 (22.8)	0.317	99 (23.4)	46 (21.0)	53 (26.1)	0.216
HLD	2114 (9.3)	1042 (9.1)	1072 (9.4)	0.493	45 (10.6)	24 (10.9)	21 (10.3)	0.838
Pulmonary HTN	108 (0.4)	45 (0.4)	63 (0.5)	0.083	1 (0.2)	1 (0.4)	0 (0.0)	0.335
COPD	474 (2.0)	218 (1.9)	256 (2.2)	0.078	1 (0.2)	0 (0.0)	1 (0.4)	0.298
Asthma	976 (4.3)	474 (4.1)	502 (4.4)	0.360	13 (3.0)	4 (1.8)	9 (4.4)	0.121
CAD	707 (3.1)	347 (3.0)	360 (3.1)	0.619	5 (1.1)	4 (1.8)	1 (0.4)	0.206
Heart Failure	1225 (5.4)	592 (5.2)	633 (5.5)	0.228	16 (3.7)	8 (3.6)	8 (3.9)	0.877
Stroke/TIA	304 (1.3)	163 (1.4)	141 (1.2)	0.204	3 (0.7)	2 (0.9)	1 (0.4)	0.607
ESRD	1032 (4.5)	513 (4.5)	519 (4.5)	0.848	18 (4.2)	9 (4.1)	9 (4.4)	0.869
Chronic Kidney Disease	1339 (5.9)	660 (5.8)	679 (5.9)	0.592	29 (6.8)	12 (5.4)	17 (8.3)	0.241

Notes: BMI in kg/m^2. p-values refer to t-test or Chi-Square test between COVID-19 and control groups. Significance at p-value < 0.05. Abbreviations and symbols: BMI = body mass index; kg = kilograms; m = meter; N = no = number; IQR = interquartile range; DKA = Diabetic Ketoacidosis; DM = Diabetes Mellitus; HTN = hypertension; HLD = hyperlipidemia; COPD = Chronic Obstructive Pulmonary Disease; CAD = coronary artery disease; TIA = Transient Ischemic Attack; ESRD = End-Stage Renal Disease.

3.1.2. Inflammatory Markers

The baseline concentrations of the available inflammatory markers are presented in Table 2. The median values of LDH, D-dimer, ferritin, and CRP were higher in patients with COVID-19 compared to patients without COVID-19 ($p < 0.001$). Significant and consistent differences in the baseline concentrations of inflammatory markers among patients with DKA/COVID-19 compared to patients with DKA but not COVID-19 were not noted.

Table 2. Laboratory values.

		COVID-19 vs. Non COVID-19				DKA with COVID-19 vs. DKA without COVID-19		
Inflammatory Markers	Total (N = 22,694)	COVID-19 Group (N = 11,347)	Control Group (N = 11,347)	p-Value	Total (N = 422)	COVID-19 Group (N = 219)	Control Group (N = 203)	p-Value
CRP (mg/L)—Median (IQR)	18.1 (5.7–602)	18.7 (6–60.1)	11.5 (2.98–61)	0.035	13.1 (4.4–52.3)	12.7 (4.4–52.3)	14.1 (6.3–20.7)	0.247
LDH (U/L)—Median (IQR)	388 (279–568)	399 (290–577)	271 (197–402)	<0.001	424 (301–619)	427 (309–631.5)	268 (169–584)	0.141
Ferritin (ng/mL)—Median (IQR)	631 (263–1310)	731 (344–1418)	212 (72–593)	<0.001	820 (454–1501)	914 (490.6–1606)	410 (158–655)	0.026
D-Dimer (ng/mL)—Median (IQR)	721 (333–2272.5)	736 (351–2314)	471 (236–1331.5)	0.008	1143 (471–2698)	1093 (481.5–2774.5)	1686.8 (294.5–2284)	0.491
Creatinine (mg/dL)—Median (IQR)	0.9 (0.7–1.3)	0.9 (0.7–1.6)	0.9 (0.7–1.2)	<0.001	0.9 (0.6–1.5)	1 (0.6–2.2)	0.8 (0.6–1.12)	<0.001
AST (U/L)—Median (IQR)	30 (20–52)	38 (25–65)	24 (17–36)	<0.001	28 (18–50)	35 (21–66)	22 (15–37)	0.017
ALT (U/L)—Median (IQR)	25 (15–47)	33 (19–60)	19 (13–32)	<0.001	22 (15–43)	24 (16–48)	20 (14–34)	0.041
HbA1c (%)—Median (IQR)	6.4 (5.7–8.2)	6.6 (5.8–8.6)	6.3 (5.6–7.9)	<0.001	12.8 (10.8–14.8)	13.1 (10.7–15.2)	12.4 (10.8–14.6)	0.371
Vitamin D (ng/mL)/Admission—Median (IQR)	21.3 (14–29.8)	20.8 (13–29.8)	22 (14.7–29.8)	0.768	14.3 (9.4–29.5)	13.6 (9.7–29)	17.8 (9–30)	0.892
Vitamin D (ng/mL)/Pre COVID-19—Median (IQR)	24.9 (16.5–33.5)	24.9 (16.5–33.5)			23.7 (15–32.3)	23.7 (15–32.3)		

Note: p-values refer to T-test between COVID-19 and control groups. Significance at p-value < 0.05. Abbreviations and symbols: N = number; IQR = interquartile range; U/L = unit/liter; mg = milligram; ng = nanogram; ml = milliliter; dL = deciliter; DKA = Diabetic Ketoacidosis; CRP = C-Reactive Protein; LDH = Lactate Dehydrogenase; AST = Aspartate Aminotransferase; ALT = Alanine Aminotransferase; HbA1c = Hemoglobin A1c.

3.1.3. Outcomes

The median LOS in patients with COVID-19 was 6 days vs. 4 days in the control group ($p < 0.001$). In total, 9.1% of patients with COVID-19 required intubation compared to 3.3% in the non-COVID-19 control group ($p < 0.001$). ICU admission happened for 23.4% of patients in the COVID-19 group vs. 14.7% of patients in the non-COVID-19 group ($p < 0.001$). A total of 8.5% of patients with COVID-19 required RRT compared to 4.2% in the control group ($p < 0.001$). In-hospital death occurred in 26.0% of patients with COVID-19 compared to 9.3% in the control group ($p < 0.001$). Outcomes are presented in Table 3 and Figure 2.

Table 3. Outcomes in COVID-19 patients vs. control group.

Outcomes		COVID-19 vs. Non COVID-19		
	Total (N = 22,694)	COVID-19 Group (N = 11,347)	Control Group (N = 11,347)	p-Value
Length of Stay—Median (IQR)	5 (2–10)	6 (3–13)	4 (2–8)	<0.001
Death—no. (%)	4007 (17.6)	2949 (25.9)	1058 (9.3)	<0.001
Intubation—no. (%)	1413 (6.2)	1034 (9.1)	379 (3.3)	<0.001
ICU Admission—no. (%)	4324 (19.0)	2658 (23.4)	1666 (14.6)	<0.001
Renal Replacement Therapy—no. (%)	1445 (6.3)	967 (8.5)	478 (4.2)	<0.001

Notes: *p*-values refer to T-test or Chi-Square test between COVID-19 and control groups. Significance at *p*-value < 0.05. Abbreviations and symbols: N = no = number; IQR = interquartile range; ICU = Intensive Care Unit.

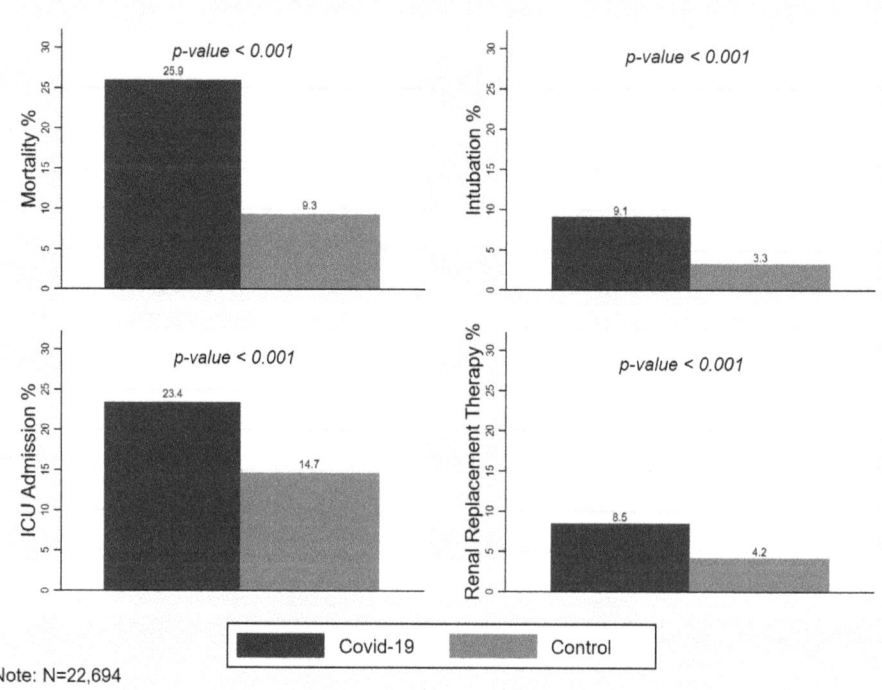

Note: N=22,694

Figure 2. Outcomes in COVID-19 vs. control groups after propensity score matching.

3.2. Subgroup Analysis for Patients with DKA

In patients with DKA and COVID-19, the LOS was 7 days compared to 4 days in patients with DKA and without COVID-19. Intubation happened for 14.6% of patients with DKA and COVID-19 vs. 5.9% of patients with DKA and without COVID-19 ($p = 0.003$). The mortality rates were 36.5% for patients with DKA and COVID-19 compared to 5.4% for patients with DKA and without COVID-19 ($p < 0.001$). The rate of requiring RRT was significantly higher in the DKA/COVID 19 group compared to the DKA/non-COVID-19 group ($p = 0.005$). There was no statistical significance of ICU admission between the two groups ($p = 0.207$). The outcomes of the subgroup analysis are presented in Table 4 and Figure 3.

Table 4. Outcomes in DKA patients with COVID-19 vs. without COVID-19.

Outcomes	DKA with COVID-19 vs. DKA without COVID-19			
	Total (N = 422)	COVID-19 Group (N = 219)	Control Group (N = 203)	*p*-Value
Length of Stay—Median (IQR)	5 (3–10)	7 (4–13)	4 (2–7)	0.003
Death—no. (%)	91 (21.5)	80 (36.5)	11 (5.4)	<0.001
Intubation—no. (%)	44 (10.4)	32 (14.6)	12 (5.9)	0.003
ICU Admission—no. (%)	242 (57.3)	132 (60.2)	110 (54.1)	0.207
Renal Replacement Therapy—no. (%)	38 (9.0)	28 (12.7)	10 (4.9)	0.005

Notes: *p*-values refer to T-test or Chi-Square test between COVID-19 and control groups. Significance at *p*-value < 0.05. Abbreviations and symbols: N = no = number; IQR = interquartile range; ICU = Intensive Care Unit; DKA = Diabetic Ketoacidosis.

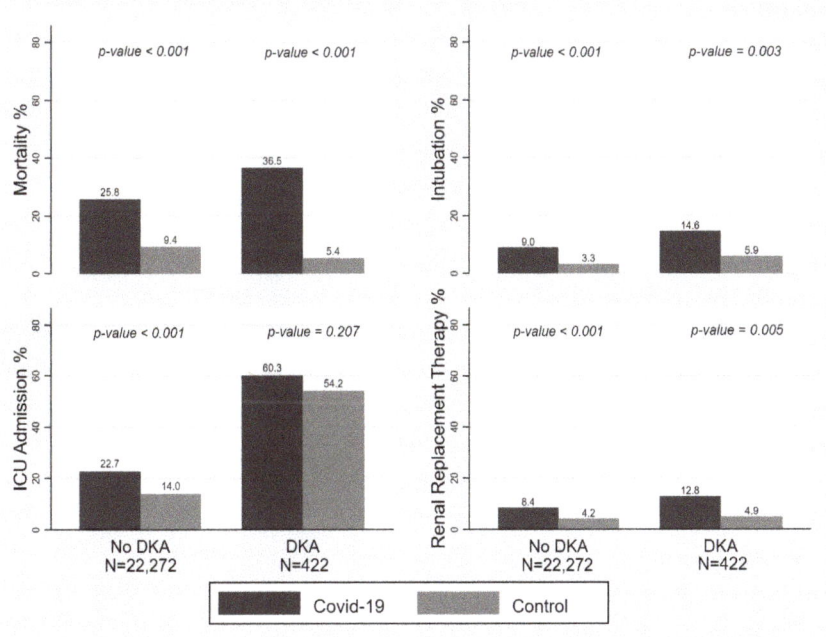

Figure 3. Outcomes in DKA vs. no DKA and COVID-19 vs. control groups after propensity score matching.

3.3. Logistic Regression Analysis

3.3.1. Matched Cohort (COVID-19 and Non-COVID-19)

Univariate associations with in-hospital mortality were examined for the available baseline demographic and clinical characteristics and are presented in Table 5. Older age, male sex, higher BMI, ESRD, COVID-19, diabetes mellitus, and DKA were all associated with a higher likelihood for in-hospital mortality in all models. Hypertension, CAD, asthma, and a history of stroke were shown to have an inverse association with in-hospital death. The use of biguanides, DPP4-inhibitors, ACE inhibitors, sulfonylureas, and statins were also shown to have an inverse association with in-hospital death.

Table 5. Baseline patient characteristics: univariate and multivariate logistic regression analysis for the outcome of mortality.

	Univariate Analysis	Multivariate Analysis Model 1	Multivariate Analysis Model 2	Multivariate Analysis Model 3	Multivariate Analysis Model 4
		n = 22,694	n = 22,694	n = 22,694	n = 22,694
Variables	OR (95% CI), p-Value	OR (95% CI), p-Value	OR (95% CI), p-Value	OR (95% CI), p-Value	OR (95% CI), p-Value
Age per 10 years	1.49 ** (1.46–1.52) $p < 0.001$	1.64 ** (1.60–1.67) $p < 0.001$	1.63 ** (1.59–1.68) $p < 0.001$	1.66 ** (1.61–1.70) $p < 0.001$	1.66 ** (1.62–1.71) $p < 0.001$
Male sex	1.18 ** (1.10–1.26) $p < 0.001$	1.42 ** (1.31–1.53) $p < 0.001$	1.40 ** (1.29–1.51) $p < 0.001$	1.42 ** (1.31–1.53) $p < 0.001$	1.33 ** (1.23–1.45) $p < 0.001$
BMI	1.00 (0.99–1.00) $p = 0.693$	1.03 ** (1.02–1.03) $p < 0.001$	1.03 ** (1.02–1.03) $p < 0.001$	1.03 ** (1.02–1.03) $p < 0.001$	1.03 ** (1.02–1.03) $p < 0.001$
COVID-19	3.41 ** (3.17–3.68) $p < 0.001$	3.95 ** (3.64–4.28) $p < 0.001$	4.11 ** (3.78–4.46) $p < 0.001$	4.10 ** (3.78–4.45) $p < 0.001$	3.62 ** (3.30–3.98) $p < 0.001$
Diabetic Ketoacidosis	1.29 * (1.02–1.63) $p = 0.034$	1.89 ** (1.47–2.43) $p < 0.001$	1.50 ** (1.14–1.96) $p = 0.003$	1.51 ** (1.15–1.99) $p = 0.003$	1.46 ** (1.10–1.94) $p = 0.009$
History of DM	2.02 ** (1.88–2.16) $p < 0.001$		1.88 ** (1.74–2.04) $p < 0.001$	2.17 ** (1.97–2.38) $p < 0.001$	1.68 ** (1.52–1.85) $p < 0.001$
Type 1 Diabetes	0.40 ** (0.22–0.74) $p = 0.004$		0.52 (0.26–1.03) $p = 0.061$	0.50 (0.25–1.00) $p = 0.051$	0.56 (0.28–1.14) $p = 0.112$
Hypertension	0.93 (0.85–1.01) $p = 0.079$		0.64 ** (0.58–0.71) $p < 0.001$	0.69 ** (0.62–0.77) $p < 0.001$	0.70 ** (0.63–0.78) $p < 0.001$
Hyperlipidemia	0.88 * (0.78–0.99) $p = 0.035$		0.77 ** (0.67–0.89) $p < 0.001$	0.87 (0.75–1.01) $p = 0.064$	0.95 (0.82–1.11) $p = 0.544$
Pulmonary Hypertension	1.56 * (1.01–2.41) $p = 0.047$		1.61 (0.95–2.73) $p = 0.079$	1.56 (0.91–2.67) $p = 0.109$	1.55 (0.87–2.77) $p = 0.138$
COPD	1.19 (0.95–1.49) $p = 0.135$		1.15 (0.89–1.49) $p = 0.275$	1.19 (0.92–1.54) $p = 0.176$	0.96 (0.73–1.26) $p = 0.781$
Asthma	0.51 ** (0.41–0.63) $p < 0.001$		0.60 ** (0.48–0.75) $p < 0.001$	0.61 ** (0.48–0.76) $p < 0.001$	0.51 ** (0.40–0.64) $p < 0.001$
CAD	1.03 (0.85–1.25) $p = 0.751$		0.74 ** (0.59–0.93) $p = 0.009$	0.78 * (0.62–0.99) $p = 0.038$	0.81 (0.63–1.03) $p = 0.085$
Heart Failure	1.31 ** (1.14–1.50) $p < 0.001$		1.00 (0.84–1.19) $p = 0.973$	1.08 (0.90–1.29) $p = 0.398$	1.21 * (1.00–1.46) $p = 0.045$
Stroke/TIA	0.87 (0.64–1.19) $p = 0.390$		0.62 ** (0.44–0.87) $p = 0.006$	0.66 * (0.46–0.93) $p = 0.019$	0.73 (0.50–1.05) $p = 0.093$
ESRD	1.84 ** (1.60–2.12) $p < 0.001$		2.11 ** (1.76–2.53) $p < 0.001$	2.03 ** (1.69–2.44) $p < 0.001$	1.76 ** (1.45–2.15) $p < 0.001$
Chronic Kidney Disease	1.47 ** (1.29–1.68) $p < 0.001$		1.06 (0.90–1.25) $p = 0.460$	1.06 (0.89–1.25) $p = 0.510$	1.12 (0.94–1.34) $p = 0.215$
Biguanides	0.65 ** (0.57–0.74) $p < 0.001$			0.63 ** (0.54–0.73) $p < 0.001$	0.72 ** (0.62–0.85) $p < 0.001$

Table 5. Cont.

Variables	Univariate Analysis OR (95% CI), p-Value	Multivariate Analysis Model 1 n = 22,694 OR (95% CI), p-Value	Multivariate Analysis Model 2 n = 22,694 OR (95% CI), p-Value	Multivariate Analysis Model 3 n = 22,694 OR (95% CI), p-Value	Multivariate Analysis Model 4 n = 22,694 OR (95% CI), p-Value
DPP4 inhibitors	0.86 * (0.76–0.99) p = 0.031			0.75 ** (0.64–0.87) p < 0.001	0.77 ** (0.65–0.91) p = 0.002
SGLT-2 inhibitors	0.60 (0.24–1.52) p = 0.278			0.93 (0.35–2.48) p = 0.881	0.83 (0.24–2.82) p = 0.764
GLP-1 agonists	0.80 (0.52–1.22) p = 0.297			0.92 (0.56–1.51) p = 0.742	0.95 (0.57–1.57) p = 0.842
Insulin	1.48 ** (1.38–1.59) p < 0.001			1.08 (0.99–1.19) p = 0.100	1.09 (0.99–1.20) p = 0.092
ACE inhibitors	0.86 ** (0.79–0.94) p = 0.001			0.71 ** (0.64–0.78) p < 0.001	0.75 ** (0.67–0.83) p < 0.001
Sulfonylureas	0.75 * (0.57–0.99) p = 0.046			0.72 * (0.53–0.97) p = 0.033	0.78 (0.56–1.08) p = 0.129
Statins	1.34 ** (1.25–1.43) p < 0.001			0.83 ** (0.76–0.90) p < 0.001	0.79 ** (0.72–0.86) p < 0.001
Heparin	2.14 ** (2.00–2.30) p < 0.001				1.51 ** (1.38–1.65) p < 0.001
Enoxaparin	1.37 ** (1.28–1.47) p < 0.001				0.92 (0.84–1.01) p = 0.096
Apixaban	1.27 ** (1.15–1.41) p < 0.001				0.61 ** (0.54–0.69) p < 0.001
Steroids	3.84 ** (3.57–4.13) p < 0.001				2.71 ** (2.48–2.97) p < 0.001
Tocilizumab	3.44 ** (2.92–4.06) p < 0.001				1.49 ** (1.22–1.82) p < 0.001
Remdesivir	1.61 ** (1.29–2.02) p < 0.001				0.54 ** (0.42–0.71) p < 0.001
Convalescent Plasma	3.97 ** (3.34–4.72) p < 0.001				1.10 (0.88–1.39) p = 0.406
Cefepime	5.63 ** (5.15–6.17) p < 0.001				3.06 ** (2.74–3.41) p < 0.001

Notes: Table 5 shows univariate analysis and four multivariate models with different definitions of our variable of interest. Model 1 includes the variables: age, sex, BMI, diabetic ketoacidosis, and COVID-19. Model 2 includes the variables: age, sex, BMI, diabetic ketoacidosis, COVID-19, and comorbidities including a history of diabetes, hypertension, hyperlipidemia, pulmonary hypertension, chronic obstructive pulmonary diseases, asthma, coronary artery disease, heart failure, stroke/TIA, end-stage renal disease, and chronic kidney disease. Model 3 includes the variables: age, aex, BMI, diabetic ketoacidosis, COVID-19, comorbidities including a history of diabetes, hypertension, hyperlipidemia, pulmonary hypertension, chronic obstructive pulmonary diseases, asthma, coronary artery disease, heart failure, stroke/TIA, end-stage renal disease, and chronic kidney disease, and antidiabetic medication classes including biguanides, DPP4 inhibitors, SGLT-2 inhibitors, GLP-1 agonists, insulin, ACE inhibitors, sulfonylureas, and statins. Model 4 includes the variables: age, sex, BMI, diabetic ketoacidosis, COVID-19, comorbidities including a history of diabetes, hypertension, hyperlipidemia, pulmonary hypertension, chronic obstructive pulmonary diseases, asthma, coronary artery disease, heart failure, stroke/TIA, end-stage renal disease, and chronic kidney disease, antidiabetic medication classes including biguanides, DPP4 inhibitors, SGLT-2 inhibitors, GLP-1 agonists, insulin, ACE inhibitors, sulfonylureas, and statins, and all the medications used during inpatient status: heparin, enoxaparin, apixaban, steroids, tocilizumab, remdesivir, convalescent plasma, and cefepime. ** $p < 0.01$, * $p < 0.05$.

Abbreviations and symbols: n = number; BMI in kg/m^2; DM = Diabetes Mellitus; DKA = Diabetic Ketoacidosis; COPD = Chronic Obstructive Pulmonary Disease; CAD = coronary artery disease; TIA = Transient Ischemic Attack; ESRD = End-Stage Renal Disease; DPP 4 = Dipeptidyl Peptidase 4; GLP 1 = Glucagon-like peptide 1; SGLT 2 = Sodium Glucose Transporter 2; ACE = Angiotensin-Converting Enzyme

3.3.2. COVID-19 Cohort

Univariate associations with in-hospital mortality for the COVID-19 cohort were examined for the available baseline demographics and clinical characteristics and are presented in Table 6. Older age, male sex, higher BMI, diabetes mellitus, and DKA were associated with a higher likelihood for in-hospital death in all models. A history of type 1 diabetes, hypertension, asthma, heart failure, and stroke/TIA were shown to have an inverse association with in-hospital mortality. The use of biguanides, DPP4-inhibitors, and ACE inhibitors was also inversely associated with in-hospital mortality.

Table 6. COVID-19 Cohort: univariate and multivariate logistic regression analysis for the outcome of mortality.

Variables	Univariate Analysis	Multivariate Analysis Model 1	Multivariate Analysis Model 2	Multivariate Analysis Model 3	Multivariate Analysis Model 4
		n = 11,371	n = 11,371	n = 11,371	n = 11,371
	OR (95% CI), p-Value	OR (95% CI), p-Value	OR (95% CI), p-Value	OR (95% CI), p-Value	OR (95% CI), p-Value
Age per 10 years	1.61 ** (1.57–1.65) $p < 0.001$	1.67 ** (1.62–1.72) $p < 0.001$	1.69 ** (1.63–1.74) $p < 0.001$	1.71 ** (1.65–1.77) $p < 0.001$	1.76 ** (1.70–1.83) $p < 0.001$
Male sex	1.18 ** (1.10–1.28) $p < 0.001$	1.47 ** (1.34–1.61) $p < 0.001$	1.46 ** (1.32–1.61) $p < 0.001$	1.47 ** (1.33–1.62) $p < 0.001$	1.34 ** (1.20–1.48) $p < 0.001$
BMI	1.00 (1.00–1.01) $p = 0.154$	1.04 ** (1.03–1.04) $p < 0.001$	1.03 ** (1.03–1.04) $p < 0.001$	1.04 ** (1.03–1.04) $p < 0.001$	1.03 ** (1.03–1.04) $p < 0.001$
Diabetic Ketoacidosis	1.94 ** (1.51–2.49) $p < 0.001$	2.57 ** (1.92–3.43) $p < 0.001$	1.95 ** (1.42–2.68) $p < 0.001$	1.95 ** (1.41–2.70) $p < 0.001$	1.95 ** (1.37–2.76) $p < 0.001$
History of DM	2.09 ** (1.93–2.26) $p < 0.001$		2.09 ** (1.90–2.30) $p < 0.001$	2.54 ** (2.28–2.85) $p < 0.001$	1.85 ** (1.64–2.09) $p < 0.001$
Type 1 Diabetes	0.65 (0.36–1.19) $p = 0.166$		0.36 * (0.16–0.81) $p = 0.014$	0.35 * (0.15–0.82) $p = 0.016$	0.37 * (0.16–0.88) $p = 0.024$
Hypertension	0.73 ** (0.66–0.80) $p < 0.001$		0.53 ** (0.46–0.60) $p < 0.001$	0.59 ** (0.51–0.68) $p < 0.001$	0.56 ** (0.48–0.65) $p < 0.001$
Hyperlipidemia	0.80 ** (0.69–0.92) $p = 0.001$		0.85 (0.71–1.01) $p = 0.064$	0.96 (0.80–1.16) $p = 0.658$	1.09 (0.90–1.33) $p = 0.376$
Pulmonary Hypertension	0.95 (0.49–1.83) $p = 0.871$		1.06 (0.47–2.35) $p = 0.895$	0.99 (0.43–2.26) $p = 0.982$	1.02 (0.37–2.83) $p = 0.962$
COPD	1.02 (0.77–1.35) $p = 0.904$		1.19 (0.86–1.65) $p = 0.288$	1.25 (0.90–1.75) $p = 0.190$	1.06 (0.73–1.53) $p = 0.773$
Asthma	0.49 ** (0.38–0.62) $p < 0.001$		0.64 ** (0.49–0.84) $p = 0.001$	0.66 ** (0.50–0.87) $p = 0.003$	0.56 ** (0.42–0.75) $p < 0.001$
CAD	0.97 (0.77–1.21) $p = 0.773$		0.85 (0.64–1.12) $p = 0.249$	0.93 (0.69–1.24) $p = 0.615$	0.98 (0.72–1.34) $p = 0.919$
Heart Failure	0.78 ** (0.65–0.94) $p = 0.010$		0.62 ** (0.49–0.79) $p < 0.001$	0.68 ** (0.54–0.87) $p = 0.002$	0.83 (0.64–1.07) $p = 0.144$
Stroke/TIA	0.66 * (0.46–0.97) $p = 0.032$		0.48 ** (0.31–0.75) $p = 0.001$	0.51 ** (0.33–0.81) $p = 0.004$	0.56 * (0.35–0.91) $p = 0.018$
ESRD	1.33 ** (1.11–1.59) $p = 0.002$		1.63 ** (1.29–2.07) $p < 0.001$	1.58 ** (1.24–2.02) $p < 0.001$	1.15 (0.89–1.49) $p = 0.295$
Chronic Kidney Disease	1.24 * (1.05–1.46) $p = 0.010$		1.05 (0.85–1.29) $p = 0.677$	1.02 (0.82–1.27) $p = 0.864$	1.08 (0.86–1.37) $p = 0.497$

Table 6. Cont.

Variables	Univariate Analysis OR (95% CI), p-Value	Multivariate Analysis Model 1 n = 11,371 OR (95% CI), p-Value	Multivariate Analysis Model 2 n = 11,371 OR (95% CI), p-Value	Multivariate Analysis Model 3 n = 11,371 OR (95% CI), p-Value	Multivariate Analysis Model 4 n = 11,371 OR (95% CI), p-Value
Biguanides	0.55 ** (0.47–0.65) p < 0.001			0.57 ** (0.47–0.69) p < 0.001	0.70 ** (0.57–0.87) p = 0.001
DPP4 inhibitors	0.75 ** (0.64–0.88) p < 0.001			0.78 * (0.64–0.95) p = 0.014	0.84 (0.68–1.03) p = 0.100
SGLT-2 inhibitors	0.77 (0.28–2.07) p = 0.601			1.13 (0.33–3.89) p = 0.847	0.86 (0.16–4.60) p = 0.858
GLP-1 agonists	1.03 (0.65–1.64) p = 0.896			1.22 (0.66–2.24) p = 0.523	1.35 (0.71–2.57) p = 0.364
Insulin	1.34 ** (1.24–1.45) p < 0.001			0.94 (0.84–1.06) p = 0.343	0.95 (0.84–1.08) p = 0.434
ACE inhibitors	0.69 ** (0.62–0.76) p < 0.001			0.58 ** (0.51–0.65) p < 0.001	0.61 ** (0.53–0.70) p < 0.001
Sulfonylureas	0.77 (0.58–1.04) p = 0.088			0.83 (0.57–1.21) p = 0.334	0.86 (0.57–1.29) p = 0.460
Statins	1.28 ** (1.19–1.39) p < 0.001			0.92 (0.82–1.02) p = 0.109	0.85 ** (0.76–0.95) p = 0.004
Heparin	2.69 ** (2.48–2.91) p < 0.001				2.02 ** (1.81–2.26) p < 0.001
Enoxaparin	0.92 * (0.85–0.99) p = 0.036				0.98 (0.87–1.11) p = 0.760
Apixaban	0.97 (0.86–1.09) p = 0.588				0.52 ** (0.44–0.61) p < 0.001
Steroids	3.51 ** (3.23–3.81) p < 0.001				3.01 ** (2.69–3.38) p < 0.001
Tocilizumab	2.07 ** (1.76–2.42) p < 0.001				1.37 ** (1.11–1.69) p = 0.003
Remdesivir	0.93 (0.74–1.17) p = 0.557				0.54 ** (0.41–0.71) p < 0.001
Convalescent Plasma	2.38 ** (2.00–2.83) p < 0.001				1.05 (0.82–1.34) p = 0.708
Cefepime	4.52 ** (4.08–5.02) p < 0.001				3.13 ** (2.74–3.58) p < 0.001

Notes: Table 6 shows univariate analysis and four multivariate models with different definitions of our variable of interest. Model 1 includes the variables: age, sex, BMI, and diabetic ketoacidosis. Model 2 includes the variables: age, sex, BMI, diabetic ketoacidosis, and comorbidities including a history of diabetes, hypertension, hyperlipidemia, pulmonary hypertension, chronic obstructive pulmonary diseases, asthma, coronary artery disease, heart failure, stroke/TIA, end-stage renal disease, and chronic kidney disease. Model 3 includes the variables: age, sex, BMI, diabetic ketoacidosis, comorbidities including a history of diabetes, hypertension, hyperlipidemia, pulmonary hypertension, chronic obstructive pulmonary diseases, asthma, coronary artery disease, heart failure, stroke/TIA, end-stage renal disease, and chronic kidney disease, and antidiabetic medication classes including biguanides, DPP4 inhibitors, SGLT-2 inhibitors, GLP-1 agonists, insulin, ACE inhibitors, sulfonylureas, and statins. Model 4 includes the variables: age, sex, BMI, diabetic ketoacidosis, comorbidities including a history of diabetes, hypertension, hyperlipidemia, pulmonary hypertension, chronic obstructive pulmonary diseases, asthma, coronary artery disease, heart failure, stroke/TIA, end-stage renal disease, and chronic kidney disease, antidiabetic medication classes including biguanides, DPP4 inhibitors, SGLT-2 inhibitors, GLP-1 agonists, insulin, ACE inhibitors, sulfonylureas, and statins, and all the medications used during inpatient status: heparin, enoxaparin, apixaban, steroids, tocilizumab, remdesivir, convalescent plasma, and cefepime. ** $p < 0.01$, * $p < 0.05$.

Abbreviations and symbols: n = number; BMI in kg/m²; DM = Diabetes Mellitus; DKA = Diabetic Ketoacidosis; COPD = Chronic Obstructive Pulmonary Disease; CAD = coronary artery disease; TIA = Transient Ischemic Attack; ESRD = End-Stage Renal Disease; DPP 4 = Dipeptidyl Peptidase 4; GLP 1 = Glucagon-like peptide 1; SGLT 2 = Sodium Glucose Transporter 2; ACE = Angiotensin-Converting Enzyme

3.3.3. DKA Cohort

Univariate associations with in-hospital mortality for the DKA cohort were examined for the available baseline demographics and clinical characteristics and are presented in Table 7. Older age, higher BMI, and hyperlipidemia were associated with a higher likelihood for in-hospital mortality in all models. COVID-19, in this cohort, was associated with an almost ten-fold likelihood for in-hospital mortality in all cohorts. In this cohort, no association between other comorbidities or the use of medications and in-hospital death was noted.

Table 7. DKA Cohort: univariate and multivariate logistic regression analysis for the outcome of mortality.

Variables	Univariate Analysis	Multivariate Analysis Model 1	Multivariate Analysis Model 2	Multivariate Analysis Model 3	Multivariate Analysis Model 4
		n = 422	n = 422	n = 422	n = 422
	OR (95% CI), p-Value	OR (95% CI), p-Value	OR (95% CI), p-Value	OR (95% CI), p-Value	OR (95% CI), p-Value
Age per 10	1.61 ** (1.38–1.88) $p < 0.001$	1.64 ** (1.38–1.94) $p < 0.001$	1.67 ** (1.37–2.05) $p < 0.001$	1.72 ** (1.40–2.12) $p < 0.001$	1.81 ** (1.44–2.27) $p < 0.001$
Male	0.87 (0.54–1.41) $p = 0.568$	1.35 (0.73–2.49) $p = 0.333$	1.47 (0.75–2.85) $p = 0.261$	1.70 (0.86–3.39) $p = 0.130$	2.08 (0.92–4.70) $p = 0.079$
BMI	1.02 (1.00–1.05) $p = 0.100$	1.05 ** (1.02–1.08) $p = 0.003$	1.05 ** (1.02–1.09) $p = 0.002$	1.05 ** (1.02–1.09) $p = 0.003$	1.04 (1.00–1.09) $p = 0.074$
COVID-19	10.05 ** (5.15–19.59) $p < 0.001$	10.08 ** (4.91–20.70) $p < 0.001$	10.31 ** (5.12–20.76) $p < 0.001$	10.26 ** (4.91–21.40) $p < 0.001$	8.56 ** (3.23–22.74) $p < 0.001$
Type 1 Diabetes	0.32 ** (0.16–0.67) $p = 0.002$		0.67 (0.28–1.62) $p = 0.379$	0.63 (0.25–1.56) $p = 0.317$	0.66 (0.23–1.90) $p = 0.440$
Hypertension	0.83 (0.47–1.46) $p = 0.513$		0.50 (0.24–1.05) $p = 0.066$	0.62 (0.29–1.32) $p = 0.216$	0.57 (0.24–1.32) $p = 0.188$
Hyperlipidemia	2.22 * (1.15–4.30) $p = 0.018$		3.13 * (1.13–8.66) $p = 0.028$	3.84 ** (1.44–10.28) $p = 0.007$	6.91 ** (2.49–19.22) $p < 0.001$
Asthma	0.65 (0.14–3.01) $p = 0.585$		1.06 (0.35–3.25) $p = 0.914$	1.04 (0.29–3.73) $p = 0.955$	0.43 (0.11–1.76) $p = 0.241$
CAD	0.91 (0.10–8.25) $p = 0.932$		0.25 (0.01–7.41) $p = 0.422$	0.18 (0.01–6.28) $p = 0.343$	0.17 (0.01–3.43) $p = 0.246$
Heart Failure	0.51 (0.11–2.28) $p = 0.378$		0.20 (0.01–2.91) $p = 0.241$	0.18 (0.01–3.64) $p = 0.261$	0.58 (0.05–6.33) $p = 0.655$
ESRD	1.04 (0.33–3.25) $p = 0.945$		2.54 (0.22–29.04) $p = 0.455$	2.98 (0.19–46.75) $p = 0.437$	5.62 (0.76–41.46) $p = 0.090$
CKD	0.74 (0.28–2.01) $p = 0.559$		0.58 (0.12–2.92) $p = 0.513$	0.60 (0.10–3.84) $p = 0.594$	0.46 (0.04–4.67) $p = 0.509$
Biguanides	0.87 (0.42–1.82) $p = 0.718$			1.00 (0.42–2.41) $p = 0.999$	1.35 (0.53–3.43) $p = 0.532$

Table 7. Cont.

Variables	Univariate Analysis	Multivariate Analysis Model 1	Multivariate Analysis Model 2	Multivariate Analysis Model 3	Multivariate Analysis Model 4
		$n = 422$	$n = 422$	$n = 422$	$n = 422$
	OR (95% CI), p-Value	OR (95% CI), p-Value	OR (95% CI), p-Value	OR (95% CI), p-Value	OR (95% CI), p-Value
DPP4 inhibitors	0.78 (0.43–1.42) $p = 0.421$			0.50 (0.22–1.12) $p = 0.094$	0.52 (0.21–1.27) $p = 0.153$
GLP-1 agonists	1.83 (0.16–20.44) $p = 0.624$			1.54 (0.26–9.04) $p = 0.634$	0.78 (0.13–4.53) $p = 0.780$
Insulin	0.67 (0.41–1.09) $p = 0.109$			0.89 (0.48–1.67) $p = 0.721$	1.05 (0.52–2.12) $p = 0.893$
ACE inhibitors	0.52 * (0.29–0.91) $p = 0.022$			0.51 (0.23–1.10) $p = 0.085$	0.46 (0.19–1.14) $p = 0.093$
Sulfonylureas	1.47 (0.28–7.69) $p = 0.652$			2.01 (0.42–9.66) $p = 0.384$	3.38 (0.46–24.84) $p = 0.232$
Statins	1.10 (0.69–1.75) $p = 0.699$			0.89 (0.48–1.63) $p = 0.706$	0.91 (0.44–1.89) $p = 0.808$
Heparin	1.78 * (1.08–2.94) $p = 0.024$				1.66 (0.79–3.46) $p = 0.178$
Enoxaparin	1.51 (0.93–2.44) $p = 0.094$				0.96 (0.40–2.32) $p = 0.929$
Apixaban	1.84 (0.86–3.94) $p = 0.116$				0.35 (0.11–1.16) $p = 0.086$
Steroids	10.44 ** (6.12–17.82) $p < 0.001$				9.15 ** (4.25–19.73) $p < 0.001$
Tocilizumab	7.16 ** (2.33–21.96) $p = 0.001$				2.39 (0.36–15.97) $p = 0.370$
Remdesivir	3.70 (0.51–26.67) $p = 0.195$				1.54 (0.13–18.66) $p = 0.735$
Convalescent Plasma	4.51 ** (1.48–13.80) $p = 0.008$				0.16 * (0.03–0.89) $p = 0.037$
Cefepime	5.87 ** (3.29–10.48) $p < 0.001$				2.85 ** (1.40–5.79) $p = 0.004$

Notes: Table 7 shows univariate analysis and four multivariate models with different definitions of our variable of interest. Model 1 includes the variables: age, sex, BMI, and COVID-19. Model 2 includes the variables: age, sex, BMI, COVID-19, and comorbidities including a history of diabetes, hypertension, hyperlipidemia, pulmonary hypertension, chronic obstructive pulmonary diseases, asthma, coronary artery disease, heart failure, stroke/TIA, end-stage renal disease, and chronic kidney disease. Model 3 includes the variables: age, sex, BMI, COVID-19 comorbidities including a history of diabetes, hypertension, hyperlipidemia, pulmonary hypertension, chronic obstructive pulmonary diseases, asthma, coronary artery disease, heart failure, stroke/TIA, end-stage renal disease, and chronic kidney disease, and antidiabetic medication classes including biguanides, DPP4 inhibitors, SGLT-2 inhibitors, GLP-1 agonists, insulin, ACE inhibitors, sulfonylureas, and statins. Model 4 includes the variables: age, sex, BMI, COVID-19, comorbidities including a history of diabetes, hypertension, hyperlipidemia, pulmonary hypertension, chronic obstructive pulmonary diseases, asthma, coronary artery disease, heart failure, stroke/TIA, end-stage renal disease, and chronic kidney disease, antidiabetic medication classes including biguanides, DPP4 inhibitors, SGLT-2 inhibitors, GLP-1 agonists, insulin, ACE inhibitors, sulfonylureas, and statins, and all the medications used during inpatient status: heparin, enoxaparin, apixaban, steroids, tocilizumab, remdesivir, convalescent plasma, and cefepime. ** $p < 0.01$, * $p < 0.05$.

Abbreviations and symbols: n = number; BMI in kg/m^2; DM = Diabetes Mellitus; DKA = Diabetic Ketoacidosis; COPD = Chronic Obstructive Pulmonary Disease; CAD = coronary artery disease; TIA = Transient Ischemic Attack; ESRD = End-Stage Renal Disease; DPP 4 = Dipeptidyl Peptidase 4; GLP 1 = Glucagon-like peptide 1; SGLT 2 = Sodium Glucose Transporter 2; ACE = Angiotensin-Converting Enzyme

4. Discussion

Diabetic ketoacidosis is a severe metabolic complication attributable to severe insulin deficiency. From previous studies, it is well established that COVID-19 is associated with ketosis, ketoacidosis, and diabetic ketoacidosis [16]. Our study investigated the association of DKA with in-hospital outcomes among patients admitted with COVID-19 in the largest public health care system of the United States. The key findings of our descriptive analysis showed that the mortality rate was seven times higher in patients with DKA and COVID-19 compared to the DKA control group, i.e., patients without COVID-19. The likelihood of death in patients with DKA and COVID-19 was found to be significantly higher compared to patients with DKA and without COVID-19.

Khan et al. reported a cohort of 14,900 patients across the eleven hospitals of New York City Health + Hospitals, which showed that the mortality rate in DKA/COVID-19 patients was almost 50% [17]. To further elucidate these findings, we adjusted for common conditions and treatments that could influence mortality. Our analysis found that diabetes was associated with a two-times-higher likelihood of death among patients with COVID-19 after adjustment for variables such as common co-morbidities, DKA, and anti-hyperglycemic medications. This is similar to the meta-analysis by Kumar et al. (33 studies, 16,003 patients) which demonstrated that diabetes in patients with COVID-19 was associated with a two-fold increase in mortality as compared to patients without diabetes [18]. This is in line with our previous meta-analysis of 18,506 patients that also showed a higher mortality in patients with diabetes and COVID-19 as compared to those without diabetes [19]. In our analysis, COVID-19 was associated with a four-times-higher likelihood for death in the matched cohort (COVID-19/control), which became ten-fold in the DKA group. Hyperosmolar hyperglycemic syndrome (HHS) and DKA can be precipitated in patients with new onset DM or with previously adequate glycemic control [20]. Some case reports described that patients with both HHS and DKA who required mechanical ventilation had a poor prognosis with 100% mortality [21]. However, the effects of long-COVID on the rates of mortality in DKA are unknown. Several plausible mechanisms have been suggested in the development of SARS-CoV-2-mediated acute diabetes and diabetic ketoacidosis. This includes damage to the pancreatic β-cell, which could either be direct, by the binding of SARS-CoV-2 to angiotensin-converting enzyme 2 (ACE2) receptors on the pancreatic islets, immune-mediated from alterations in the self-antigens, or by β-cell death resulting from the release of inflammatory markers such as tumor-necrosis factor-α (TNFα) and interferon-γ by a SARS-CoV/SARS-CoV-2-infected exocrine pancreas [22–24]. Damage to the pancreatic β-cell in the setting of relative (Type 2 DM) or absolute (Type 1 DM) insulin deficiency can lead to an imbalance in the insulin:glucagon ratio. This imbalance causes an increase in glucose synthesis, reduced glucose utilization, and excessive lipolysis, leading to hyperglycemic ketoacidosis [25,26]. The production of interferon (IFN) gamma can lead to resistance to insulin on muscles, leading to hyperinsulinemia in order to maintain a euglycemic state. However, patients with a reduced production of insulin or an increased resistance to insulin might fail this compensatory mechanism if they are affected by COVID-19 [27].

Diabetes in COVID-19 can lead to severe disease and increase the overall mortality. Some of the possible explanations for this include: (a) compromised innate immunity, which is the first line of defense against COVID-19. Uncontrolled diabetes leads to reduced innate immunity, which gives rise to the unhindered proliferation of the virus [28,29]. (b) Exaggerated cytokine storm response: even in the absence of immune stimulation, diabetes is associated with a pro-inflammatory state characterized by increased levels of interleukin (IL)-1, IL-6, tumor-necrosis factor (TNF)-α, and ferritin. This cytokine response is exaggerated when there is an appropriate stimulus such as COVID-19 viral infection leading to acute respiratory distress syndrome (ARDS) and rapid deterioration [30–32]. (c) Increased oxidative stress: ACE2 is a membrane glycoprotein expressed in the lungs, kidneys, intestine, and blood vessels. It is known to break down angiotensin II and angiotensin I to smaller peptides such as angiotensin (Ang) (1–7) and angiotensin (1–9), respectively. ACE2/Ang (1–7) plays a crucial role as anti-inflammatory mechanism and antioxidant protecting lungs against ARDS. ACE2 is under-expressed in diabetes patients, possibly due to glycosylation, which explains the increased susceptibility to severe lung injury and ARDS in COVID-19 patients [33,34]. However, even the over-expression of ACE2 would be detrimental, as SARS-CoV-2 utilizes ACE2 as a receptor for entry into the host pneumocytes [35]. It is also interesting to note that there have been a few cases of patients presenting with DKA after being vaccinated against COVID-19 [36,37]. These authors have attributed DKA after vaccination to poor oral intake or the inability to titrate insulin requirements, especially in patients with T1DM combined with the vaccine-induced enhancement of a robust systemic immune-inflammatory response [36,38].

To our knowledge, this study is the largest to date assessing the impact of DKA on the in-hospital outcomes of patients with COVID-19 of different sexes, age groups, and racial/ethnic backgrounds. We should acknowledge that our study has several limitations. First, this was a retrospective cohort involving electronic medical records; hence, there are risks related to observational bias and unmeasured confounding. Second, our cohort is unique in that it is enriched with immigrant populations, Medicaid-Medicare recipients, and the uninsured, which may have unique unidentified confounding factors; therefore, our findings cannot be easily generalized to patient populations with other characteristics.

5. Conclusions

In summary, our study of a large cohort of hospitalized patients with COVID-19 in a public healthcare system showed that DKA and diabetes were associated with increased in-hospital death after adjusting for DKA/diabetes-related potentially confounding factors. This demonstrates that the presence of DKA is associated with worse outcomes of coronavirus infection. We propose that the enhanced prevention of COVID-19 infection in persons with diabetes by known preventive measures such as masks, social distancing, and vaccination—and, more importantly, the enhanced monitoring of COVID-19 patients with DKA/diabetes during their hospitalization—may help reduce mortality.

Supplementary Materials: The following supporting information can be downloaded at: https://www.mdpi.com/article/10.3390/diabetology3030036/s1, Graphs concerning the quality of the matching technique used: Figure S1. Extent of covariate imbalance in terms of standardized percentage differences before and after matching. Figure S2. Propensity scores, subject-specific probability of mortality (A) before matching and (B) after matching. Statistics: Table S1. Correlation matrix of disorders. Table S2. Correlation matrix of disorders in the DKA cohort. Regression analysis for the outcome of intubation: Table S3. Baseline patient characteristics: univariate and multivariate logistic regression analysis for the outcome of intubation. Table S4. COVID-19 cohort: univariate and multivariate logistic regression analysis for the outcome of intubation. Table S5. DKA cohort: univariate and multivariate logistic regression analysis for the outcome of intubation. Regression analysis for the outcome of ICU admission: Table S6. Baseline patient characteristics: univariate and multivariate logistic regression analysis for the outcome of ICU admission. Table S7. COVID-19 cohort: univariate and multivariate logistic regression analysis for the outcome of ICU admission. Table S8. DKA cohort: univariate and multivariate logistic regression analysis for the outcome of ICU admission. Regression analysis for the outcome of Renal Replacement Therapy: Table S9. Baseline patient characteristics: univariate and multivariate logistic regression analysis for the outcome of Renal Replacement Therapy. Table S10. COVID-19 cohort: univariate and multivariate logistic regression analysis for the outcome of Renal Replacement Therapy. Table S11. DKA cohort: univariate and multivariate logistic regression analysis for the outcome of Renal Replacement Therapy.

Author Contributions: Conceptualization—N.C.-P., S.P., C.C., K.H.H., D.B. and P.K. Methodology—S.P., N.C.-P., D.K., L.P. and P.K. Formal analysis—D.K., L.P., N.C.-P. and S.P. Resources—P.K. and R.F. Data curation—S.P. and N.C.-P. Writing—original draft preparation—S.P. and N.C.-P. Writing—review and editing—N.C.-P., S.P., A.K., N.C.-P., K.H.H., J.C., D.B., D.K., R.F., L.P. and P.K. Supervision—P.K. and L.P. Project administration—P.K. All authors have read and agreed to the published version of the manuscript.

Funding: This research received no external funding.

Institutional Review Board Statement: The study was approved by the Biomedical Research Alliance of New York Institutional Review Board with a waiver of informed consent (IRB #20-12-318-373).

Informed Consent Statement: Patient consent was waived by the IRB, as the data were fully de-identified and anonymized before the data were accessed.

Data Availability Statement: The data is available upon reasonable request.

Acknowledgments: We acknowledge the contribution of Fela Oyeneyin for his assistance with data extraction.

Conflicts of Interest: The authors declare no conflict of interest.

References

1. Rubino, F.; Amiel, S.A.; Zimmet, P.; Alberti, G.; Bornstein, S.; Eckel, R.H.; Mingrone, G.; Boehm, B.; Cooper, M.E.; Chai, Z.; et al. New-onset diabetes in Covid-19. *N. Engl. J. Med.* **2020**, *383*, 789–790. [CrossRef] [PubMed]
2. Newton, C.A.; Raskin, P. Diabetic ketoacidosis in type 1 and type 2 diabetes mellitus: Clinical and biochemical differences. *Arch. Intern. Med.* **2004**, *164*, 1925–1931. [CrossRef]
3. Kamata, Y.; Takano, K.; Kishihara, E.; Watanabe, M.; Ichikawa, R.; Shichiri, M. Distinct clinical characteristics and therapeutic modalities for diabetic ketoacidosis in type 1 and type 2 diabetes mellitus. *J. Diabetes Complicat.* **2017**, *31*, 468–472. [CrossRef]
4. Sathish, T.; Kapoor, N.; Cao, Y.; Tapp, R.J.; Zimmet, P. Proportion of newly diagnosed diabetes in COVID-19 patients: A systematic review and meta-analysis. *Diabetes Obes. Metab.* **2021**, *23*, 870–874. [CrossRef] [PubMed]
5. de Sá-Ferreira, C.O.; da Costa, C.H.M.; Guimarães, J.C.W.; Sampaio, N.S.; Silva, L.M.L.; de Mascarenhas, L.P.; Rodrigues, N.G.; Dos Santos, T.L.; Campos, S.; Young, E.C. Diabetic ketoacidosis and COVID-19: What have we learned so far? *Am. J. Physiol. Endocrinol. Metab.* **2022**, *322*, E44–E53. [CrossRef] [PubMed]
6. Kiran, R.; Saroch, A.; Pannu, A.K.; Sharma, N.; Dutta, P.; Kumar, M. Clinical profile and outcomes of diabetic ketoacidosis during COVID-19 pandemic in north India. *Trop. Dr.* **2022**, *18*, 494755221076896. [CrossRef]
7. Alhumaid, S.; Al Mutair, A.; Al Alawi, Z.; Rabaan, A.A.; Alomari, M.A.; Al Salman, S.A.; Al-Alawi, A.S.; Al Hassan, M.H.; Alhamad, H.; Al-Kamees, M.A.; et al. Diabetic ketoacidosis in patients with SARS-CoV-2: A systematic review and meta-analysis. *Diabetol. Metab. Syndr.* **2021**, *13*, 120. [CrossRef] [PubMed]
8. Stevens, J.S.; Bogun, M.M.; McMahon, D.J.; Zucker, J.; Kurlansky, P.; Mohan, S.; Yin, M.T.; Nickolas, T.L.; Pajvani, U.B. Diabetic ketoacidosis and mortality in COVID-19 infection. *Diabetes Metab.* **2021**, *47*, 101267. [CrossRef] [PubMed]
9. Muhammad, A.; Hakim, M.; Afaq, S.; Khattak, F.A.; Shakireen, N.; Jawad, M.; Saeed, R.; Haq, Z.U. Diabetic ketoacidosis amongst patients with COVID-19: A retrospective chart review of 220 patients in Pakistan. *Endocrinol. Diabetes Metab.* **2022**, *5*, e00331. [CrossRef]
10. Kempegowda, P.; Melson, E.; Johnson, A.; Wallett, L.; Thomas, L.; Zhou, D.; Holmes, C.; Juszczak, A.; Karamat, M.A.; Ghosh, S.; et al. Effect of COVID-19 on the clinical course of diabetic ketoacidosis (DKA) in people with type 1 and type 2 diabetes. *Endocr. Connect.* **2021**, *10*, 371–377. [CrossRef]
11. Chamorro-Pareja, N.; Parthasarathy, S.; Annam, J.; Hoffman, J.; Coyle, C.; Kishore, P. Letter to the editor: Unexpected high mortality in COVID-19 and diabetic ketoacidosis. *Metab. Clin. Exp.* **2020**, *110*, 154301. [CrossRef] [PubMed]
12. Available online: https://www.aafp.org/pubs/afp/issues/2005/0501/p1705.html#:~{}:text=A%20diagnosis%20of%20diabetic%20ketoacidosis,mEq%20per%20L%20or%20less (accessed on 12 May 2022).
13. Austin, P.C. An introduction to propensity score methods for reducing the effects of confounding in observational studies. *Multivar. Behav. Res.* **2011**, *46*, 399–424. [CrossRef] [PubMed]
14. Austin, P.C. Optimal caliper widths for propensity-score matching when estimating differences in means and differences in proportions in observational studies. *Pharm. Stat.* **2011**, *10*, 150–161. [CrossRef] [PubMed]
15. Wang, Y.; Cai, H.; Li, C.; Jiang, Z.; Wang, L.; Song, J.; Xia, J. Optimal caliper width for propensity score matching of three treatment groups: A Monte Carlo study. *PLoS ONE* **2013**, *8*, e81045.
16. Li, J.; Wang, X.; Chen, J.; Zuo, X.; Zhang, H.; Deng, A. COVID-19 infection may cause ketosis and ketoacidosis. *Diabetes Obes. Metab.* **2020**, *22*, 1935–1941. [CrossRef]
17. Khan, F.; Paladino, L.; Sinert, R. The impact of COVID-19 on Diabetic Ketoacidosis patients. *Diabetes Metab. Syndr.* **2022**, *16*, 102389. [CrossRef]

18. Kumar, A.; Arora, A.; Sharma, P.; Anikhindi, S.A.; Bansal, N.; Singla, V.; Khare, S.; Srivastava, A. Is diabetes mellitus associated with mortality and severity of COVID-19? *A meta-analysis. Diabetes Metab. Syndr.* **2020**, *14*, 535–545, Epub 2020 May 6. PMCID:PMC7200339. [CrossRef] [PubMed]
19. Palaiodimos, L.; Chamorro-Pareja, N.; Karamanis, D.; Li, W.; Zavras, P.D.; Chang, K.M.; Mathias, P.; Kokkinidis, D.G. Diabetes is associated with increased risk for in-hospital mortality in patients with COVID-19: A systematic review and meta-analysis comprising 18,506 patients. *Hormones* **2021**, *20*, 305–314, Epub 2020 Oct 29. PMCID:PMC7595056. [CrossRef] [PubMed]
20. Rafique, S.; Ahmed, F.W. A Case of combined diabetic ketoacidosis and hyperosmolar hyperglycemic state in a patient with COVID-19. *Cureus* **2020**, *12*, e8965. [CrossRef]
21. Singh, B.; Kaur, P.; Majachani, N.; Patel, P.; Reid, R.-J.R.; Maroules, M. COVID-19 and combined diabetic ketoacidosis and hyperglycemic hyperosmolar nonketotic coma: Report of 11 cases. *J. Investig. Med. High Impact Case Reports.* **2021**, *9*, 23247096211021231. [CrossRef]
22. Yang, J.K.; Lin, S.S.; Ji, X.J.; Guo, L.M. Binding of SARS coronavirus to its receptor damages islets and causes acute diabetes. *Acta Diabetol.* **2010**, *47*, 193–199, Epub 2009 Mar 31. PMCID:PMC7088164. [CrossRef] [PubMed]
23. Wu, C.T.; Lidsky, P.V.; Xiao, Y.; Lee, I.T.; Cheng, R.; Nakayama, T.; Jiang, S.; Demeter, J.; Bevacqua, R.J.; Chang, C.A.; et al. SARS-CoV-2 infects human pancreatic β cells and elicits β cell impairment. *Cell Metab.* **2021**, *33*, 1565–1576.e5, Epub 2021 May 18. PMCID:PMC8130512. [CrossRef] [PubMed]
24. Al-Kuraishy, H.M.; Al-Gareeb, A.I.; Alblihed, M.; Guerreiro, S.G.; Cruz-Martins, N.; Batiha, G.E. COVID-19 in Relation to Hyperglycemia and Diabetes Mellitus. *Front Cardiovasc. Med.* **2021**, *8*, 644095, PMCID:PMC8189260. [CrossRef] [PubMed]
25. Ghimire, P.; Dhamoon, A.S. Ketoacidosis. In *StatPearls*; StatPearls Publishing: Treasure Island, FL, USA, 2022. Available online: https://www.ncbi.nlm.nih.gov/books/NBK534848/ (accessed on 2 June 2022).
26. Chiasson, J.L.; Aris-Jilwan, N.; Bélanger, R.; Bertrand, S.; Beauregard, H.; Ekoé, J.M.; Fournier, H.; Havrankova, J. Diagnosis and treatment of diabetic ketoacidosis and the hyperglycemic hyperosmolar state. *CMAJ* **2003**, *168*, 859–866, Erratum in: CMAJ. 2003 May 13;168, 1241. PMCID:PMC151994. [PubMed]
27. Lim, S.; Bae, J.H.; Kwon, H.-S.; Nauck, M.A. COVID-19 and diabetes mellitus: From pathophysiology to clinical management. *Nat. Rev. Endocrinol.* **2021**, *17*, 11–30. [CrossRef]
28. Ma, R.C.W.; Holt, R.I.G. COVID-19 and diabetes. *Diabet. Med.* **2020**, *37*, 723–725, Epub 2020 Apr 3. PMCID:PMC7228343. [CrossRef] [PubMed]
29. Jafar, N.; Edriss, H.; Nugent, K. The effect of short-term hyperglycemia on the innate immune system. *Am. J. Med. Sci.* **2016**, *351*, 201–211. [CrossRef] [PubMed]
30. Geerlings, S.E.; Hoepelman, A.I. Immune dysfunction in patients with diabetes mellitus (DM). *FEMS Immunol. Med. Microbiol.* **1999**, *26*, 259–265. [CrossRef] [PubMed]
31. Mehta, P.; McAuley, D.F.; Brown, M.; Sanchez, E.; Tattersall, R.S.; Manson, J.J. HLH across speciality collaboration, UK. COVID-19: Consider cytokine storm syndromes and immunosuppression. *Lancet* **2020**, *395*, 1033–1034, Epub 2020 Mar 16. PMCID:PMC7270045. [CrossRef] [PubMed]
32. Huang, I.; Lim, M.A.; Pranata, R. Diabetes mellitus is associated with increased mortality and severity of disease in COVID-19 pneumonia—A systematic review, meta-analysis, and meta-regression. *Diabetes Metab. Syndr.* **2020**, *14*, 395–403, Epub 2020 Apr 17. PMCID:PMC7162793. [CrossRef] [PubMed]
33. Wu, C.; Chen, X.; Cai, Y.; Xia, J.; Zhou, X.; Xu, S.; Huang, H.; Zhang, L.; Zhou, X.; Du, C.; et al. Risk Factors associated with acute respiratory distress syndrome and death in patients with coronavirus disease 2019 pneumonia in Wuhan, China. *JAMA Intern. Med.* **2020**, *180*, 934–943, Erratum in: JAMA Intern Med. 2020 Jul 1;180, 1031. PMCID:PMC7070509. [CrossRef] [PubMed]
34. Tikellis, C.; Thomas, M.C. Angiotensin-converting enzyme 2 (ACE2) is a key modulator of the renin angiotensin system in health and disease. *Int. J. Pept.* **2012**, *2012*, 256294, Epub 2012 Mar 20. PMCID:PMC3321295. [CrossRef] [PubMed]
35. Pal, R.; Bhansali, A. COVID-19, diabetes mellitus and ACE2: The conundrum. *Diabetes Res. Clin. Pract.* **2020**, *162*, 108132, Epub 2020 Mar 29. PMCID:PMC7118535. [CrossRef] [PubMed]
36. Yakou, F.; Saburi, M.; Hirose, A.; Akaoka, H.; Hirota, Y.; Kobayashi, T.; Awane, N.; Asahi, N.; Amagawa, T.; Ozawa, S.; et al. A case series of ketoacidosis after coronavirus disease 2019 vaccination in patients with type 1 diabetes. front endocrinol (Lausanne). *Front. Endocrinol.* **2022**, *13*, 840580, PMCID:PMC8971718. [CrossRef] [PubMed]
37. Makiguchi, T.; Fukushima, T.; Tanaka, H.; Taima, K.; Takayasu, S.; Tasaka, S. Diabetic ketoacidosis shortly after COVID-19 vaccination in a non–small-cell lung cancer patient receiving combination of PD-1 and CTLA-4 inhibitors: A case report. *Thorac. Cancer* **2022**, *13*, 1220–1223. [CrossRef]
38. Lee, H.J.; Sajan, A.; Tomer, Y. Hyperglycemic emergencies associated with COVID-19 vaccination: A Case series and discussion. *J. Endocr. Soc.* **2021**, *5*, bvab141. [CrossRef]

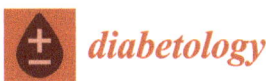

Article

Narrative Review: Obesity, Type 2 DM and Obstructive Sleep Apnoea—Common Bedfellows

Dimitar Sajkov [1,2], Bliegh Mupunga [1,2], Jeffrey J. Bowden [2], Christopher Langton [1,2] and Nikolai Petrovsky [1,3,*]

[1] Australian Respiratory and Sleep Medicine Institute (ARASMI), Bedford Park, SA 5042, Australia
[2] Department of Respiratory and Sleep Medicine, Flinders Medical Centre, Flinders Drive, Bedford Park, SA 5042, Australia
[3] Department of Endocrinology, College of Medicine and Public Health, Flinders University, Flinders Drive, Bedford Park, SA 5042, Australia
* Correspondence: nikolai.petrovsky@flinders.edu.au; Tel.: +61-8-8204-4572; Fax: +61-8-8204-5987

Abstract: Obstructive sleep apnoea (OSA) and type 2 DM mellitus (T2DM) share obesity as a major risk factor. Furthermore, these conditions share overlapping mechanisms including inflammation, activation of the autonomic nervous system, and hypoxia-linked endocrinopathy. Hence, the pathogenesis of the two conditions may be more closely related than previously recognised. This raises the question of whether treatment of OSA might assist resolution of obesity and/or T2DM. Here, we present a narrative review of the literature to identify clinical and scientific data on the relationship between obstructive sleep apnoea and T2DM control. We found there is a paucity of adequately powered well-controlled clinical trials to directly test for a causal association. While routine screening of all T2DM patients with polysomnography cannot currently be justified, given the high prevalence of sleep disordered breathing in the overweight/obese population, all T2DM patients should at a minimum have a clinical assessment of potential obstructive sleep apnoea risk as part of their routine clinical care. In particular, screening questionnaires can be used to identify T2DM subjects at higher risk of OSA for consideration of formal polysomnography studies. Due to morbid obesity being a common feature in both T2DM and OSA, polysomnography should be considered as a screening tool in such high-risk individuals.

Keywords: obstructive sleep apnoea; DM; obesity; inflammation; polysomnography

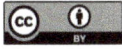

1. Introduction

An overlap in morphological and metabolic features in patients with obstructive sleep apnoea (OSA) and type 2 DM mellitus (T2DM) has been recognised and described since 1993 [1–3], with most patients with T2DM being overweight or obese with excessive visceral fat, features commonly seen in OSA. T2DM is characterised by insulin resistance with relative insulin deficiency and accounts for 90–95% of the total DM population [4]. It is a chronic progressive condition associated with both microvascular and macrovascular complications resulting in high morbidity and mortality. The global incidence of DM has been rising rapidly in parallel with the increasing prevalence of obesity. Recent studies have shown DM to affect 537 million people (https://DMatlas.org/ accessed 14 July 2022). A recent study showed that the prevalence of overweight and obese children combined between 1980 and 2013 rose by 47.1%, with the total number of overweight and obese children and adults increasing from 857 million in 1980 to 2.1 billion globally in 2013 [5].

OSA is a multi-system disorder, affecting cardiovascular and neuro-endocrine systems and lipid metabolism. OSA affects between 20 and 25% of adult men in some populations and its incidence rises with obesity [6], a concerning fact given that over 37% of the world population is currently classed as obese (BMI > 30 kg/m^2) [5]. OSA is characterised by repetitive episodes of hypoxia and hyper-oxygenation with sleep fragmentation. Various mechanisms contribute to the sequelae of OSA including fragmented sleep and loss of sleep, activation of the sympathetic nervous system, recurrent intermittent hypoxia, endothelial dysfunction, systemic inflammation, and hormonal imbalance. The prevalence of OSA (defined as Apnoea–Hypopnea Index(AHI) > 5/hr) is influenced by gender and age, with males and postmenopausal women at highest risk. Evidence of an association between T2DM and OSA is mounting, raising questions as to whether there might be a causal relationship in either direction. A clearer understanding of the pathophysiological pathways and interrelationships between T2DM and OSA may help target common mechanisms and improve outcomes in these patients. In this review, we summarise evidence for possible causal associations between OSA and T2DM and address several practical questions, namely, does treatment of OSA improve diabetic control, does improved DM control improve OSA and should all patients with T2DM be routinely screened for OSA?

2. Potential Pathophysiological Links between T2DM and OSA

2.1. Inflammation

A model for the common origins of OSA and T2DM is presented in Figure 1. Increased inflammatory markers are seen in both T2DM and OSA, thereby suggesting that low-grade inflammation may be a possible link between the two conditions. Patients with T2DM have increased inflammatory markers including serum levels of fibrinogen, C-reactive protein (CRP), and IL-6 [7], with raised serum CRP and TNFα also reported in OSA [8–11]. Inflammatory cytokines can impair glucose metabolism with TNFα, conferring insulin resistance in animal studies via impairment of insulin receptor function [12,13]. TNFα also acts on adipocytes through transcription factors such as NF-kB and hypoxia-inducible factor-1 [14]. The concept of oxidative stress characterised by an imbalance between oxidant-producing systems and antioxidant defence mechanisms (redox balance), resulting in excessive formation of reactive oxygen species (ROS), is well documented in OSA [15]. Chronic repetitive hypoxic episodes increase the formation of ROS and cytokines, suppressing insulin secretion and worsening insulin sensitivity [16–18]. ROS can contribute to dysregulation of adipo-cytokines, thereby increasing insulin resistance. Moreover, some cytokines have sleep regulatory properties with TNFα, IL-6, and IL-1 promoting NREM sleep, whereas IL-1 antagonists inhibit NREM sleep [18,19]. Inflammation may lead to increased production of advanced glycation end-products (AGE) from oxidation and glycation of reducing sugars and amino acids [20]. High levels of AGEs have been detected in both T2DM and non-diabetic patients with OSA [21]. These compounds may play a role in diabetic vascular disease [22]. In non-diabetic patients with OSA, levels of AGEs were significantly higher than those without OSA and positively correlated with an AHI ≥ 5/h, while there was no relationship with measures of insulin sensitivity [23]. In 18 patients in this cohort with moderate to severe OSA treated with CPAP, there was a significant decrease in AGEs from 5.1 to 4.9 ($p = 0.017$) after 3 months of treatment. Nonetheless, the role of AGEs in the pathophysiology of OSA and DM requires further study. Sleep deprived obese patients with OSA were observed to have higher levels of pro-inflammatory markers (IL-2, IL-4, IL-5, IL-6, IL-8, IL-13, and IFN-gamma) in OSA subjects compared to controls without OSA [24].

2.2. Autonomic Nervous System

Increased sympathetic activity may lead to altered glucose metabolism in OSA. Sympathetic activity increases muscle glycogen breakdown and hepatic gluconeogenesis. Activation of the sympathetic nervous system with catecholamine release may raise cholesterol, triglycerides, and insulin and cause glucose intolerance and insulin resistance through lipolysis [25,26]. Insulin resistance is aggravated by increased lipolysis and raised levels of free fatty acids [27].

2.3. Endocrinopathy

Several hormones have been identified in the development of insulin resistance and DM in OSA. In animal studies, leptin-deficient mice exposed to hypoxic environments were observed to develop elevated insulin levels and impaired glucose tolerance [28]. The same observation was replicated in non-obese mice exposed to intermittent hypoxia (IH) under euglycemic environment with reduction in insulin sensitivity and reduced muscle glucose uptake despite pharmacologic blockade of the sympathetic system [29,30]. A study of glucose-induced insulin secretion and gene expression showed that IH reduced β-cell insulin secretion, potentially through downregulation of CD38 [31], with the ecto-cyclase activity of CD38 to produce intracellular cyclic ADP-ribose being critical for insulin secretion [32].

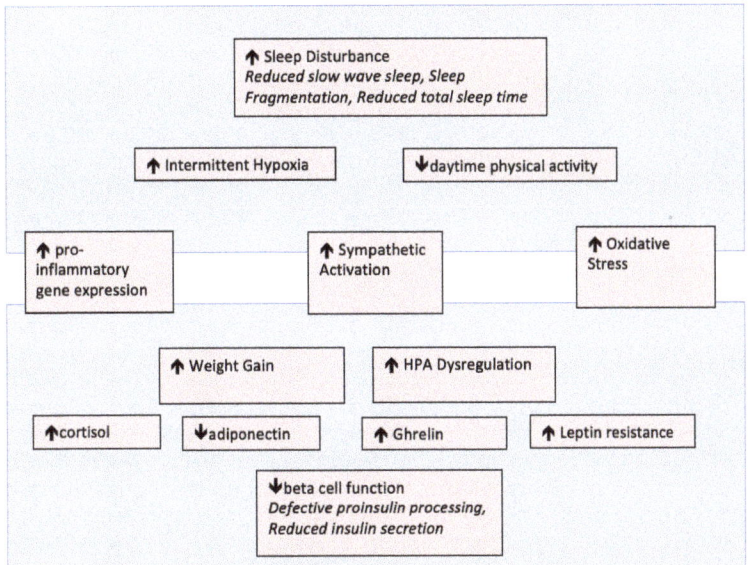

Figure 1. This figure depicts the many disordered pathways observed in OSA and DM and the potential important links between them. Up and down arrows indicate increases or decreases in the relevant condition/marker in either OSA (top grey panel) or DM (bottom grey panel) or both (pink boxes linking the two grey panels).

Adipose tissue is not only an energy storage tissue but an active endocrine organ secreting adipokines including leptin, adiponectin, and cytokines [14,33,34]. Leptin is secreted by white adipocytes and acts as an appetite suppressant at the hypothalamic level as well as acting peripherally through skeletal muscles and pancreatic B cells [35–37]. Levels of leptin in some studies correlate with the percentage of body fat and have been observed to be higher in obese patients suggesting leptin resistance [38,39]. Leptin is not only involved in regulation of insulin secretion and glucose metabolism but has a role in the regulation of both the sympathetic system and inflammatory responses [18]. Leptin has been implicated in ventilatory control. Hypercapnic obese and non-obese patients have been found to have high levels of leptin, which improved with non-invasive ventilation, particularly in patients with obesity hypoventilation syndrome [40–43]. High leptin levels are associated with reduced ventilatory drive, regardless of the amount of body fat in some studies [44]. Nocturnal awakening and arousals are associated with altered levels of leptin, leptin resistance, pulsatile cortisol release, and autonomic activation, which can lead to dysregulation of the hypothalamic–pituitary–adrenal axis and glucose impairment fostering the development of T2DM [45]. Leptin was also found to be elevated in OSA due to repeated episodes of hypoxia. Therefore, it remains unresolved as to whether leptin elevation is a result of sleep disordered breathing or the cause of it. Reduced circulating leptin levels were detected after treatment with CPAP, particularly in non-obese patients [46–48]. However, some studies have found no relationship between leptin and AHI after adjustments for obesity [49,50].

Adiponectin increases fatty acid metabolism and inhibits gluconeogenesis in the liver [51]. Levels are reduced in insulin resistance, DM, and visceral obesity among other conditions [52,53]. The relationship between adiponectin and OSA remains unresolved. Levels of adiponectin are significantly reduced in OSA patients compared to simple snorers, but other studies have reported no difference [54,55]. CPAP therapy reduced adiponectin levels after only two days of treatment in one study, whereas in a randomised trial, no change was observed between subjects treated with CPAP and sham CPAP after 3 months of treatment [56,57]. Compliance with CPAP was a compounding effect in previous studies on the effect of CPAP on hormonal changes.

Glucagon-like peptide (GLP)-1 receptor agonist therapy is highly effective for weight loss and glycaemic control in T2DM and has similarly been shown to have positive benefits for OSA [58,59]. Severe OSA has been shown to be associated with a lower GLP-1 response to glucose challenge, which could be yet another mechanism by which OSA affects glucose metabolism.

2.4. Pancreatic Effects of Chronic Intermittent Hypoxia

Examination of a possible association between DM and OSA cannot avoid addressing the role of the pancreas. Pancreatic endocrine dysfunction is central to the pathophysiology of DM, as while insulin resistance drives type 2 DM, it only when the pancreas no longer keep up with the demand for more insulin that hyperglycaemia eventuates. In studies of pancreatic β-cell function in rodents exposed to intermittent hypoxia (IH), impaired insulin synthesis was demonstrated, speculated to be due to reduced activity of the enzyme that converts pro-insulin to active insulin. β-cell apoptosis results from exposure to IH [60]. Sherwani et al. noted IH exposed mice had significantly higher plasma levels of glucose associated with lower insulin levels compared to animals exposed to intermittent air. IH resulted in reduced insulin release in addition to decreased islet cell viability thought to be mediated by increased release of long chain fatty acids such as palmitic and stearic acid [61]. Polak et al., showed in mice that even after discontinuation of IH, the impaired glucose metabolism persisted to varying degrees [62]. Reactive oxygen species (ROS) from mitochondria have also been implicated in the endocrinopathy with resultant β-cell injury following exposure to IH. This effect is mediated via downregulation of insulin secretion promoting genes such as CD38 [31,32].

3. Sleep Loss and Fragmentation

Sleep deprivation and short sleep are risk factors for impaired glucose metabolism and adverse cardiovascular events. Sleep fragmentation and reduced total sleep time in the absence of significant OSA independently increase the risk of T2DM [63]. Cappuccio et al. in 2010 in a systematic review and meta-analysis of over 100,000 patients assessed the relationship between sleep habits and incidence of DM. Quantity and quality of sleep predicted the risk of development of DM with sleep maintenance insomnia conferring the highest risk (RR was 1.84; 1.39–2.43, $p < 0.0001$) [64]. Xu et al. reported on the effect of day napping or short night sleeping and concluded that both conditions were associated with an increased risk of DM [65]. Sleep fragmentation results in reduced proportion of slow wave sleep and increased sympathetic activity, both of which may adversely affect glucose metabolism. Selective suppression of slow wave sleep in healthy adults has been reported to reduce insulin sensitivity [66,67]. Two laboratory-based studies examined these concepts. One compared 4 and 12 h sleep and noted that the rate of clearance of glucose post-challenge was slower in the sleep restricted group, suggesting reduced sensitivity to insulin. The second crossover study compared 4 and 10 h in bed and demonstrated higher morning glucose levels in the sleep-deprived patients [68]. In an animal study, Gharib et al. observed that mice exposed to sleep fragmentation developed insulin resistance and impaired glucose metabolism through up-regulation of transcription factors and other pathways [69]. A study by Fendri et al. examined the overnight glucose profiles of patients with diagnosed T2DM who were being investigated for symptomatic sleep disordered breathing. All the patients had continuous glucose monitoring during polysomnography [70]. The mean nocturnal glucose level was 31% higher in the sleep apnoea patients ($p = 0.05$) and more marked during REM (38% greater, $p = 0.008$) compared to the non-sleep apnoea patients. In a study examining the effect of sleep duration on the risk of DM and preDM, excluding patients with high-risk features for OSA, Chao et al. found that both short and long sleepers (<6 h, $\geq$8.5 h) had higher risk of newly diagnosed DM with OR 1.55 (CI 1.07–2.24) and 2.83 (1.19–6.73), respectively [71]. No effect was observed with the pre-DM state. Similarly, insufficient and excessive sleep among obese adolescents was associated with acute and chronic glucose intolerance [72]. In a cohort of 96 obese sleep-deprived adolescents, 58 had sleep apnoea (RDI > 5/h, portable overnight polysomnography) and 42% had abnormal glucose metabolism based on abnormal HOMA, fasting glucose levels, and OGTT; higher fasting levels of glucose were observed with higher severity of OSA, suggesting an interplay between disordered sleep, inflammation, and abnormal glucose metabolism.

4. Population Studies of Relationship between OSA and T2DM

Although many studies have established a causal link between obesity and T2DM, as well as between obesity and OSA, no clear association has been demonstrated between T2DM and OSA. The latter association has been implied by indirect observation studies, and there is still a significant knowledge gap in this area. A large-scale multi-ethnic study of adults demonstrated abnormal fasting glucose and T2DM was strongly associated with moderate–severe OSA [73]. Studies suggest 30% of all patients with OSA have T2DM and 86% of obese OSA patients have T2DM [74,75]. In the Sleep Health Heart Study, fasting and 2 h glucose levels were significantly higher in the moderate–severe OSA patients than those with no sleep-disordered breathing [75]. In the same study, nocturnal hypoxemia was independently associated with markers of impaired glucose metabolism [76]. Seicean et al. in their study of 2588 subjects with sleep-disordered breathing (RDI $\geq$ 10, unattended polysomnography) found that OSA was associated with T2DM and impaired glucose tolerance with an adjusted odds ratio of 1.4 (1.1–2.7) for impaired fasting glucose and impaired glucose tolerance and 1.7 (1.1–2.7) for occult DM [77]. The Wisconsin Sleep Cohort Study OSA (AHI $\geq$ 15) reported similar results with a higher risk for T2DM after adjusting for age, sex, and waist girth [78]. Marshall et al. reported on a smaller population of 399 patients in Western Australia of whom 10 had moderate–severe OSA (RDI $\geq$15) and 2 (20%) had incident T2DM at 4 years [79]. A small prospective case–control study compared markers of glucose intolerance following a glucose load between young men with OSA to matched controls and found that OSA was associated with lower insulin sensitivity and higher total insulin secretion to maintain normoglycemia [80]. Bulcun et al., in a study of 112 patients with OSA and 12 snorers, found that glucose disorders were much higher in OSA patients than snorers (50.8% versus 15.7%; $p = 0.055$), and in addition observed significant positive correlations between insulin resistance and both AHI ($p = 0.005$) and arousal index ($p = 0.01$) [81]. In 137 patients with diagnosed T2DM and preDM with extreme obesity (BMI > 40 kg/m^2), the ORs for associated OSA were 3.18 (95% CI; 1.00, 10.07) and 4.17 (CI; 1.09, 15.88), respectively, after adjustment for age, obesity, and insulin levels [82]. The European Sleep Apnoea Cohort Study demonstrated that for all levels of obesity, the presence of OSA increased the risk of T2DM and was associated with worse glycaemic control [83]. Moreover, a metanalysis of 25 studies covering 154,948 OSA patients showed an association between OSA and increased risk of impaired fasting glucose and T2DM development [84].

The Sleep AHEAD study showed that baseline apnoea–hypopnea index (AHI) and weight loss were the most important predictors of AHI change [85]. Notably, weight loss by diet or bariatric surgery has a positive effect both on OSA severity and diabetic control [86], indicating the central role that excess body adiposity plays in the pathogenesis of both conditions. Additional prospective studies are needed to better characterise the mechanistic relationship between T2DM and OSA.

5. Effect of CPAP on T2DM

CPAP treatment has been associated with improvement in insulin sensitivity, although clinical trials have revealed conflicting results. In general, most trials have been uncontrolled and un-blinded studies examining the effect of treatment of OSA with CPAP on markers of glucose metabolism. Various studies have identified improvement with use of CPAP in post-prandial glucose levels [87], hyperinsulinemic euglycemic clamp HBA1c, and mean sleep glucose levels [87–90]. However, outcomes from other studies on the effect of CPAP therapy on long-term glucose control in T2DM with OSA have not shown consistent benefit [57,91]. In eight randomised controlled trials (five with non-DM and three with DM), no significant difference was observed with CPAP on fasting glucose or HbA1c [92]. However, a retrospective analysis of patients with DM and OSA treated with CPAP showed a significant improvement in HbA1c after 5 years when compared with matched controls not receiving CPAP [93]. Moreover, a recent meta-analysis of seven trials of patients with DM and OSA treated with CPAP suggested improvement in glycaemic control and insulin resistance [94]. Nonetheless, there was considerable heterogeneity in the response to CPAP in these trials being considered.

The potential reasons for the disparity of these results are complex. The outcomes of CPAP therapy on OSA will depend on the effectiveness of treatment and compliance with therapy. Importantly, even with effective CPAP therapy, there may not be normalisation of all physiological parameters. Satisfactory compliance with CPAP is generally considered to require at least 4 h of treatment per night, though this figure is arbitrary [95]. Even with greater than 4 h use of CPAP per night, a significant number of patients still complain of daytime tiredness [96].

Nonetheless effective use of CPAP may improve some parameters. Steiropoulos et al. noted that only those subjects utilising CPAP for more than 4 h per night showed a decrease in HbA1c [97]. In the study by West et al., which did not demonstrate an effect on HbA1c, average compliance was only 3.6 h on 75% of nights per night [57]. In a study by Oktay et al., no effect of CPAP was observed on fasting blood glucose, although no measures of compliance were monitored [91]. The type of CPAP therapy does not appear to influence the outcome. No demonstrable benefit was identified when auto-titrating CPAP was compared to fixed pressure machines in treatment of sleep disordered breathing in diabetics [98]. In a recent publication, nightly eight-hour CPAP for 2 weeks resulted in improved glucose levels by 1276.9 mg/dL (p = 0.03) and improved insulin sensitivity compared to placebo in prediabetic patients [99].

The severity of OSA in these studies has been similar, on the basis of the Respiratory Disturbance index or AHI, although it should be recognised that these measures, which are widely used to categorise OSA, describe the frequency of respiratory events, but not the severity of such events. These are aggregate markers which include hypopneic and apnoeic events terminated by arousal and also those leading to hypoxemia. More recently, it has been recognised that there are different phenotypes of OSA, and it is not a uniform disorder [100]. It is conceivable that those subjects with more frequent and severe hypoxic episodes may benefit to a greater degree than those with milder degrees of respiratory disturbance or hypoxemia. Some studies have suggested that OSA severity may be better defined by examining the percent of time spent per night with oxygen saturations below 90%.

CVD is a leading cause of death in patients with T2DM or OSA. Multiple studies on the effect of CPAP therapy on cardiovascular outcomes in general population and patients with T2DM has been undertaken [101], with some ongoing controversies in the field. CPAP therapy has been shown to improve control of arrhythmias and blood pressure [102]; however, its effect on mortality rate was not established in SAVE RCT, which was attributed to established comorbidities and poor long-term adherence to CPAP therapy [103]. Notably, a recent study confirmed a dose–response relationship between positive airway pressure therapy and major adverse CV events [104]. Further studies are still required to clarify the relative contributions of hypoxemia and sleep fragmentation to disordered glucose control and effect of OSA treatment on complications (hypertension, vascular disease, CKD).

6. Should All Patients with T2DM Be Screened for OSA?

Although obesity, T2DM, and OSA are interrelated, it must be remembered that lean and young patients also can suffer from OSA attributed to cardiovascular autonomic neuropathy [105], and some lean individuals may also exhibit insulin-resistant DM. Metabolic syndrome has been observed in approximately one in three patients with OSA and BMI < 25 kg/m^2 and approximately two of every three lean non-obese patients with OSA had at least two markers of the metabolic syndrome [106].

One way to separate out effect of DM from obesity with respect to the link to OSA is to study sleep disturbances in those with type 1 DM (T1DM) where obesity is not normally a causal factor, although it may still be present in some individuals with T1DM. A recent review of T1DM and sleep highlights that sleep disorders with subsequent metabolic disturbances occur with increased frequency in normal weight individuals with T1DM [107]. Notably, sleep disturbances in T1DM can result in secondary disturbances in glucose control and neuroendocrine function including elevated night-time levels of growth hormone, epinephrine, and ACTH [108]. Normal weight children with T1DM were shown to have a higher apnoea index when compared to age- and weight-matched non-diabetic children, with the higher apnoea index correlating with poorer glycaemic control [109]. A small study in adults with T1DM found 40% to have OSA [110], and another study similarly showed that daytime sleepiness and OSA was more common in those with T1D than non-diabetic controls, with evidence that cardiovascular autonomic neuropathy was contributing to this [105]. These T1DM studies, while preliminary, clearly support the existence of a link between DM and sleep disorders independent of obesity.

Given that a uniform benefit of treatment of OSA in DM has not been demonstrated, routine screening of the T2DM population with laboratory polysomnography currently cannot be justified in all patients. Ambulatory polysomnography has increasingly replaced laboratory-based polysomnography, and more simplified multiple channel recording devises have been developed to investigate patients with high risk of OSA. Given the high prevalence of sleep disordered breathing in this population, all patients should have an assessment of their potential risk of OSA as part of their routine clinical care. Several questionnaires have been developed for OSA screening. Widely used are the Berlin questionnaire (BQ), STOP-BANG questionnaire (SBQ), Epworth sleepiness scale (ESS), and OSA-50 questionnaire (OSA50) [111–114]. Compared with the BQ, STOP, and ESS, the SBQ is a more accurate tool for detecting mild, moderate, and severe OSA. In subjects with suspected OSA, the SBQ, BQ, and OSA-50 questionnaires, combined with the ESS, can be used to rule in, but not to rule out, clinically relevant OSA [115]. Combined use of the STOP-BANG with different cut-off scores and the ESS facilitates a flexible balance between sensitivity and specificity.

On the basis of current data, treatment of OSA cannot be assured to improve diabetic control although it may be beneficial in some circumstances. These screening tools allow for more effective targeting of investigations and cost-effective treatment in those with T2DM identified with OSA to reduce daytime sleepiness and cardiovascular comorbidities in patients with T2DM.

Much research is needed to better characterise the links between DM, obesity, metabolic dysfunction, and sleep disorders. Many of the existing studies of these relationships are based on relatively small numbers of subjects, raising the possibility of sampling and other biases and confounders. Hence, it would be very useful to try and separate out these variables in large study populations to explore the relationship between discrete factors. For example, studies of sleep patterns in the presence of hyperglycemia or euglycemia in normal weight individuals would assist in determining whether hyperglycemia by itself has a detrimental effect on sleep. Similarly, cardiovascular and sleep studies in normal weight individuals with autonomic neuropathy would remove obesity as a confounder when determining the relationship between autonomic neuropathy, OSA, and cardiovascular disease. Finally, causal relationships would be best established by longitudinal intervention studies where a variable such as glycaemic control or OSA is treated and then the impacts of this treatment measured on the other variables.

7. Conclusions

T2DM and OSA are closely associated and share multiple common mechanisms, including activation of the autonomic nervous system, the inflammatory cascade, and hypoxia-linked endocrinopathy. Evidence is emerging that visceral fat accumulation may be the important element in the development of these conditions. Differences in measurement of fat excess may account for some of the discrepancies in various studies. The role of race and ethnicity is important to maintain consistency as definitions of obesity used in studies of the relationship between OSA and T2DM may differ in different parts of the world. A further challenge is to find a way to control for the effects of variability of CPAP use among patients in different studies. The long-term benefits of CPAP therapy on diabetic control remain questionable. Ultimately, additional studies are needed to better understand the mechanistic cellular and gene pathways underlying OSA and T2DM, which may then allow the intersections between these diseases to be better understood, which might then provide the opportunity to develop novel treatments able to address both conditions at the same time.

Author Contributions: Conceptualization, N.P.; writing—original draft preparation, B.M., D.S., N.P.; writing—review and editing, B.M., J.J.B., C.L. and N.P. All authors have read and agreed to the published version of the manuscript.

Funding: This research received no external funding.

Conflicts of Interest: The authors declare no conflict of interest.

References

1. Jennum, P.; Schultz-Larsen, K.; Christensen, N. Snoring, sympathetic activity and cardiovascular risk factors in a 70 year old population. *Eur. J. Epidemiol.* **1993**, *9*, 477–482. [CrossRef] [PubMed]
2. Grunstein, R.R.; Stenlof, K.; Hedner, J.; Sjostrom, L. Impact of obstructive sleep apnea and sleepiness on metabolic and cardiovascular risk factors in the Swedish Obese Subjects (SOS) Study. *Int. J. Obes. Relat. Metab. Disord.* **1995**, *19*, 410–418. [PubMed]
3. Enright, P.L.; Newman, A.B.; Wahl, P.W.; Manolio, T.A.; Haponik, E.F.; Boyle, P.J. Prevalence and correlates of snoring and observed apneas in 5201 older adults. *Sleep* **1996**, *19*, 531–538. [CrossRef]
4. American Diabetes Association. Diagnosis and classification of diabetes. *Diabetes Care* **2014**, *37* (Suppl. 1), S81–S90. [CrossRef] [PubMed]
5. Ng, M.; Fleming, T.; Robinson, M.; Thomson, B.; Graetz, N.; Margono, C.; Mullany, E.C.; Biryukov, S.; Abbafati, C.; Abera, S.F.; et al. Global, regional, and national prevalence of overweight and obesity in children and adults during 1980–2013: A systematic analysis for the Global Burden of Disease Study 2013. *Lancet* **2014**, *384*, 766–781. [CrossRef]
6. Shah, N.; Roux, F. The relationship of obesity and obstructive sleep apnea. *Clin. Chest Med.* **2009**, *30*, 455–465. [CrossRef]
7. Shoelson, S.E.; Lee, J.; Goldfine, A.B. Inflammation and insulin resistance. *J. Clin. Investig.* **2006**, *116*, 1793–1801. [CrossRef]
8. Vgontzas, A.N.; Papanicolaou, D.A.; Bixler, E.O.; Kales, A.; Tyson, K.; Chrousos, G.P. Elevation of plasma cytokines in disorders of excessive daytime sleepiness: Role of sleep disturbance and obesity. *J. Clin. Endocrinol. Metab.* **1997**, *82*, 1313–1316. [CrossRef]
9. Vgontzas, A.N.; Papanicolaou, D.A.; Bixler, E.O.; Hopper, K.; Lotsikas, A.; Lin, H.M.; Kales, A.; Chrousos, G.P. Sleep apnea and daytime sleepiness and fatigue: Relation to visceral obesity, insulin resistance, and hypercytokinemia. *J. Clin. Endocrinol. Metab.* **2000**, *85*, 1151–1158. [CrossRef]
10. Ciftci, T.U.; Kokturk, O.; Bukan, N.; Bilgihan, A. The relationship between serum cytokine levels with obesity and obstructive sleep apnea syndrome. *Cytokine* **2004**, *28*, 87–91. [CrossRef]

11. Minoguchi, K.; Tazaki, T.; Yokoe, T.; Minoguchi, H.; Watanabe, Y.; Yamamoto, M.; Adachi, M. Elevated production of tumor necrosis factor-alpha by monocytes in patients with obstructive sleep apnea syndrome. *Chest* **2004**, *126*, 1473–1479. [CrossRef] [PubMed]
12. Hotamisligil, G.S.; Shargill, N.S.; Spiegelman, B.M. Adipose expression of tumor necrosis factor-alpha: Direct role in obesity-linked insulin resistance. *Science* **1993**, *259*, 87–91. [CrossRef] [PubMed]
13. Hotamisligil, G.S. Mechanisms of TNF-alpha-induced insulin resistance. *Exp. Clin. Endocrinol. DM* **1999**, *107*, 119–125. [CrossRef] [PubMed]
14. Trayhurn, P.; Wang, B.; Wood, I.S. Hypoxia in adipose tissue: A basis for the dysregulation of tissue function in obesity? *Br. J. Nutr.* **2008**, *100*, 227–235. [CrossRef] [PubMed]
15. Lavie, L. Intermittent hypoxia: The culprit of oxidative stress, vascular inflammation and dyslipidemia in obstructive sleep apnea. *Expert Rev. Respir. Med.* **2008**, *2*, 75–84. [CrossRef] [PubMed]
16. Bloch-Damti, A.; Bashan, N. Proposed mechanisms for the induction of insulin resistance by oxidative stress. *Antioxid. Redox Signal.* **2005**, *7*, 1553–1567. [CrossRef] [PubMed]
17. Robertson, R.P. Oxidative stress and impaired insulin secretion in type 2 DM. *Curr. Opin. Pharmacol.* **2006**, *6*, 615–619. [CrossRef]
18. Lurie, A. Metabolic disorders associated with obstructive sleep apnea in adults. *Adv. Cardiol.* **2011**, *46*, 67–138.
19. Vgontzas, A.N.; Zoumakis, E.; Lin, H.M.; Bixler, E.O.; Trakada, G.; Chrousos, G.P. Marked decrease in sleepiness in patients with sleep apnea by etanercept, a tumor necrosis factor-alpha antagonist. *J. Clin. Endocrinol. Metab.* **2004**, *89*, 4409–4413. [CrossRef]
20. Thornalley, P.J.; Battah, S.; Ahmed, N.; Karachalias, N.; Agalou, S.; Babaei-Jadidi, R.; Dawnay, A. Quantitative screening of advanced glycation endproducts in cellular and extracellular proteins by tandem mass spectrometry. *Biochem. J.* **2003**, *375*, 581–592. [CrossRef]
21. Tan, K.C.; Chow, W.S.; Lam, J.C.; Lam, B.; Bucala, R.; Betteridge, J.; M Ip, M.S. Advanced glycation endproducts in nondiabetic patients with obstructive sleep apnea. *Sleep* **2006**, *29*, 329–333. [CrossRef] [PubMed]
22. Friedman, E.A. Advanced glycosylated end products and hyperglycemia in the pathogenesis of diabetic complications. *Diabetes Care* **1999**, *22* (Suppl. 2), B65–B71. [PubMed]
23. Lam, J.C.; Tan, K.C.; Lai, A.Y.; Lam, D.C.; Ip, M.S. Increased serum levels of advanced glycation end-products is associated with severity of sleep disordered breathing but not insulin sensitivity in non-diabetic men with obstructive sleep apnoea. *Sleep Med.* **2012**, *13*, 15–20. [CrossRef]
24. Cizza, G.; Piaggi, P.; Lucassen, E.A.; de Jonge, L.; Walter, M.; Mattingly, M.S.; Kalish, H.; Csako, G.; Rother, K.I.; Study Group, S.E. Obstructive sleep apnea is a predictor of abnormal glucose metabolism in chronically sleep deprived obese adults. *PLoS ONE* **2013**, *8*, e65400.
25. Kjeldsen, S.E.; Rostrup, M.; Moan, A.; Mundal, H.H.; Gjesdal, K.; Eide, I.K. The sympathetic nervous system may modulate the metabolic cardiovascular syndrome in essential hypertension. *J. Cardiovasc. Pharmacol.* **1992**, *20* (Suppl. 8), S32–S39. [CrossRef]
26. Dimsdale, J.E.; Coy, T.; Ziegler, M.G.; Ancoli-Israel, S.; Clausen, J. The effect of sleep apnea on plasma and urinary catecholamines. *Sleep* **1995**, *18*, 377–381.
27. Kruszynska, Y.T.; Worrall, D.S.; Ofrecio, J.; Frias, J.P.; Macaraeg, G.; Olefsky, J.M. Fatty acid-induced insulin resistance: Decreased muscle PI3K activation but unchanged Akt phosphorylation. *J. Clin. Endocrinol. Metab.* **2002**, *87*, 226–234. [CrossRef]
28. Polotsky, V.Y.; Li, J.; Punjabi, N.M.; Rubin, A.E.; Smith, P.L.; Schwartz, A.R.; O'Donnell, C.P. Intermittent hypoxia increases insulin resistance in genetically obese mice. *J. Physiol.* **2003**, *552*, 253–264. [CrossRef]
29. Iiyori, N.; Alonso, L.C.; Li, J.; Sanders, M.H.; Garcia-Ocana, A.; O'Doherty, R.M.; Polotsky, V.Y.; O'Donnell, C.P. Intermittent hypoxia causes insulin resistance in lean mice independent of autonomic activity. *Am. J. Respir. Crit. Care Med.* **2007**, *175*, 851–857. [CrossRef]
30. Tasali, E.; Leproult, R.; Ehrmann, D.A.; Van Cauter, E. Slow-wave sleep and the risk of type 2 diabetes in humans. *Proc. Natl. Acad. Sci. USA* **2008**, *105*, 1044–1049. [CrossRef]
31. Ota, H.; Tamaki, S.; Itaya-Hironaka, A.; Yamauchi, A.; Sakuramoto-Tsuchida, S.; Morioka, T.; Takasawa, S.; Kimura, H. Attenuation of glucose-induced insulin secretion by intermittent hypoxia via down-regulation of CD38. *Life Sci.* **2012**, *90*, 206–211. [CrossRef] [PubMed]
32. An, N.H.; Han, M.K.; Um, C.; Park, B.H.; Park, B.J.; Kim, H.K.; Kim, U.H. Significance of ecto-cyclase activity of CD38 in insulin secretion of mouse pancreatic islet cells. *Biochem. Biophys. Res. Commun.* **2001**, *282*, 781–786. [CrossRef]
33. Hopkins, T.A.; Ouchi, N.; Shibata, R.; Walsh, K. Adiponectin actions in the cardiovascular system. *Cardiovasc. Res.* **2007**, *74*, 11–18. [CrossRef] [PubMed]
34. Ye, J.; Gao, Z.; Yin, J.; He, Q. Hypoxia is a potential risk factor for chronic inflammation and adiponectin reduction in adipose tissue of ob/ob and dietary obese mice. *Am. J. Physiol. Endocrinol. Metab.* **2007**, *293*, E1118–E1128. [CrossRef] [PubMed]
35. Jequier, E. Leptin signaling, adiposity, and energy balance. *Ann. N. Y. Acad. Sci.* **2002**, *967*, 379–388. [CrossRef]
36. Paracchini, V.; Pedotti, P.; Taioli, E. Genetics of leptin and obesity: A HuGE review. *Am. J. Epidemiol.* **2005**, *162*, 101–114. [CrossRef]
37. Yildiz, B.O.; Haznedaroglu, I.C. Rethinking leptin and insulin action: Therapeutic opportunities for diabetes. *Int. J. Biochem. Cell. Biol.* **2006**, *38*, 820–830. [CrossRef]
38. Considine, R.V.; Sinha, M.K.; Heiman, M.L.; Kriauciunas, A.; Stephens, T.W.; Nyce, M.R.; Ohannesian, J.P.; Marco, C.C.; McKee, L.J.; Bauer, T.L.; et al. Serum immunoreactive-leptin concentrations in normal-weight and obese humans. *N. Engl. J. Med.* **1996**, *334*, 292–295. [CrossRef]

39. Shimizu, H.; Oh, I.S.; Okada, S.; Mori, M. Leptin resistance and obesity. *Endocr. J.* **2007**, *54*, 17–26. [CrossRef]
40. O'Donnell, C.P.; Schaub, C.D.; Haines, A.S.; Berkowitz, D.E.; Tankersley, C.G.; Schwartz, A.R.; Smith, P.L. Leptin prevents respiratory depression in obesity. *Am. J. Respir. Crit. Care Med.* **1999**, *159*, 1477–1484. [CrossRef]
41. O'Donnell, C.P.; Tankersley, C.G.; Polotsky, V.P.; Schwartz, A.R.; Smith, P.L. Leptin, obesity, and respiratory function. *Respir. Physiol.* **2000**, *119*, 163–170. [CrossRef]
42. Yee, B.J.; Cheung, J.; Phipps, P.; Banerjee, D.; Piper, A.J.; Grunstein, R.R. Treatment of obesity hypoventilation syndrome and serum leptin. *Respiration* **2006**, *73*, 209–212. [CrossRef] [PubMed]
43. Redolfi, S.; Corda, L.; La Piana, G.; Spandrio, S.; Prometti, P.; Tantucci, C. Long-term non-invasive ventilation increases chemosensitivity and leptin in obesity-hypoventilation syndrome. *Respir. Med.* **2007**, *101*, 1191–1195. [CrossRef]
44. Campo, A.; Fruhbeck, G.; Zulueta, J.J.; Iriarte, J.; Seijo, L.M.; Alcaide, A.B.; Galdiz, J.B.; Salvador, J. Hyperleptinaemia, respiratory drive and hypercapnic response in obese patients. *Eur. Respir. J.* **2007**, *30*, 223–231. [CrossRef]
45. Feng, Y.; Zhang, Z.; Dong, Z.Z. Effects of continuous positive airway pressure therapy on glycaemic control, insulin sensitivity and body mass index in patients with obstructive sleep apnoea and type 2 diabetes: A systematic review and meta-analysis. *NPJ Prim. Care Respir. Med.* **2015**, *25*, 15005. [CrossRef]
46. Chin, K.; Shimizu, K.; Nakamura, T.; Narai, N.; Masuzaki, H.; Ogawa, Y.; Mishima, N.; Nakamura, T.; Nakao, K.; Ohi, O. Changes in intra-abdominal visceral fat and serum leptin levels in patients with obstructive sleep apnea syndrome following nasal continuous positive airway pressure therapy. *Circulation* **1999**, *100*, 706–712. [CrossRef] [PubMed]
47. Sanner, B.M.; Kollhosser, P.; Buechner, N.; Zidek, W.; Tepel, M. Influence of treatment on leptin levels in patients with obstructive sleep apnoea. *Eur. Respir. J.* **2004**, *23*, 601–604. [CrossRef] [PubMed]
48. Kapsimalis, F.; Varouchakis, G.; Manousaki, A.; Daskas, S.; Nikita, D.; Kryger, M.; Gourgoulianis, K. Association of sleep apnea severity and obesity with insulin resistance, C-reactive protein, and leptin levels in male patients with obstructive sleep apnea. *Lung* **2008**, *186*, 209–217. [CrossRef]
49. Patel, S.R.; Palmer, L.J.; Larkin, E.K.; Jenny, N.S.; White, D.P.; Redline, S. Relationship between obstructive sleep apnea and diurnal leptin rhythms. *Sleep* **2004**, *27*, 235–239. [CrossRef]
50. Tatsumi, K.; Kasahara, Y.; Kurosu, K.; Tanabe, N.; Takiguchi, Y.; Kuriyama, T. Sleep oxygen desaturation and circulating leptin in obstructive sleep apnea-hypopnea syndrome. *Chest* **2005**, *127*, 716–721. [CrossRef]
51. Chiarugi, P.; Fiaschi, T. Adiponectin in health and diseases: From metabolic syndrome to tissue regeneration. *Expert Opin. Ther. Targets* **2010**, *14*, 193–206. [CrossRef] [PubMed]
52. Goldstein, B.J.; Scalia, R.G.; Ma, X.L. Protective vascular and myocardial effects of adiponectin. *Nat. Clin. Pract. Cardiovasc. Med.* **2009**, *6*, 27–35. [CrossRef] [PubMed]
53. Kawano, J.; Arora, R. The role of adiponectin in obesity, DM, and cardiovascular disease. *J. Cardiometabolic Syndr.* **2009**, *4*, 44–49. [CrossRef] [PubMed]
54. Sharma, S.K.; Kumpawat, S.; Goel, A.; Banga, A.; Ramakrishnan, L.; Chaturvedi, P. Obesity, and not obstructive sleep apnea, is responsible for metabolic abnormalities in a cohort with sleep-disordered breathing. *Sleep Med.* **2007**, *8*, 12–17. [CrossRef] [PubMed]
55. Tokuda, F.; Sando, Y.; Matsui, H.; Koike, H.; Yokoyama, T. Serum levels of adipocytokines, adiponectin and leptin, in patients with obstructive sleep apnea syndrome. *Intern. Med.* **2008**, *47*, 1843–1849. [CrossRef] [PubMed]
56. Harsch, I.A.; Bergmann, T.; Koebnick, C.; Wiedmann, R.; Ruderich, F.; Hahn, E.G.; Konturek, P.C. Adiponectin, resistin and subclinical inflammation—The metabolic burden in Launois Bensaude Syndrome, a rare form of obesity. *J. Physiol. Pharmacol.* **2007**, *58* (Suppl. 1), 65–76. [PubMed]
57. West, S.D.; Nicoll, D.J.; Wallace, T.M.; Matthews, D.R.; Stradling, J.R. Effect of CPAP on insulin resistance and HbA1c in men with obstructive sleep apnoea and type 2 diabetes. *Thorax* **2007**, *62*, 969–974. [CrossRef]
58. Sprung, V.S.; Kemp, G.J.; Wilding, J.P.; Adams, V.; Murphy, K.; Burgess, M.; Emegbo, S.; Thomas, M.; Needham, A.J.; Weimken, A.; et al. Randomised, cOntrolled Multicentre trial of 26 weeks subcutaneous liraglutide (a glucagon-like peptide-1 receptor Agonist), with or without contiNuous positive airway pressure (CPAP), in patients with type 2 diabetes mellitus (T2DM) and obstructive sleep apnoEa (OSA) (ROMANCE): Study protocol assessing the effects of weight loss on the apnea-hypnoea index (AHI). *BMJ Open* **2020**, *10*, e038856. [CrossRef]
59. Blackman, A.; Foster, G.D.; Zammit, G.; Rosenberg, R.; Aronne, L.; Wadden, T.; Claudius, B.; Jensen, C.B.; Mignot, E. Effect of liraglutide 3.0 mg in individuals with obesity and moderate or severe obstructive sleep apnea: The SCALE Sleep Apnea randomized clinical trial. *Int. J. Obes.* **2016**, *40*, 1310–1319. [CrossRef]
60. Wang, N.; Khan, S.A.; Prabhakar, N.R.; Nanduri, J. Impairment of pancreatic beta-cell function by chronic intermittent hypoxia. *Exp. Physiol.* **2013**, *98*, 1376–1385. [CrossRef]
61. Sherwani, S.I.; Aldana, C.; Usmani, S.; Adin, C.; Kotha, S.; Khan, M.; Eubank, T.; Scherer, P.E.; Parinandi, N.; Magalang, U.J. Intermittent hypoxia exacerbates pancreatic beta-cell dysfunction in a mouse model of diabetes mellitus. *Sleep* **2013**, *36*, 1849–1858. [CrossRef] [PubMed]
62. Polak, J.; Shimoda, L.A.; Drager, L.F.; Undem, C.; McHugh, H.; Polotsky, V.Y.; Punjabi, N.M. Intermittent hypoxia impairs glucose homeostasis in C57BL6/J mice: Partial improvement with cessation of the exposure. *Sleep* **2013**, *36*, 1483–1490. [CrossRef] [PubMed]

63. Spiegel, K.; Tasali, E.; Leproult, R.; Van Cauter, E. Effects of poor and short sleep on glucose metabolism and obesity risk. *Nat. Rev. Endocrinol.* 2009, *5*, 253–261. [CrossRef] [PubMed]
64. Cappuccio, F.P.; D'Elia, L.; Strazzullo, P.; Miller, M.A. Quantity and quality of sleep and incidence of type 2 diabetes: A systematic review and meta-analysis. *Diabetes Care* 2010, *33*, 414–420. [CrossRef]
65. Xu, Q.; Song, Y.; Hollenbeck, A.; Blair, A.; Schatzkin, A.; Chen, H. Day napping and short night sleeping are associated with higher risk of diabetes in older adults. *Diabetes Care* 2010, *33*, 78–83. [CrossRef]
66. Ayas, N.T.; White, D.P.; Al-Delaimy, W.K.; Manson, J.E.; Stampfer, M.J.; Speizer, F.E.; Patel, S.; Hu, F.B. A prospective study of self-reported sleep duration and incident diabetes in women. *Diabetes Care* 2003, *26*, 380–384. [CrossRef] [PubMed]
67. Mallon, L.; Broman, J.E.; Hetta, J. High incidence of diabetes in men with sleep complaints or short sleep duration: A 12-year follow-up study of a middle-aged population. *Diabetes Care* 2005, *28*, 2762–2767. [CrossRef] [PubMed]
68. Spiegel, K.; Knutson, K.; Leproult, R.; Tasali, E.; Van Cauter, E. Sleep loss: A novel risk factor for insulin resistance and Type 2 diabetes. *J. Appl. Physiol.* 2005, *99*, 2008–2019. [CrossRef]
69. Gharib, S.A.; Khalyfa, A.; Abdelkarim, A.; Bhushan, B.; Gozal, D. Integrative miRNA-mRNA profiling of adipose tissue unravels transcriptional circuits induced by sleep fragmentation. *PLoS ONE* 2012, *7*, e37669.
70. Fendri, S.; Rose, D.; Myambu, S.; Jeanne, S.; Lalau, J.D. Nocturnal hyperglycaemia in type 2 diabetes with sleep apnoea syndrome. *Diabetes Res. Clin. Pract.* 2011, *91*, e21–e23. [CrossRef]
71. Chao, C.Y.; Wu, J.S.; Yang, Y.C.; Shih, C.C.; Wang, R.H.; Lu, F.H.; Chang, C.J. Sleep duration is a potential risk factor for newly diagnosed type 2 diabetes mellitus. *Metabolism* 2011, *60*, 799–804. [CrossRef] [PubMed]
72. Koren, D.; Levitt Katz, L.E.; Brar, P.C.; Gallagher, P.R.; Berkowitz, R.I.; Brooks, L.J. Sleep architecture and glucose and insulin homeostasis in obese adolescents. *Diabetes Care* 2011, *34*, 2442–2447. [CrossRef] [PubMed]
73. Bakker, J.P.; Weng, J.; Wang, R.; Redline, S.; Punjabi, N.M.; Patel, S.R. Associations between Obstructive Sleep Apnea, Sleep Duration, and Abnormal Fasting Glucose. The Multi-Ethnic Study of Atherosclerosis. *Am. J. Respir. Crit. Care Med.* 2015, *192*, 745–753. [CrossRef]
74. Einhorn, D.; Stewart, D.A.; Erman, M.K.; Gordon, N.; Philis-Tsimikas, A.; Casal, E. Prevalence of sleep apnea in a population of adults with type 2 diabetes mellitus. *Endocr. Pract.* 2007, *13*, 355–362. [CrossRef] [PubMed]
75. Laaban, J.P.; Daenen, S.; Leger, D.; Pascal, S.; Bayon, V.; Slama, G.; Elgrably, F. Prevalence and predictive factors of sleep apnoea syndrome in type 2 diabetic patients. *Diabetes Metab.* 2009, *35*, 372–377. [CrossRef] [PubMed]
76. Punjabi, N.M.; Shahar, E.; Redline, S.; Gottlieb, D.J.; Givelber, R.; Resnick, H.E. Sleep-disordered breathing, glucose intolerance, and insulin resistance: The Sleep Heart Health Study. *Am. J. Epidemiol.* 2004, *160*, 521–530. [CrossRef]
77. Seicean, S.; Kirchner, H.L.; Gottlieb, D.J.; Punjabi, N.M.; Resnick, H.; Sanders, M.; Budhiraja, R.; Singer, M.; Redline, S. Sleep-disordered breathing and impaired glucose metabolism in normal-weight and overweight/obese individuals: The Sleep Heart Health Study. *Diabetes Care* 2008, *31*, 1001–1006. [CrossRef]
78. Reichmuth, K.J.; Austin, D.; Skatrud, J.B.; Young, T. Association of sleep apnea and type II diabetes: A population-based study. *Am. J. Respir. Crit. Care Med.* 2005, *172*, 1590–1595. [CrossRef]
79. Marshall, N.S.; Wong, K.K.; Phillips, C.L.; Liu, P.Y.; Knuiman, M.W.; Grunstein, R.R. Is sleep apnea an independent risk factor for prevalent and incident diabetes in the Busselton Health Study? *J. Clin. Sleep Med.* 2009, *5*, 15–20. [CrossRef]
80. Pamidi, S.; Wroblewski, K.; Broussard, J.; Day, A.; Hanlon, E.C.; Abraham, V.; Tasali, E. Obstructive sleep apnea in young lean men: Impact on insulin sensitivity and secretion. *Diabetes Care* 2012, *35*, 2384–2389. [CrossRef] [PubMed]
81. Bulcun, E.; Ekici, M.; Ekici, A. Disorders of glucose metabolism and insulin resistance in patients with obstructive sleep apnoea syndrome. *Int. J. Clin. Pract.* 2012, *66*, 91–97. [CrossRef] [PubMed]
82. Fredheim, J.M.; Rollheim, J.; Omland, T.; Hofso, D.; Roislien, J.; Vegsgaard, K.; Hjelmesæth, J. Type 2 diabetes and pre-diabetes are associated with obstructive sleep apnea in extremely obese subjects: A cross-sectional study. *Cardiovasc. Diabetol.* 2011, *10*, 84. [CrossRef]
83. Kent, B.D.; Grote, L.; Ryan, S.; Pepin, J.L.; Bonsignore, M.R.; Tkacova, R.; Saaresranta, T.; Verbraecken, J.; Lévy, P.; Hedner, J.; et al. Diabetes mellitus prevalence and control in sleep-disordered breathing: The European Sleep Apnea Cohort (ESADA) study. *Chest* 2014, *146*, 982–990. [CrossRef]
84. Wang, C.; Tan, J.; Miao, Y.; Zhang, Q. Obstructive sleep apnea, prediabetes and progression of type 2 diabetes: A systematic review and meta-analysis. *J. Diabetes Investig.* 2022, *13*, 1396–1411. [CrossRef]
85. Kuna, S.T.; Reboussin, D.M.; Strotmeyer, E.S.; Millman, R.P.; Zammit, G.; Walkup, M.P.; Wadden, T.A.; Wing, R.R.; Pi-Sunyer, F.X.; Spira, A.P.; et al. Effects of Weight Loss on Obstructive Sleep Apnea Severity. Ten-Year Results of the Sleep AHEAD Study. *Am. J. Respir. Crit. Care Med.* 2021, *203*, 221–229. [CrossRef] [PubMed]
86. Carneiro-Barrera, A.; Diaz-Roman, A.; Guillen-Riquelme, A.; Buela-Casal, G. Weight loss and lifestyle interventions for obstructive sleep apnoea in adults: Systematic review and meta-analysis. *Obes. Rev.* 2019, *20*, 750–762. [CrossRef] [PubMed]
87. Babu, A.R.; Herdegen, J.; Fogelfeld, L.; Shott, S.; Mazzone, T. Type 2 diabetes, glycemic control, and continuous positive airway pressure in obstructive sleep apnea. *Arch. Intern. Med.* 2005, *165*, 447–452. [CrossRef]
88. Harsch, I.A.; Schahin, S.P.; Radespiel-Troger, M.; Weintz, O.; Jahreiss, H.; Fuchs, F.S.; Wiest, G.H.; Hahn, E.G.; Lohmann, T.; Konturek, P.C.; et al. Continuous positive airway pressure treatment rapidly improves insulin sensitivity in patients with obstructive sleep apnea syndrome. *Am. J. Respir. Crit. Care Med.* 2004, *169*, 156–162. [CrossRef]

89. Hassaballa, H.A.; Tulaimat, A.; Herdegen, J.J.; Mokhlesi, B. The effect of continuous positive airway pressure on glucose control in diabetic patients with severe obstructive sleep apnea. *Sleep Breath.* **2005**, *9*, 176–180. [CrossRef]
90. Dawson, A.; Abel, S.L.; Loving, R.T.; Dailey, G.; Shadan, F.F.; Cronin, J.W.; Kripke, D.F.; Kline, L.E. CPAP therapy of obstructive sleep apnea in type 2 diabetics improves glycemic control during sleep. *J. Clin. Sleep Med.* **2008**, *4*, 538–542. [CrossRef]
91. Oktay, B.; Akbal, E.; Firat, H.; Ardic, S.; Kizilgun, M. CPAP treatment in the coexistence of obstructive sleep apnea syndrome and metabolic syndrome, results of one year follow up. *Acta Clin. Belg.* **2009**, *64*, 329–334. [CrossRef] [PubMed]
92. Patil, S.P.; Ayappa, I.A.; Caples, S.M.; Kimoff, R.J.; Patel, S.R.; Harrod, C.G. Treatment of Adult Obstructive Sleep Apnea With Positive Airway Pressure: An American Academy of Sleep Medicine Systematic Review, Meta-Analysis, and GRADE Assessment. *J. Clin. Sleep Med.* **2019**, *15*, 301–334. [CrossRef] [PubMed]
93. Guest, J.F.; Panca, M.; Sladkevicius, E.; Taheri, S.; Stradling, J. Clinical outcomes and cost-effectiveness of continuous positive airway pressure to manage obstructive sleep apnea in patients with type 2 diabetes in the U.K. *Diabetes Care* **2014**, *37*, 1263–1271. [CrossRef] [PubMed]
94. Shang, W.; Zhang, Y.; Wang, G.; Han, D. Benefits of continuous positive airway pressure on glycaemic control and insulin resistance in patients with type 2 diabetes and obstructive sleep apnoea: A meta-analysis. *Diabetes Obes. Metab.* **2021**, *23*, 540–548. [CrossRef] [PubMed]
95. Weaver, T.E.; Sawyer, A.M. Adherence to continuous positive airway pressure treatment for obstructive sleep apnoea: Implications for future interventions. *Indian J. Med. Res.* **2010**, *131*, 245–258.
96. Pepin, J.L.; Viot-Blanc, V.; Escourrou, P.; Racineux, J.L.; Sapene, M.; Levy, P.; Dervaux, B.; Lenne, X.; Mallart, A. Prevalence of residual excessive sleepiness in CPAP-treated sleep apnoea patients: The French multicentre study. *Eur. Respir. J.* **2009**, *33*, 1062–1067. [CrossRef]
97. Steiropoulos, P.; Papanas, N.; Nena, E.; Tsara, V.; Fitili, C.; Tzouvelekis, A.; Christaki, P.; Maltezos, E.; Bouros, D. Markers of glycemic control and insulin resistance in non-diabetic patients with Obstructive Sleep Apnea Hypopnea Syndrome: Does adherence to CPAP treatment improve glycemic control? *Sleep Med.* **2009**, *10*, 887–891. [CrossRef]
98. Patruno, V.; Aiolfi, S.; Costantino, G.; Murgia, R.; Selmi, C.; Malliani, A.; Montano, N. Fixed and autoadjusting continuous positive airway pressure treatments are not similar in reducing cardiovascular risk factors in patients with obstructive sleep apnea. *Chest* **2007**, *131*, 1393–1399. [CrossRef]
99. Pamidi, S.; Wroblewski, K.; Stepien, M.; Sharif-Sidi, K.; Kilkus, J.; Whitmore, H.; Tasali, E. Eight Hours of Nightly Continuous Positive Airway Pressure Treatment of Obstructive Sleep Apnea Improves Glucose Metabolism in Patients with Prediabetes. A Randomized Controlled Trial. *Am. J. Respir. Crit. Care Med.* **2015**, *192*, 96–105. [CrossRef]
100. Eckert, D.J. Phenotypic approaches to obstructive sleep apnoea—New pathways for targeted therapy. *Sleep Med. Rev.* **2018**, *37*, 45–59. [CrossRef]
101. Wang, X.; Zhang, Y.; Dong, Z.; Fan, J.; Nie, S.; Wei, Y. Effect of continuous positive airway pressure on long-term cardiovascular outcomes in patients with coronary artery disease and obstructive sleep apnea: A systematic review and meta-analysis. *Respir. Res.* **2018**, *19*, 1–9. [CrossRef] [PubMed]
102. Lam, J.C.M.; Lai, A.Y.K.; Tam, T.C.C.; Yuen, M.M.A.; Lam, K.S.L.; Ip, M.S.M. CPAP therapy for patients with sleep apnea and type 2 diabetes mellitus improves control of blood pressure. *Sleep Breath.* **2017**, *21*, 377–386. [CrossRef] [PubMed]
103. McEvoy, R.D.; Antic, N.A.; Heeley, E.; Luo, Y.; Ou, Q.; Zhang, X.; Mediano, O.; Chen, R.; Drager, L.F.; Liu, Z.; et al. CPAP for Prevention of Cardiovascular Events in Obstructive Sleep Apnea. *N. Engl. J. Med.* **2016**, *375*, 919–931. [CrossRef]
104. Gervès-Pinquié, C.; Bailly, S.; Goupil, F.; Pigeanne, T.; Launois, S.; Leclair-Visonneau, L.; Masson, P.; Bizieux-Thaminy, A.; Blanchard, M.; Sabil, A.; et al. Positive Airway Pressure Adherence, Mortality and Cardio-Vascular Events in Sleep Apnea Patients. *Am. J. Respir. Crit. Care Med.* **2022**, *11*, 1–9. [CrossRef] [PubMed]
105. Janovsky, C.C.; Rolim, L.C.; de Sa, J.R.; Poyares, D.; Tufik, S.; Silva, A.B.; Dib, S.A. Cardiovascular autonomic neuropathy contributes to sleep apnea in young and lean type 1 diabetes mellitus patients. *Front. Endocrinol.* **2014**, *5*, 119. [CrossRef]
106. Chaudhary, P.; Goyal, A.; Pakhare, A.; Goel, S.K.; Kumar, A.; Reddy, M.A.; Anoohya, V. Metabolic syndrome in non-obese patients with OSA: Learning points of a cross-sectional study from a tertiary care hospital in Central India. *Sleep Breath.* **2022**, *26*, 681–688. [CrossRef]
107. Farabi, S.S. Type 1 diabetes and Sleep. *Diabetes Spectr.* **2016**, *29*, 10–13. [CrossRef] [PubMed]
108. Jauch-Chara, K.; Schmid, S.M.; Hallschmid, M.; Born, J.; Schultes, B. Altered neuroendocrine sleep architecture in patients with type 1 diabetes. *Diabetes Care* **2008**, *31*, 1183–1188. [CrossRef]
109. Villa, M.P.; Multari, G.; Montesano, M.; Pagani, J.; Cervoni, M.; Midulla, F.; Cerone, E.; Ronchetti, R. Sleep apnoea in children with diabetes mellitus: Effect of glycaemic control. *Diabetologia* **2000**, *43*, 696–702. [CrossRef]
110. Borel, A.L.; Benhamou, P.Y.; Baguet, J.P.; Halimi, S.; Levy, P.; Mallion, J.M.; Pepin, J.L. High prevalence of obstructive sleep apnoea syndrome in a Type 1 diabetic adult population: A pilot study. *Diabet Med.* **2010**, *27*, 1328–1329. [CrossRef]
111. Chai-Coetzer, C.L.; Antic, N.A.; Rowland, L.S.; Catcheside, P.G.; Esterman, A.; Reed, R.L.; Williams, H.; Dunn, S.; McEvoy, R.D. A simplified model of screening questionnaire and home monitoring for obstructive sleep apnoea in primary care. *Thorax* **2011**, *66*, 213–219. [CrossRef] [PubMed]
112. Chai-Coetzer, C.L.; Antic, N.A.; Rowland, L.S.; Reed, R.L.; Esterman, A.; Catcheside, P.G.; Eckermann, S.; Vowles, N.; Williams, H.; Dunn, S. Primary care vs specialist sleep center management of obstructive sleep apnea and daytime sleepiness and quality of life: A randomized trial. *JAMA* **2013**, *309*, 997–1004. [CrossRef] [PubMed]

113. Chiu, H.Y.; Chen, P.Y.; Chuang, L.P.; Chen, N.H.; Tu, Y.K.; Hsieh, Y.J.; Wang, Y.C.; Guilleminault, C. Diagnostic accuracy of the Berlin questionnaire, STOP-BANG, STOP, and Epworth sleepiness scale in detecting obstructive sleep apnea: A bivariate meta-analysis. *Sleep Med. Rev.* **2017**, *36*, 57–70. [CrossRef] [PubMed]
114. Kee, K.; Dixon, J.; Shaw, J.; Vulikh, E.; Schlaich, M.; Kaye, D.M.; Zimmet, P.; Naughton, M.T. Comparison of Commonly Used Questionnaires to Identify Obstructive Sleep Apnea in a High-Risk Population. *J. Clin. Sleep Med.* **2018**, *14*, 2057–2064. [CrossRef] [PubMed]
115. Senaratna, C.V.; Perret, J.L.; Lowe, A.; Bowatte, G.; Abramson, M.J.; Thompson, B.; Lodge, C.; Russell, M.; Hamilton, G.S.; Dharmage, S.C. Detecting sleep apnoea syndrome in primary care with screening questionnaires and the Epworth sleepiness scale. *Med. J. Aust.* **2019**, *211*, 65–70. [CrossRef] [PubMed]

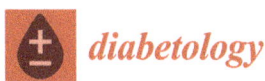

Article

Implementation of Chronic Care Model for Diabetes Self-Management: A Quantitative Analysis

Rashid M. Ansari [1,*], Mark F. Harris [2], Hassan Hosseinzadeh [3] and Nicholas Zwar [4]

1. School of Population Health, Faculty of Medicine, University of New South Wales, Sydney 2052, Australia
2. Centre for Primary Health Care and Equity, University of New South Wales, Sydney 2052, Australia; m.f.harris@unsw.edu.au
3. School of Health Sciences, University of Wollongong, Sydney 2522, Australia; hassanh@uow.edu.au
4. Faculty of Health Sciences and Medicine, Bond University, Gold Coast 4229, Australia; nzwar@bond.edu.au
* Correspondence: rashid.ansari@uqconnect.edu.au

Abstract: Objective: The main aim of this study was to implement the Chronic Care Model (CCM) for the self-management of type 2 diabetes in primary health care settings of rural areas of Pakistan and identify its effectiveness and develop strategies for overcoming its challenges. The two core elements of the Chronic Care Model: patient Self-Management Support (SMS) and Delivery System Design (DSD), were implemented to improve the quality of life and risk behaviour of type 2 diabetes patients in the middle-aged population of rural Pakistan. Methods: Thirty patients with type 2 diabetes and 20 healthcare professionals were included in this study consisting of 10 general practitioners and 10 nurses recruited from various clinics (medical centres) of Al-Rehman Hospital in Abbottabad, Pakistan. The quantitative content analysis method was used to identify the frequency of the most recurring statements. A *t*-test was performed to see the mean difference of HbA1c at baseline after 3-months and 6-months follow-up between male and female patients with diabetes. The hypothesis was tested to identify that diabetes self-management has a gendered dimension in rural areas of Pakistan. Results: The quantitative analysis demonstrated that diabetes self-management has a gendered dimension in the rural areas of Pakistan as the mean difference of HbA1c after a 6-month intervention of the two components of the chronic care model between male and female patients of diabetes was 0.83 ($p = 0.039$) with 95% CI ($-0.05; -1.61$). The mean difference in BMI after the intervention of 6 months between males and females was significant ($p < 0.05$). The mean difference was 4.97 kg/m^2, $p = 0.040$ with 95% CI ($-0.24; -9.69$). The results have shown that the two components of CCM were effective and improved clinical outcomes for diabetes patients of the rural areas of Pakistan. Conclusions: The application of the two Chronic Care Model's components provided a viable structure for diabetes self-management education and assistance. As a result, developing systems that incorporate long-term diabetes self-management education has an effect on the health care system's outcomes.

Keywords: Chronic Care Model; self-management of type 2 diabetes; chronic disease; healthcare system of Pakistan; patients' quality of life

Citation: Ansari, R.M.; Harris, M.F.; Hosseinzadeh, H.; Zwar, N. Implementation of Chronic Care Model for Diabetes Self-Management: A Quantitative Analysis. *Diabetology* 2022, 3, 407–422. https://doi.org/10.3390/diabetology3030031

Academic Editor: Sathish Thirunavukkarasu

Received: 16 June 2022
Accepted: 28 June 2022
Published: 6 July 2022

Publisher's Note: MDPI stays neutral with regard to jurisdictional claims in published maps and institutional affiliations.

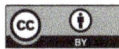

Copyright: © 2022 by the authors. Licensee MDPI, Basel, Switzerland. This article is an open access article distributed under the terms and conditions of the Creative Commons Attribution (CC BY) license (https://creativecommons.org/licenses/by/4.0/).

1. Introduction

Diabetes is one of the most prevalent metabolic illnesses worldwide, resulting in a high rate of morbidity and mortality in Pakistan (WHO, 2003 [1]; Jafar et al., 2006 [2]; Akhtar et al., 2019 [3]). According to data, Pakistan is one of the top ten countries in the world for people with diabetes aged 20 to 79 years (Whiting et al., 2011 [4]). As a result, type 2 diabetes mellitus is a serious health concern in Pakistan. Adnan and Aasim (2020 [5]) conducted a pooled analysis (meta-analysis) of the prevalence of Type 2 diabetes in the adult population of Pakistan and reported a higher pool estimate of diabetes in males than in females (13.1% vs. 12.4%).

The Chronic Care Model (CCM) was created with the primary objective of enhancing the healthcare system and facilitating individual and population health interventions. The Chronic Care Model's applications helped to emphasize patient-centred care and an interdisciplinary approach (AGDHA, 2006 [6]; Anderson et al., 1986 [7]). This study discusses the CCM, providing evidence of its efficacy and describing in detail the two key elements of the model that are used to address self-management of type 2 diabetes in the middle-aged population of the rural areas of Pakistan.

The knowledge and skills in diabetes self-management are critical to effective diabetes management and self-care (Burke et al., 2014 [8]). The Chronic Care Models emphasize patient-centred care, patient empowerment, and support for self-management. There is evidence that therapies based on these principles enhance health status in chronic disorders (Bojadzievski and Gabbay, 2011 [9]; Stellefson et al., 2013 [10]).

Diabetes educators and healthcare professionals employ evidence-based healthcare delivery models such as the Chronic Care Model to improve outcomes for persons with diabetes. It was revealed from the literature reviews that out of 12 studies, six studies showed evidence of the effectiveness of the CCM for type 2 diabetes self-management in primary care settings as well as significant improvements in clinical outcomes (Piatt et al., 2006 [11]; Hiss et al., 2007 [12]; Piatt et al., 2010 [13]; Carter et al., 2011 [14]; Foy et al., 2011 [15]; Lee et al., 2011 [16]).

This study examines two critical components of the Chronic Care Model: patient self-management support (SMS) and delivery system design (DSD) for middle-aged patients with type 2 diabetes in rural Pakistan. It evaluates the effectiveness of these CCM components in improving patients' diabetes self-management approach, quality of life, risk behaviour, knowledge and awareness of diabetes and its complications, and treatment adherence.

The International Diabetes Federation estimates that 463 million people had diabetes in 2019 and 700 million by 2040. Thus, diabetes mellitus is clearly one of the most rapidly evolving health concerns of the twenty-first century. Type 2 diabetes accounts for approximately 90% of all diabetes cases worldwide. Type 2 diabetes is anticipated to cost the global economy USD 760 billion in 2019 and USD 845 billion by 2045 [17] (IDF, 2019).

The incidence rate of diabetes in Pakistan is expected to increase to 15% (13.8 million people) by 2030. (WHO, 2003 [1], WHO, 2014 [18]). As a result, Pakistan is rated seventh in terms of diabetes prevalence (Jafar et al., 2006 [2]). This increases the risk of developing type 2 diabetes in the community (Jafar et al., 2005 [2]; Ansari, 2009 [19]; Whiting et al., 2011 [4]).

The CCM is the most often utilized care model (Wagner, 1996 [20]). The model is composed of six components (Figure 1): delivery system design (DSD), self-management support (SMS), decision support, clinical information systems (all implemented at the practice level), and at the community level, there are two components such as community resources and health care organizations (Bodenheimer et al., 2002 [21]; Wagner, 1996 [20]).

The two important components of CCM were studied in this article and applied to primary health care to see how effective the two elements of the CCM, patient "Self-Management Support" (SMS) and "Delivery System Design" (DSD), were in improving the quality of life and risk behaviour of Type 2 diabetes patients.

The literature review revealed that attempts had been made to examine the efficacy of the CCM on chronic illness outcomes and the extent to which the CCM's components have benefited primary health care (Bodenheimer et al., 2002 [22]; Tsai et al., 2005 [23]). The findings indicated that including one or more CCM elements resulted in improved patient or process outcomes for a number of chronic conditions (Wagner et al., 1996 [20]). Diabetes (lower HbA1c levels), heart failure, asthma, and depression all had the strongest evidence (Tsai et al., 2005 [23]).

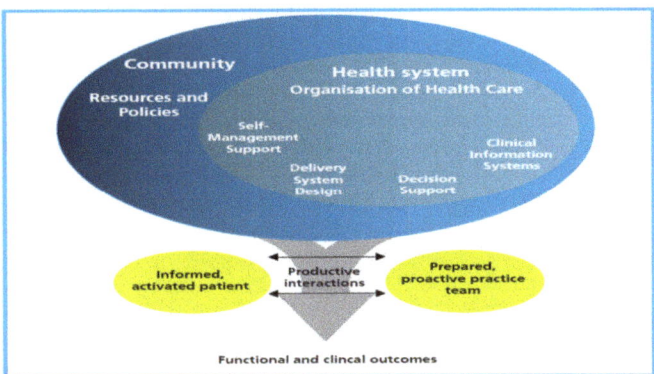

Figure 1. The Wagner Chronic Care Model with its elements: Source: Wagner et al. (1996) [20].

A study was conducted by Zwar et al. (2006) [24] aimed at examining the efficacy of the components of CCM on chronic illness outcomes and the extent to which the CCMs components have benefited primary healthcare. The usefulness of the four elements of CCM was identified by Zwar et al. (2006) [24] following the results of 23 systematic reviews.

In addition, there were six reviews on type 2 diabetes (Deakin et al., 2005 [25]; Norris et al., 2001 [26]; Norris et al., 2002 [27]; Fass et al., 1997 [28]; Loveman et al., 2003 [29]; Van Dam et al., 2003 [30]), two reviews on asthma (Powell and Gibson, 2002 [31]; Toelle and Ram, 2004 [32]), one on chronic obstructive pulmonary disease (Turnock et al., 2005 [33]), one on hypertension (Boulware et al., 2001 [34]) and one on arthritis (Stellefson et al., 2013 [10]).

It has been reported that out of six reviews on diabetes, only four reviews showed that patients with diabetes were in a position to understand the importance of diabetes self-management (Deakin et al., 2005 [25]; Norris et al., 2001 [26]; Norris et al., 2002 [27]; Loveman et al., 2003 [29]). The other two reviews established a link between increased knowledge and improved patient outcomes for diabetes group training (Deakin et al., 2005 [25]) and for self-management education in community meeting places (Norris et al., 2002 [27]).

2. Application of Chronic Care Model in Pakistan

In Pakistan, there is no teamwork approach to self-management support, and delivery system design does not have an adequate structure (Rafique and Shaikh, 2000 [35]) as recommended by the American Diabetes Association (ADA, 2016 [36]). There is no evidence in Pakistan for implementing the Chronic Care Model in the primary health care system besides the fact that diabetes is the main priority in the country (Hakeem and Fawwad, 2010 [37]; Ansari et al., 2016 [38]).

2.1. Self-Management Support (SMS)

The Chronic Care Model's self-management support component was included in this study for diabetics in rural Pakistan. The research shows that self-management support improves patient-level outcomes such as physiological disease markers, quality of life, health status, and satisfaction (Zwar et al., 2016 [24]). Overall, patient self-management support (SMS) was the most commonly used intervention, followed by clinician decision support (Page et al., 2005 [39]) and delivery system design (Turnock et al., 2005 [33]).

These results support a previous analysis of the elements of the CCM by Tsai et al. (2005) [23] and further analysis of patient and provider interventions by Weingarten et al. (2002) [40]. The effectiveness of the CCM for type 2 diabetes self-management in primary care settings, as well as significant improvements in clinical outcomes, was also identified by Baptista et al. (2016) [41] in their systematic review. The systematic review conducted by Reynolds et al. (2018) [42] confirmed that self-management support is the most frequent Chronic Care Model intervention, and it is associated with statistically significant improvement, predominantly for diabetes. Despite the benefits associated with self-management of diabetes, most patients in the middle-aged population of Pakistan do not adhere to self-management recommendations (IDF, 2014 [43]; Jafar et al., 2006 [2]).

Following the recommendations and barriers are both troublesome for lifestyle behaviours such as food habits and physical exercise, rather than modifying adherence (WHO, 2003 [1]; Narayan, 2005 [44]; Jafar et al., 2006 [2]; Ansari, 2009 [19]). This is evident in the culture, history, and lifestyle behaviour of rural Pakistanis, whose dietary habits and physical activity present significant challenges for the middle-aged population in managing type 2 diabetes (Hasan et al., 2000 [45]; Rafique and Shaikh, 2000 [35]).

2.2. Delivery System Design (DSD)

Delivery system design (DSD) entails collaboration among diverse groups of health professionals. Interventions that addressed delivery system design improved adherence to guidelines, patient service utilization, and disease-related physiological measures (Zwar et al., 2006 [24]). Numerous scholars have argued in favour of modifying the design of the delivery system in order to improve patient health care services (Coleman et al., 1998 [46]; Norris et al., 2002 [27]; Rich et al., 1995 [47]; Shojania et al., 2006 [48]).

Among delivery models, case management has frequently been highlighted as an effective strategy (Rich et al., 1995 [47]). Coleman et al. (1998) [46] asserted that case management is successful at mitigating the negative consequences of lower resources. Case management is positively associated with the improvement of patients' healthcare services (Norris et al., 2002 [27]).

3. Material and Methods

3.1. Study Design

The quantitative content analysis method was used to specifically identify the frequency of the most frequent responses or statements. The findings of qualitative thematic analysis based on the interviews and its analysis provided useful information for this study to carry out the quantitative analysis (Ansari et al., 2021 [49]).

In the literature, there was no evidence of similar types of previous studies (qualitative or quantitative) with the same idea and sample composition exploring different perspectives of diabetes patients and healthcare professionals as described in this study. This is a retrospective study that uses the same database which was used in our previous publication related to qualitative studies (Ansari et al., 2021 [49]). The study was approved by the ethics committee of the University of New South Wales, Australia (ref: HC16882), and by Ayub Medical Institutions, Abbottabad, Pakistan, from the office of the Chairman Medical Ethics Committee. Moreover, written consent to participate in this study was obtained from the participants using the UNSW participant information statement and consent form.

3.2. Research Participants

Thirty people with type 2 diabetes were chosen from the total group of participants. Male and female involvement was kept equal (50 percent each). The individuals' mean age was 52 years (range 40–65 years, SD = 6.83), and the mean time from diagnosis was 8.5 years (range 3–12 years, SD = 2.7). The HbA1c levels for both men and women patients were 9.26 (range from 7 to 13 percent, SD = 1.80) in the hospital's medical records. The BMI was 28 kg/m^2 (range: 17.8–46.1, SD = 7.18).

The other group of volunteers included 20 healthcare professionals, including 10 nurses and 10 doctors. Males and females were evenly represented. The same authors described the recruitment process, study teams, and qualitative analysis (Ansari et al., 2019 [19]). The study was conducted in rural Abbottabad. Abbottabad had 1.1719 million residents in 2010. (NIPS, 2013). The city is 110 km north of Islamabad (the capital city). Around 80% of the population lives in rural areas with 19 basic healthcare clinics, five of which are affiliated with the hospital where the study was done (UNDP, 2013; NIPS, 2013).

3.3. Statistical Analysis

The statistical analysis was performed using STATA 15 software (StataCorp. 2015. Stata Statistical Software: Release 15. College Station, TX: StataCorp LP). A p-value < 0.05 was considered as the criterion for statistical significance. In order to assess the demographic characteristics and clinical measurements between the variables, a t-test was performed and used to evaluate the predictors and their association with glycaemic control. The hypothesis was tested to identify that diabetes self-management has a gendered dimension in rural areas of Pakistan.

3.4. Data Collection

Face-to-face interviews with 30 type 2 diabetes patients and 20 healthcare workers (10 general practitioners and 10 nurses) were done in the Urdu language in a clinical environment at several Al-Rehman hospital medical facilities in Pakistan.

The primary author and an auxiliary nurse from the medical centre participated in semi-structured interviews. The interviewees were moderated by the primary author, who encouraged individuals to express their perspectives. Participants were urged to offer their perspectives on the issues raised. Each interview lasted between 30 and 40 min. The interviews, which were semi-structured, were transcribed and translated from the Urdu language. Following an initial check to confirm that data collection was complete, all participant identifying information was erased, and objective identifiers were put on the transcripts to ensure participant anonymity. The questionnaire utilized in this study was aligned with the Chronic Care Model's components, and the questions were identical for patients and healthcare providers.

4. Results

The two major themes of CCM at the practice level (Table 1) have been discussed in detail below for patients with diabetes in the middle-aged population of rural areas of Pakistan. These are the themes of self-management support (SMS) and delivery systems (DSD) design. These themes were discussed in detail by the same authors (Ansari et al., 2021 [49]) as part of qualitative analysis. The statements provided by participants throughout the interviews were categorized into subthemes according to the Chronic Care Model's components. The examination of data from 30 patients and 20 healthcare professionals yielded 340 statements from all 50 participants (n = 50), which were classified into six major Chronic Care Model themes. Male and female patients with Type 2 diabetes made a total of 226 statements, as indicated in Table 1. A total of 114 statements were made by healthcare professionals.

Table 1. The number of factors affecting the self-management of type 2 diabetes outcome (n = 50) (Ansari et al., 2021 [49]).

Themes (CCM)	Type 2 Diabetes Patients (Statements)		Health Professionals (Statements)	Total (Statements)
Practice Level	Male	Female		N (%)
Delivery System (DSD)	20	10	30	60 (18)
Self-management (SMS)	22	25	21	68 (20)
Decision Support	19	10	20	49 (14)
Clinical Information	20	19	11	50 (15)
Community and System Level				
Community Resources	20	40	20	80 (23)
Health Care System	10	11	12	33 (10)
Total Statements	111	115	114	340 (100)

4.1. Quantitative Analysis

The quantitative analysis was carried out considering the two important components of CCM and applied to the primary health care system with an objective to study how effective the two components of the CCM (Self-Management Support and Delivery System Design) were in improving the self-management approach and risk behaviour of patients with type 2 diabetes in the middle-aged population of rural Pakistan.

The American Diabetes Association (ADA) recommended a collaborative approach to self-management assistance and delivery system design (Rafique and Shaikh, 2000 [35,36]; ADA, 2016). However, there was a gap in recommended evidence-based diabetes care and practice in the rural areas of Pakistan (Rafique and Shaikh, 2000 [35,36]; ADA, 2016), and hence, quality improvement strategies and key performance indicators used to measure the improvement of the quality of diabetes care delivered were misaligned.

This quantitative research aimed at addressing the above-mentioned gap through the application of the two main components of the CCM model, which allowed for better measurement of care outcomes against quality improvement strategies.

The specific question related to this research was:

Do the components of the Chronic Care Model improve clinical outcomes for patients with type 2 diabetes in the rural areas of Pakistan?

This study identified that diabetes self-management has a gendered dimension in rural areas of Pakistan, and this research gap was addressed in this study by using the two components of CCM.

We hypothesized that the mean difference of HbA1c (%) between males and females at the follow-up after 6-months would be equal in the two groups of participants.

The two subthemes of the self-management support (SMS), patients' central role in managing type 2 diabetes and effective self-management support strategies, were implemented based on the various statements made by the patients during qualitative analysis (Ansari et al., 2021 [49]). There was a lack of knowledge about diabetes, and patients did not view themselves as actively managing their disease. The other important aspect was the patients' desire to attend the educational/information classes on diabetes self-management in the local language.

The educational classes were arranged for the patients providing information about the diabetes self-management approach and explaining the complications of diabetes in case the disease is not controlled. Nurses played an important role and prompted great interest among the patients in attending the classes regularly. The nurses conducted the educational classes for six months, 3 days a week, and one hour with each group of 15 patients with diabetes.

The overall impact of the lectures was evident as the patients reported going to the walk regularly, being more careful with their eating habits and selecting healthy food to eat, and showing more interest in monitoring blood glucose. The patients were using their prescribed medications as usual.

The self-management support (SMS) component was most effective, which allowed for better measurement of care outcomes, that is, improved and better management and control of blood sugar. However, the implementation of the other core element of the Chronic Care Model, "Delivery System Design", helped to influence the self-management activities of the middle-aged population of rural areas.

This core element of CCM facilitated routine, proactive scheduled visits of general practitioners incorporating the patients' goals and assisting individuals in maintaining optimal health and enabled the health system to manage its resources more effectively.

The database of the patients participating in this research was updated in the electronic system of the primary health clinic. The baseline medical record was already available before the start of the research work. The results of metabolic indicators tests were recorded in the electronic system after 3 months and 6 months intervals of implementation of the two components of the Chronic Care Model.

4.2. Application of the Two Components of CCM

4.2.1. Baseline Analysis of HbA1c

The *t*-test in Table 2 shows that the mean difference of HbA1c at baseline analysis between male and female patients with diabetes is 0.43 and that difference is statistically non-significant ($p = 0.519$) with 95% CI (0.92; 1.79). Figure 2 shows the scatter plot of HbA1c and age variables by sex at baseline analysis while Figure 3 shows the histograms of the distribution of data for male and female patients. The histogram in Figure 3 for females is right-skewed, that is, the mode (7.0) is less than the median (9.0), and the median is less than the mean (9.2). The histogram for males is approximately normal. The following Figure 4 shows these statistics on the histograms.

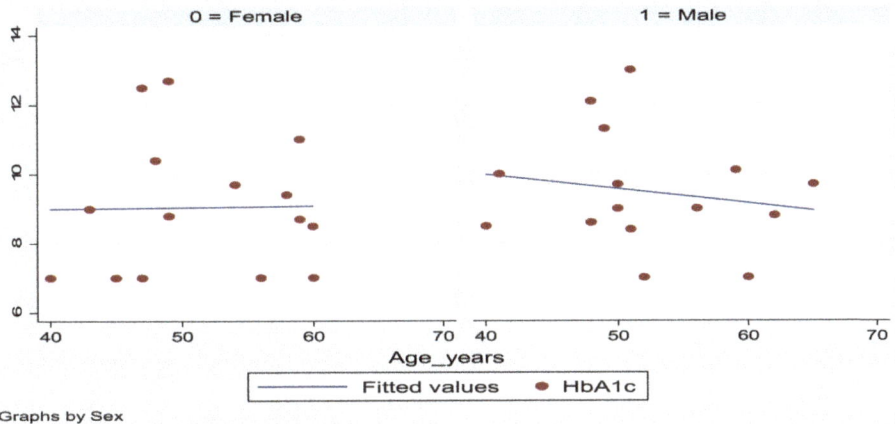

Figure 2. Scatter plots of HbA1c and age variables by sex at baseline analysis.

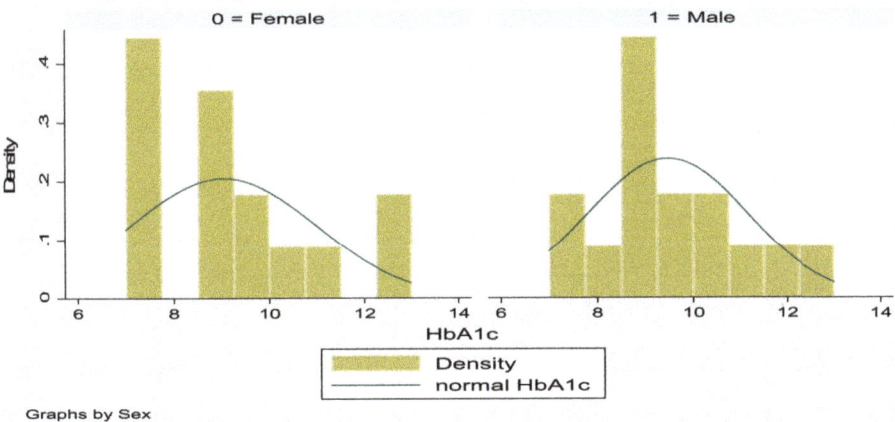

Figure 3. The histograms of HbA1c variable by sex at baseline analysis.

Table 2. Summary statistics of two-sample *t*-test of HbA1c by sex in the sample of the population at baseline analysis.

Sex	N	Mean (HbA1c %)	SD (HbA1c)	Confidence Interval (CI)		
Male	15	9.48	1.68	8.55–10.41		
Female	15	9.05	1.94	7.97–10.12		
Combined	30	9.26	1.80	8.59–9.93		
Difference		Mean	*t*-value	CI		*p*-value
(Male-Female)		0.43	−0.654	0.92–1.79		0.519

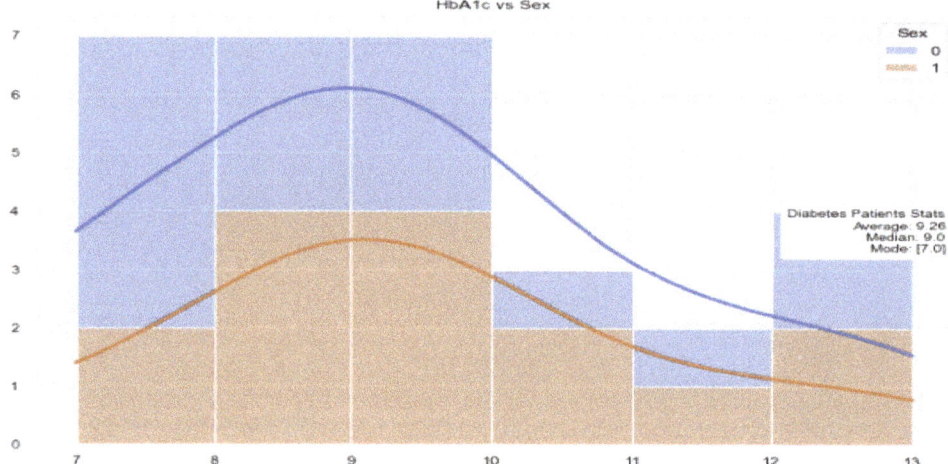

Figure 4. The histograms of HbA1c by sex show statistics at baseline analysis.

4.2.2. After the 3-months intervention of CCM components

The *t*-test in Table 3 shows that the mean difference of HbA1c after a 3-month intervention of the two components of the Chronic Care Model in the sample population between male and female patients with diabetes is 1.06, and that difference is statistically significant ($p = 0.041$) with 95% CI (−0.05; −2.09). Figure 5 shows plots of HbA1c and age variables by sex after 3 months.

Table 3. Summary statistics of two-sample *t*-test of HbA1c by sex in the sample. of population after 3-months follow-up.

Sex	N	Mean (HbA1c %)	SD	Confidence Interval (CI)		
Male	15	9.19	1.33	8.45–9.92		
Female	15	8.12	1.40	7.35–8.89		
Combined	30	8.65	1.44	8.11–9.19		
Difference		Mean	*t*-value	CI		*p*-value
(Male-Female)		1.06	−2.144	−0.05–−2.09		0.041

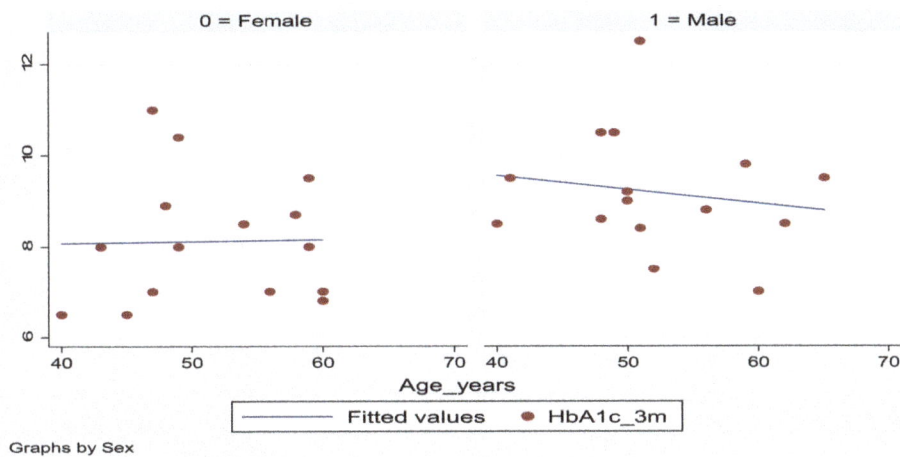

Figure 5. Scatter plots of HbA1c and age variables by sex after 3 months.

The histogram in Figure 6 for female patients is right-skewed, that is, the median (8.55) is less than the mean (8.65). The histogram for male patients in Figure 6 is approximately normal. Figure 7 shows these statistics on the histograms.

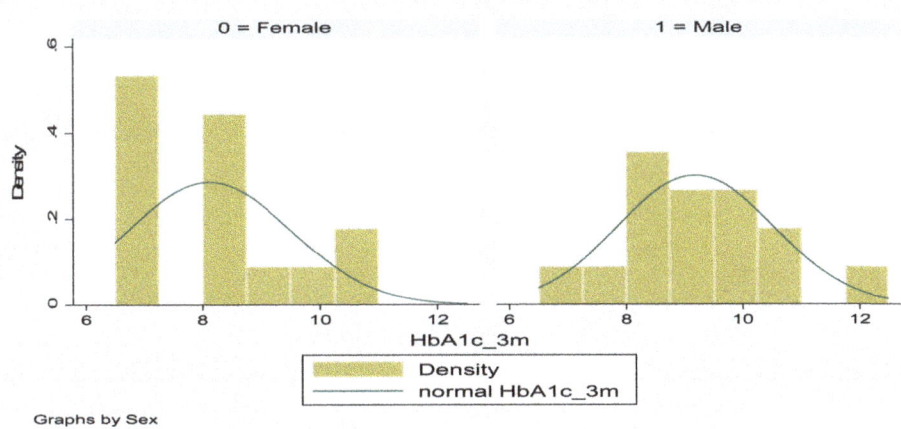

Figure 6. The histograms of HbA1c variable by sex after 3-months intervention.

4.2.3. After the 6-Month Intervention of CCM Components

The *t*-test in Table 4 showed that the mean difference of HbA1c after a 6-month intervention of the two components of the Chronic Care Model in the sample of the population between male and female patients with diabetes is 0.83. It was observed from the hypothesis test (that the two-sided *p*-value was 0.039 ($p < 0.05$). We rejected the null hypothesis and concluded that the mean difference of HbA1c (%) between males and females was not equal. The statistics *t*-value = -2.168, df = 28 and with 95% CI (-0.046; -1.61).

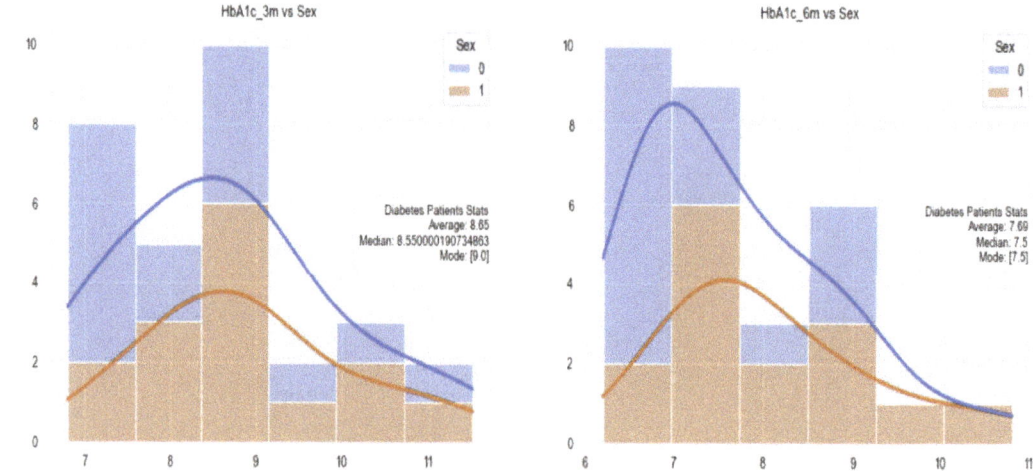

Figure 7. The histograms of HbA1c by sex show statistics after 3-months and 6-months intervention.

Table 4. Summary statistics of two-sample *t*-test of HbA1c by sex in the sample population after 6-months follow-up.

Sex	N	Mean (HbA1c %)	SD	Confidence Interval (CI)	
Male	15	8.11	1.16	7.46–8.75	
Female	15	7.28	0.91	6.77–7.79	
Combined	30	7.69	1.11	7.28–8.11	
Difference		Mean	*t*-value	CI	*p*-value
(Male-Female)		0.83	−2.168	−0.04−−1.61	0.039

Figure 8 shows the scatter plots of HbA1c and age variables by sex after 6 months. The histogram for female patients in Figure 9 is right-skewed and for male patients is approximately normal with a symmetrical distribution (mode = median = 7.5). Figure 7 shows these statistics on the histograms.

The overall results of the quantitative analysis showed that the variable HbA1c was reduced from 9.48% from the baseline analysis to 8.11% after a 6-months intervention of the two components of the Chronic Care Model; for male patients with type 2 diabetes and for female patients, the results were more promising as HbA1C was reduced from 9.05% to 7.28% after a six-months follow-up. Table 5 gives the summary statistics of a two-sample *t*-test of BMI by sex in the sample population after a 6-months follow-up.

Table 5 provides the results of the sample t-test of BMI by sex. For body mass index, the sample *t*-test after 3 months showed the mean difference in BMI was not significant between males and females at the baseline ($p > 0.05$). The mean difference was 4.15 kg/m^2, $p = 0.115$ with 95% CI (−9.37; 1.08). However, after the 6-months intervention of the two components of the Chronic Care Model in the sample of the population, the mean difference in BMI between males and females was significant ($p < 0.05$). The mean difference was 4.97 kg/m^2, $p = 0.040$ with 95% CI (−0.243; −9.690).

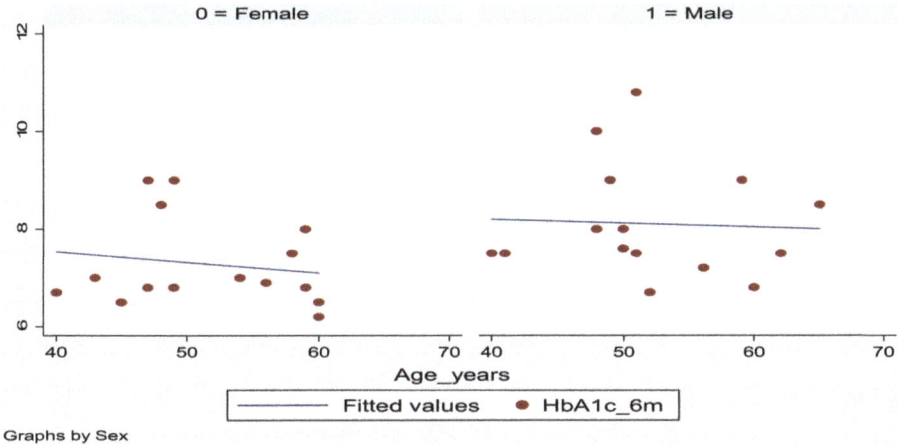

Figure 8. Scatter plots of HbA1c and age variables by sex after 6 months.

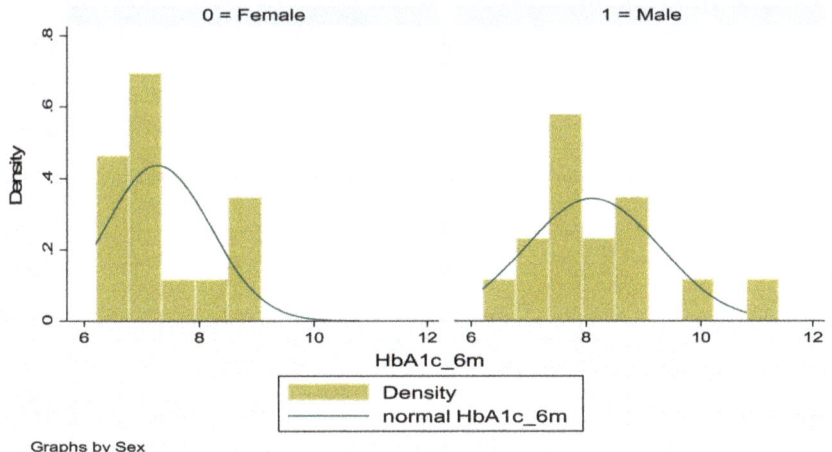

Figure 9. The histograms of HbA1c variable by sex after the 6-month intervention.

Table 5. Summary statistics of two-sample *t*-test of BMI by sex in the sample of population after a 6-months follow-up.

Sex	N	Mean BMI (Kg/m^2)	SD	Confidence Interval (CI)	
Male	15	29.43	5.67	25.61–33.26	
Female	15	24.43	6.90	21.33–27.60	
Combined	30	26.95	1.22	24.45–29.45	
Difference		Mean	*t*-value	CI	*p*-value
(Male-Female)		4.97	−2.154	−0.243–(−9.69)	0.040

5. Discussion

Implementation of the Chronic Care Model aimed to manage the predicted increase in chronic disease by emphasizing a patient-centred approach that focuses on the individual managing and living with chronic disease, illness, and disability (Plumb et al., 2012 [50]). Furthermore, the successful implementation of the Chronic Care Model provided general practitioners with an effective framework for supporting diabetes self-management education and support (Roberto et al., 2012 [51]).

Davy et al. (2015) [52] demonstrated the necessity of including human aspects, including the influence that various stakeholders have on the success or failure of adopting a CCM, through a systematic review. Successful implementation of complex interventions such as a CCM may rely not only on adequate resources and the establishment of effective systems and processes but also on a diverse variety of different stakeholders who will understand and influence the process.

Timpel et al. (2020) [53] developed an evidence-based and expert-driven chronic care management model for patients with diabetes. The Manage Care Model provided guidance for the development and implementation of chronic care programmes, regional networks, and national strategies. They have also suggested that future research will be required to validate the model as an instrument of regional chronic care management.

The two key components of the Chronic Care Model in this study assessed their relevance, feasibility, acceptability, and effectiveness in the primary healthcare system of rural Pakistan. Studies that assessed the effectiveness of the Chronic Care Model also revealed some progress in terms of health outcomes for people living with chronic diseases when delivery system design and self-management assistance were used, and the results of these studies corroborate our findings (Baptista et al., 2016 [41]; Molayaghobi et al., 2019 [54]).

The studies on diabetes knowledge, beliefs, and practices among people with diabetes provided further evidence that there was a lack of information available to people with diabetes in Pakistan as the large population has never received any diabetes education (Rafique and Shaikh, 2000 [35]; Afridi and Khan, 2003 [55]).

Implementation of the two core elements of the Chronic Care Model, "Delivery System Design" and "Self-management Support", helped to influence the self-management activities of the middle-aged population of rural areas. The quantitative analysis demonstrated that, when compared to standard diabetes care, multi-faceted care delivered via CCM components improved HbA1c levels in all type 2 diabetes patients. This finding is in line with several healthcare settings internationally with a specific focus on diabetes, where implementation of the CCM model was found to be the most effective in clinical practice (Busetto et al., 2016 [56]).

The results of the analysis revealed that all the patients who participated in this study had shown a significant reduction in HbA1c ranging from 0.5% to 1% without experiencing hypoglycaemia as per the electronic record of the clinic. The results have addressed the research question and demonstrated that the two components of CCM were effective and improved clinical outcomes for patients with type 2 diabetes in the rural areas of Pakistan. These results are significant as reducing the HbA1c level by 0.2% could lower the mortality due to diabetes by 10% (S herwani et al., 2016 [57]). These findings are in agreement with the studies carried out by Stratton et al. (2000) [58] that a reduction in HbA1c is likely to reduce the risk of complications.

The quantitative analysis demonstrated that diabetes self-management has a gendered dimension as the mean of HbA1c among male patients of type 2 diabetes was 8.11% after a 6-months intervention of the two components of the Chronic Care Model, compared to female patients, whose mean HbA1C was 7.28%, there was a promising difference of 0.83%. Similar results were obtained for body mass index as the mean BMI among male patients was 29.43 kg/m^2 after a 6-months intervention of the two components of the Chronic Care Model, compared to female patients, whose mean BMI was 24.43 kg/m^2, there was a difference of 4.97 kg/m^2. These results are in agreement with other studies reporting the aspect of gender differences in the self-management of type 2 diabetes (Ansari et al., 2019 [19]).

The two subthemes of "Delivery System Design" that received the most attention from participants and health professionals were task distribution among team members and planned interactions to support evidence-based care. The approach of collaboration was deemed to be the most beneficial in terms of optimizing general practitioners' time, as there is a shortage of general practitioners in rural areas of Pakistan, and therefore, more patients will have access to the physicians through a teamwork approach (Shaikh and Hatcher, 2004 [59]; Ansari et al., 2016 [60]).

The previous studies using the two main components of the Chronic Care Model such as patient self-management and delivery system design were found to be the most effective interventions (Fisher et al., 2005 [61]; Foy et al., 2011 [15]; Lee et al., 2011 [16]; Molayaghobi et al., 2019 [54]). The results of these studies are in agreement with our findings, suggesting that in the context of primary healthcare in Pakistan, the two components of CCM were found to be most suitable and effective.

6. Strength and Limitations

The study's strength was in evaluating the two critical components of the Chronic Care Model's relevance, feasibility, acceptability, and effectiveness in rural Pakistan's primary healthcare system. The study emphasized the healthcare system's influence on diabetes self-management outcomes. Previous studies did not address this issue and instead focused exclusively on patient-related factors.

The limitation is related to the delivery system, that is, the absence of workforce structure in rural locations: the absence of dietitians, social workers, and diabetes health educators. In addition, involving family members in this study might have been beneficial, providing significant insight into their perspectives of diabetes self-management practices.

7. Relevance to Clinical Practice

The two main themes of CCM at the practice level, namely, the self-management support (SMS) and delivery system design (DSD), have shown their effectiveness in primary healthcare settings in rural areas of Pakistan. Additionally, family participation in such organizations is critical for the members' own diabetes education and for receiving information on the best ways to support a family member with type 2 diabetes. Diabetes self-management education, preventive and monitoring programmes that consider gender-specific methods, and recommendations would be more suitable and successful in the rural areas of Pakistan.

8. Conclusions

The two elements of the Chronic Care Model were found to be most suitable, feasible, and effective after their implementation in a primary healthcare clinic, and implementation of all the components of CCM in the future will improve the overall efficiency of the health care system of the rural areas of Pakistan. The implementation of the two core elements of CCM in a primary healthcare clinic setting reflected that evidence-based approaches to dealing with this culturally diverse community are effective.

Author Contributions: R.M.A. conducted the semi-structured interviews, and recorded, and transcribed the data. R.M.A. and H.H. analyzed and interpreted the patient data regarding the self-management of type 2 diabetes and drafted the manuscript. M.F.H. reviewed the work and provided extensive comments to improve the article. H.H. and N.Z. reviewed the manuscript and provided comments to enhance the overall presentation of the results. All authors have read and agreed to the published version of the manuscript.

Funding: This research did not receive any specific funding.

Institutional Review Board Statement: The study was conducted according to the guidelines of the Declaration of Helsinki, and approved by the ethics committee of the University of New South Wales, Australia, and Ayub Medical Institution of Pakistan (protocol code HC16882, 6 April 2017).

Informed Consent Statement: Informed consent was obtained from all subjects involved in the study.

Data Availability Statement: The data used to generate the results in the paper are not available to share.

Acknowledgments: The authors are thankful to the director of Al-Rehman hospital, Abbottabad, Pakistan, for facilitating the interviews and data collection activities.

Conflicts of Interest: The authors declare no conflict of interest.

References

1. World Health Organization. WHO Framework Convention on Tobacco Control. 2003. Available online: https://www.who.int/tobacco/resources/publication/fctc/en/index.html (accessed on 10 May 2022).
2. Jafar, T.H.; Chaturvedi, N.; Pappas, G. Prevalence of overweight and obesity and their association with hypertension and diabetes mellitus in an Indo-Asian population. *CMAJ* **2006**, *175*, 1071–1077. [CrossRef] [PubMed]
3. Akhtar, S.; Nasir, J.A.; Abbas, T.; Sarwar, A. Diabetes in Pakistan: A systematic review and meta-analysis. *Pak. J. Med. Sci.* **2019**, *35*, 1173–1178. [CrossRef]
4. Whiting, D.R.; Guariguata, L.; Weil, C.; Shaw, J. IDF Diabetes Atlas: Global estimates of the prevalence of diabetes for 2011–2030. *Diabetes Res. Clin. Pract.* **2011**, *94*, 311–321. [CrossRef] [PubMed]
5. Adnan, M.; Aasim, M. Prevalence of Type 2 Diabetes Mellitus in Adult Population of Pakistan: A Meta-Analysis of Prospective Cross-Sectional Surveys. *Ann. Glob. Health* **2020**, *86*, 7. [CrossRef]
6. Australian Government Department of Health and Ageing (AGDHA). National Chronic Disease Strategy. 2006. Available online: www.health.gov.au/internet/main/publised (accessed on 10 May 2022).
7. Anderson, N.A.; Bridges-Webb, C.; Chancellor, A.H.B. *General Practice in Australia*; Sydney University Press: Sydney, Australia, 1986; pp. 3–4.
8. Burke, S.D.; Sherr, D.; Lipman, R.D. Partnering with diabetes educators to improve patient outcomes. *Diabetol. Metab. Syndr. Obes.* **2014**, *7*, 45–53. [CrossRef]
9. Bojadzievski, T.; Gabbay, R.A. Patient-centered medical home and diabetes. *Diabetes Care* **2011**, *34*, 1047–1053. [CrossRef]
10. Stellefson, M.; Dipnarine, K.; Stopka, C. The Chronic Care Model and Diabetes Management in US Primary Care Settings: A Systematic Review. *Prev. Chronic Dis.* **2013**, *10*, 120–180. [CrossRef]
11. Piatt, G.A.; Orchard, T.J.; Emerson, S.; Simmons, D.; Songer, T.J.; Brooks, M.M.; Zgibor, J.C.; Ahmad, U.; Siminerio, L.M.; Korytkowski, M. Translating the chronic care model into the community: Results from a randomized controlled trial of a multifaceted diabetes care intervention. *Diabetes Care* **2006**, *29*, 811–817. [CrossRef]
12. Hiss, R.G.; Armbruster, B.A.; Gillard, M.L.; McClure, L.A. Nurse care manager collaboration with community-based physicians providing diabetes care: A randomized controlled trial. *Diabetes Educ.* **2007**, *33*, 493–502. [CrossRef]
13. Piatt, G.A.; Anderson, R.M.; Brooks, M.M.; Songer, T.; Siminerio, L.M.; Korytkowski, M.M.; Zgibor, J.C. 3-year follow-up of clinical and behavioral improvements following a multifaceted diabetes care intervention: Results of a randomized controlled trial. *Diabetes Educ.* **2010**, *36*, 301–309. [CrossRef]
14. Carter, E.L.; Nunlee-Bland, G.; Callender, C. A patient-centric, provider-assisted diabetes telehealth self-management intervention for urban minorities. *Perspect. Health Inf. Manag.* **2011**, *8*, 1b. [PubMed]
15. Foy, R.; Eccles, M.P.; Hrisos, S.; Hawthorne, G.; Steen, N.; Gibb, I.; Grimshaw, J.; Croal, B. A cluster randomized trial of educational messages to improve the primary care of diabetes. *Implement. Sci.* **2011**, *6*, 129. [CrossRef] [PubMed]
16. Lee, A.; Siu, C.F.; Leung, K.T.; Lau, L.C.H.; Chan, C.C.M.; Wong, K.-K. General practice and social service partnership for better clinical outcomes, patient self-efficacy and lifestyle behaviours of diabetic care: Randomized control trial of a chronic care model. *Postgrad. Med. J.* **2011**, *87*, 688–693.
17. International Diabetes Federation. Diabetes Prevalence. 2019. Available online: http://www.idf.org/home/index.cfm (accessed on 15 June 2021).
18. World Health Organization. Non-Communicable Diseases, Geneva: World Health Organization. 2013. Available online: http://www.who.int/mediacentre/factsheet/en (accessed on 10 May 2022).
19. Ansari, R.M. Effect of physical activity and obesity on type 2 diabetes in middle-aged population. *J. Environ. Public Health* **2009**, *2009*, 4–9. [CrossRef] [PubMed]
20. Wagner, E.H.; Austin, B.T.; Von Korff, M. Organizing care for patients with chronic illness. *Milbank Q.* **1996**, *74*, 511–544. [CrossRef]
21. Bodenheimer, T.; Wagner, E.H.; Grumbach, K. Improving primary care for patients with chronic illness: The chronic care model, Part 2. *JAMA* **2002**, *288*, 1909–1914. [CrossRef] [PubMed]
22. Bodenheimer, T.; Wagner, E.H.; Grumbach, K. Improving primary care for patients with chronic illness. *JAMA* **2002**, *288*, 1775–1779. [CrossRef]

23. Tsai, A.C.; Morton, S.C.; Mangione, C.M.; Keeler, E.B. A Meta-analysis of Interventions to Improve Care for Chronic Illnesses. *Am. J. Manag. Care* **2005**, *11*, 478–488.
24. Zwar, N.; Harris, M.; Griffiths, R.; Roland, M.; Dennis, S.; Powell Davies, G.; Hasan, I. *A Systematic Review of Chronic Disease Management*; Research Centre for Primary Health Care and Equity, School of Public Health and Community Medicine, UNSW: Sydney, Australia, 2006.
25. Deakin, T.; McShane, C.E.; Cade, J.E.; Williams, R. Group based training for self-management strategies in people with type 2 diabetes mellitus. *Cochrane Database Syst. Rev.* **2005**, *6*, CD003417. [CrossRef]
26. Norris, S.L.; Engelgau, M.M.; Narayan, K.M. Effectiveness of self-management training in type 2 diabetes: A systematic review of randomized controlled trials. *Diabetes Care* **2001**, *24*, 561–587. [CrossRef]
27. Norris, S.L.; Nichols, P.J.; Caspersen, C.J.; Glasgow, R.E.; Engelgau, M.M.; Jack, L.; Snyder, S.R.; Carande-Kulis, V.G.; Isham, G.J.; Garfield, S. Increasing diabetes self-management education in community settings: A systematic review. *Am. J. Prev. Med.* **2002**, *22* (Suppl. S4), 39–66. [CrossRef]
28. Faas, A.; Schellevis, F.G.; Van Eijk, J.T. The efficacy of self-monitoring of blood glucose in NIDDM subjects: A criteria-based literature review. *Diabetes Care* **1997**, *20*, 1482–1486. [CrossRef] [PubMed]
29. Loveman, E.; Cave, C.; Green, C.; Royle, P.; Dunn, N.; Waugh, N. The clinical and cost-effectiveness of patient education models for diabetes: A systematic review and economic evaluation. *Health Technol. Assess.* **2003**, *7*, iii-1. [CrossRef] [PubMed]
30. van Dam, H.A.; van der Horst, F.; van den Borne, B.; Ryckman, R.; Crebolder, H. Provider-patient interaction in diabetes care: Effects on patient self-care and outcomes. A systematic review. *Patient Educ. Couns.* **2003**, *51*, 17–28. [CrossRef]
31. Powell, H.; Gibson, P.G. Options for self-management education for adults with asthma. *Cochrane Database Syst. Rev.* **2002**, *2010*, CD004107. [CrossRef]
32. Toelle, B.G.; Ram, F.S.F. Written individualized management plans for asthma in children and adults. *Cochrane Database Syst. Rev.* **2004**, CD002171. [CrossRef]
33. Turnock, A.C.; Walters, E.H.; Walters, J.A.E.; Wood-Baker, R. Action plans for chronic obstructive pulmonary disease. *Cochrane Database Syst. Rev.* **2005**, CD005074. [CrossRef]
34. Boulware, L.E.; Daumit, G.L.; Frick, K.D.; Minkovitz, C.S.; Lawrence, R.S.; Powe, N.R. An evidence based review of patient-centered behavioral interventions for hypertension. *Am. J. Prev. Med.* **2001**, *21*, 221–232. [CrossRef]
35. Rafique, G.; Shaikh, F. Identifying needs and barriers to diabetes education in patients with diabetes. *J. Pak. Med. Assoc.* **2000**, *56*, 347–352.
36. American Diabetes Association Standards of Medical Care in Diabetes. *J. Clin. Appl. Res. Educ. Diabetes Care* **2016**, *39* (Suppl. S1). Available online: www.diabetes.org/diabetescare (accessed on 15 June 2021).
37. Hakeem, R.; Fawwad, A. Diabetes in Pakistan, Epidemiology, Determinants and Prevention. *J. Diabetol.* **2010**, *3*, 4.
38. Ansari, R.M.; Hosseinzadeh, H.; Zwar, N. Primary Healthcare System of Pakistan: Challenges to Self-Management of Type 2 Diabetes. *Open J. Endocr. Metab. Dis.* **2016**, *6*, 173–182. [CrossRef]
39. Page, T.; Lockwood, C.; Conroy-Hiller, T. Effectiveness of nurse-led cardiac clinics in adult patients with a diagnosis of coronary heart disease. *Int. J. Evid.-Based Healthc.* **2005**, *3*, 2–26. [PubMed]
40. Weingarten, S.R.; Henning, J.M.; Badamgarav, E.; Knight, K.; Hasselblad, V.; Gano, A., Jr.; Ofman, J.J. Interventions used in disease management programmes for patients with chronic illness-which one's work? Meta-analysis of published reports. *BMJ* **2002**, *325*, 925. [CrossRef]
41. Baptista, D.R.; Wiens, A.; Pontarolo, R.; Regis, L.; Reis, W.C.T.; Correr, C.J. The chronic care model for type 2 diabetes: A systematic review. *Diabetol. Metab. Syndr.* **2016**, *8*, 7. [CrossRef] [PubMed]
42. Reynolds, R.; Dennis, S.; Hasan, I.; Slewa, J.; Chen, W.; Tian, D.; Bobba, S.; Zwar, N. A systematic review of chronic disease management intervention in primary care. *BMC Fam. Pract.* **2018**, *19*, 11. [CrossRef] [PubMed]
43. International Diabetes Federation. Diabetes Prevalence. 2014. Available online: http://www.idf.org/home/index.cfm (accessed on 10 May 2022).
44. Narayan, K.M.V. The Diabetes Pandemic: Looking for the silver lining. *Clin. Diabetes* **2005**, *23*, 51–52. [CrossRef]
45. Hasan, Z.U.; Zia, S.; Maracy, M. Baseline disease knowledge assessment in patients with type 2 diabetes in a rural area of northwest of Pakistan. *J. Pak. Med. Ass.* **2000**, *54*, 67–73.
46. Coleman, K.; Austin, B.T.; Brach, C.; Wagner, E.H. Evidence on the Chronic Care Model in the new millennium. *Health Aff.* **2009**, *28*, 75–85. [CrossRef]
47. Rich, M.W.; Beckham, V.; Wittenberg, C.; Leven, C.L.; Freedland, K.E.; Carney, R.M. A multidisciplinary intervention to prevent the readmission of elderly patients with congestive heart failure. *N. Engl. J. Med.* **1995**, *1*, 1190–1195. [CrossRef]
48. Shojania, K.G.; Ranji, S.R.; McDonald, K.M.; Grimshaw, J.M.; Sundaram, V.; Rushakoff, R.J.; Owens, D.K. Effects of quality improvement strategies for type 2 diabetes on glycemic control: A meta-regression analysis. *JAMA* **2006**, *4*, 427–440. [CrossRef] [PubMed]
49. Ansari, R.M.; Harris, M.F.; Hosseinzadeh, H.; Zwar, N. Applications of a Chronic Care Model for Self-Management of Type 2 Diabetes: A Qualitative Analysis. *Int. J. Environ. Res. Public Health* **2021**, *18*, 10840. [CrossRef]
50. Plumb, J.; Weinsten, L.C.; Brawer, R.; Scott, K. Community-Based Partnerships for Improving Chronic Disease Management. *Prim. Care Clin. Off. Pract.* **2012**, *39*, 433–447. [CrossRef]

51. Roberto, N.; Katie, C.; Rafael, B.; Sauto, R. Integrated care for Chronic Conditions: The contribution of the ICCC framework. *Health Policy* **2012**, *105*, 55–64.
52. Davy, C.; Bleasel, J.; Liu, H.; Tchan, M.; Ponniah, S.; Brown, A. Factors influencing the implementation of chronic care models: A systematic literature review. *BMC Fam. Pract.* **2015**, *16*, 102. [CrossRef] [PubMed]
53. Timpel, P.; Lang, C.; Wens, J.; Contel, J.C.; Schwarz, P.E.H.; On behalf of the MANAGE CARE Study Group. The Manage Care Model–Developing an Evidence-Based and Expert-Driven Chronic Care Management Model for Patients with Diabetes. *Int. J. Integr. Care* **2020**, *20*, 2. [CrossRef]
54. Molayaghobi, N.S.; Abazari, P.; Taleghani, F.; Iraj, B.; Etesampour, A.; Zarei, A.; Hashemi, H.; Abasi, F. Overcoming challenges of implementing chronic care model in diabetes management: An action research approach. *Int. J. Prev. Med.* **2019**, *10*, 13.
55. Afridi, M.A.; Khan, M.N. Role of Health Education in the Management of Diabetes Mellitus. *J. Coll. Physicians Surg.—Pak.* **2003**, *13*, 558–561.
56. Busetto, L.; Luijkx, K.; Elissen, A.; Vrijhoef, H. Intervention types and outcomes of integrated care for diabetes mellitus type 2, A systematic review. *J. Eval. Clin. Pract.* **2016**, *22*, 299–310. [CrossRef]
57. Sherwani, S.I.; Khan, H.A.; Ekhzaimy, A.; Masood, A.; Sakharkar, M.K. Significance of HbA1c Test in Diagnosis and Prognosis of Diabetic Patients. *Biomark. Insights* **2016**, *11*, 95–104. [CrossRef]
58. Stratton, I.M.; Alder, A.I.; Neil, H.A.W.; Matthews, D.R.; Manley, S.E.; Cull, C.A.; Holman, R.R.; Turner, R.C.; Hadden, D. Association of glycemic with macro vascular and microvascular complications of type 2 diabetes: Prospective observational studies. *BMJ* **2000**, *321*, 405–412. [CrossRef] [PubMed]
59. Shaikh, B.T.; Hatcher, J. Health Seeking Behaviour and Health Service Utilization in Pakistan, Challenging the Policy Makers. *J. Public Health* **2004**, *27*, 49–54. [CrossRef] [PubMed]
60. Ansari, R.M.; Hosseinzadeh, H.; Zwar, N. Application of Chronic Care Model for self-management of type 2 diabetes: Focus on the middle-aged population of Pakistan. *Int. J. Med. Res. Pharm. Sci.* **2016**, *3*, 1–7. [CrossRef]
61. Fisher, E.B.; Brownson, C.A.; O'Tool, M.L.; Shetty, G.; Anwuri, V.V.; Glasgow, R.E. Ecological approaches to self-ma agement: The case of diabetes. *Am. J. Public Health* **2005**, *95*, 1523–1535. [CrossRef] [PubMed]

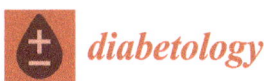

Review

Verapamil and Its Role in Diabetes

Paul Zimmermann [1,2], Felix Aberer [3], Max L. Eckstein [1], Sandra Haupt [1], Maximilian P. Erlmann [1] and Othmar Moser [1,3,*]

[1] Division of Exercise Physiology and Metabolism, Department of Sport Science, University of Bayreuth, 95440 Bayreuth, Germany; paul.zimmermann@arcormail.de (P.Z.); max.eckstein@uni-bayreuth.de (M.L.E.); sandra.haupt@uni-bayreuth.de (S.H.); maximilian.erlmann@uni-bayreuth.de (M.P.E.)

[2] Department of Cardiology, Klinikum Bamberg, 96049 Bamberg, Germany

[3] Division of Endocrinology and Diabetology, Medical University of Graz, 8010 Graz, Austria; felix.aberer@medunigraz.at

* Correspondence: othmar.moser@uni-bayreuth.de

Abstract: Autoimmune pancreatic β-cell loss and destruction play a key role in the pathogenesis and development of type 1 diabetes, with a prospective increased risk for developing micro- and macrovascular complications. In this regard, orally administered verapamil, a calcium channel antagonist, usually intended for use as an anti-arrhythmic drug, has previously shown potential beneficial effects on β-cell preservation in new-onset type 1 diabetes. Furthermore, observational data suggest a reduced risk of type 2 diabetes development. The underlying pathophysiological mechanisms are not well investigated and remain widely inconclusive. The aim of this narrative review was to detail the role of verapamil in promoting endogenous β-cell function, potentially eligible for early treatment in type 1 diabetes, and to summarize existing evidence on its effect on glycemia in individuals with type 2 diabetes.

Keywords: type 1 diabetes; type 2 diabetes; insulin; beta cell preservation; verapamil; thioredoxin-interacting protein (TXNIP)

1. Introduction

Approximately 537 million people globally suffer from type 1 (T1D) and type 2 diabetes mellitus (T2D) and prevalence of both is substantially increasing [1,2]. Without sufficient action to address this situation, the number of people suffering from diabetes is predicted to be 643 million in 2030 [2]. The key factor in developing T1D and advanced T2D is the loss or impairment of the insulin-secreting β-cells of the pancreas. In the last 100 years daily insulin injections have been established as the life-saving treatment for most people with T1D and some with T2D. Nevertheless, despite emerging advancements in insulin development and diabetes technology, the majority of people living with diabetes do not achieve individual therapy goals, increasing their risk of acute and late complications [3].

Pancreatic β-cell loss and destruction play a key role in the pathogenesis and development of T1D. In the pancreatic tissue, islets of Langerhans secrete several different hormones, which are responsible for maintenance of glucose homeostasis. Insulin, the only hormone able to lower blood glucose concentration, is secreted by the β-cells, which represent the major cellular component of the pancreatic isles [4]. The primary physiological stimulus for insulin secretion is known to be the increase of circulating glucose concentration. The direct insulin secretion by glucose involves a "triggering" and an "amplifying" pathway. The "triggering" pathway is activated by several biochemical signals, involving the adenosine triphosphate (ATP) generation by glucose metabolism, the closure of ATP-sensitive potassium (K_{ATP}) channels resulting in membrane depolarization and consequent activation of voltage-gated calcium channels. The subsequent sharp rise of intracellular calcium levels contributes to the triggered exocytosis of readily releasable pooled insulin secretory granules by membrane fusion and release to the cell exterior. After the "first phase" of insulin release resulting in a sharp peak, the amplifying pathway provides lower but sustained insulin release for several hours in the "second phase" of insulin secretion. The amplifying pathway is activated in the presence of maximal intracellular Ca^{2+} levels and is largely independent of K_{ATP} driven mechanisms [5].

Residual c-peptide levels representing a consistent and sensitive measure of β-cell function [6] and being detected in many people for years following the diagnosis of T1D, contribute to β-cell responsiveness to hyperglycemia and α-cell responsiveness by reciprocal regulation of glucagon secretion to hypoglycemia for glycemic control in individuals with T1D [7]. Carr et al. demonstrated that detectable c-peptide is associated with an increased time spent in the normal glucose range and with less hyperglycemic episodes, but not with the risk of hypoglycemia in those with newly diagnosed T1D [8]. Preserved c-peptide levels in T1D were associated with a more pronounced counter regulation in response to clamp-induced hypoglycemia [9]. On the one hand, regular physical exercise contributes to β-cell preservation, improved insulin sensitivity and less requirements of exogenous insulin administration [10]; on the other hand, in T1D subjects undertaking high levels of physical exercise, the honeymoon period, which is defined by an absence of insulin requirements early after onset of diabetes, is five times longer compared to matched sedentary controls [11]. Next to physical activity, conscious macronutrient intake, such as gluten deprivation or reduced consumption of refined grains may have beneficial effects on β-cell preservation in people affected by new-onset T1D [12,13].

Individuals with T1D are exposed to an increased risk for developing micro- and macrovascular complications, which are associated with episodes of dysglycemia. In this context, residual β-cell secretion, evaluated by measuring fasting c-peptide levels, has been shown to be prospectively associated with reduced incidence of microvascular complications in T1D [14]. Even modestly detectable β-cell levels correlated with a reduced incidence of diabetes-related complications, such as retinopathy and nephropathy [15].

By the fact that autoimmune-mediated β-cell destruction is unavoidably progressing, sooner or later, complex insulin therapy is required for the lifetime. The time from T1D diagnosis to complete lack of measurable insulin (c-peptide) is highly individual as shown by Davies et al., who demonstrated that after 6–9 years of diabetes diagnosis, insulin remained detectable in 60% of individuals, while after 10–20 years of diabetes duration only 35% of the individuals remained c-peptide positive, as defined by detectable fasting c-peptide ≥ 0.017 nmol/L and non-fasting c-peptide ≥ 0.2 nmol/L [16]. Recent research on T1D enables us to refine our understanding in pathogenesis and subsequent development of insulin deficiency in T1D and potentially establish novel prevention and therapy strategies [17]. The impairment of β-cells leads to long-term immune-mediated destruction, low insulin secretory capacity and autoantigen presentation [17]. However, up to now, evidence on effective therapies to delay or halt this process is largely lacking [18].

For these reasons, β-cell rescue and preservation strategies are hot topics on current and future therapeutic strategies in T1D. Exploring beneficial actions for the treatment of T1D, clinical data are suggesting positive effects for peptides or medication reducing the β-cell stress, such as verapamil [17,19,20]. Verapamil was the first non-dihydropyridine calcium channel blocker (CCB) that was approved by the Food and Drug Administration (FDA) in 1981 for clinical use [21]. In several clinical implications, such as cardiac arrhythmias or combination treatment of hypertension, it has proven efficacy in everyday clinical practice due to its good safety profile and pharmacodynamic properties [22,23].

Next to the previously described impact of preserved endogenous insulin secretion, measured by c-peptide levels in T1D individuals, the role of c-peptide is not well defined in T2D, a disease that is considered to be associated with insulin resistance and a reduced β-cell function [24]. Therefore, preserving β-cells function is one of the principle aims in the treatment of T2D to delay the natural course of the disease, necessitating the introduction of insulin therapy in the majority of patients [14]. In T2D patients, regular moderate physical activity and physical health represent well accepted key factors next to regular orally administrated antidiabetic medication and finally additional exogenous insulin application combined with conscious macronutrient intake in order to prospectively hold back the progress of β-cell decline and insulin resistance. In this matter, several clinical observational studies in general reported about decreased risk of new onset diabetes and lower fasting blood glucose levels in diabetes patients receiving orally administered verapamil [25–27]. Dietary factors are estimated to contribute to maintaining insulin secretion and sensitivity by reduced consumption of refined grains and meat products in T2D [13]. Some prospective studies reported a positive association between residual insulin secretion in T2D patients and less microvascular complications [28], but up to now, to our knowledge, no data regarding the association between residual insulin secretion and major outcomes, such as all-cause mortality and mortality due to cardiovascular diseases, are available in T2D patients [29].

In this regard, we review the role of orally administered verapamil in diabetes positively influencing β-cell function and glycemic control as well as its potential properties to prevent diabetes development.

2. Method Section
Scientific Research

We selected relevant scientific research published from October 1984 until May 2022 by searching PubMed. Potentially eligible studies were considered to be included in our narrative review after searching by combined-term medial subject headings and keywords, such as type 1 diabetes (T1D), type 2 diabetes (T2D), insulin secretion, β-cell preservation, verapamil, and Thioredoxin-interacting protein (TXNIP). After completing the search, 69 papers and one web source were included to detail the systemic and cellular effects of orally administrated CCB verapamil in T1D and T2D subjects.

3. Insulin Secretion in Pancreatic β-Cells and the Role of TXNIP—Influence of Verapamil and Clinical Implications

3.1. The Role of Pancreatic β-Cells in T1D and T2D

T1D is an autoimmune-mediated disease characterized by progressive destruction of the pancreatic β-cells resulting in long term lack of the hormone insulin [30]. Pancreatic β-cells play a pivotal role in the synthetization and secretion of insulin, as the body's solo source [31]. In this regard, insulin represents the main player for promotion and maintenance of metabolism [32]. In the scientific community it is an accepted fact that diabetes is associated with a reduction in β-cell mass and to date there is no approved drug treatment that targets damage to these cells [33,34]. Pancreatic β-cells have, as reported in several studies, a weak antioxidant capacity and are very sensitive to oxidative stress interactions occurring within the cells [31,33]. Although several trials have studied the mechanisms of β-cell loss in the different types of diabetes, there is less information referring to the residual β-cells in autoimmune T1D [35].

Different mechanisms are postulated for β-cell failure as demonstrated especially for T2D individuals [36]. β-cells in T2D patients are reported to be secretory-functionally inactive for decades and their potential and preserving might contribute to new therapeutical approaches [35]. A heated discussion is ongoing whether a β-cell reduction occurs in every person with T2D. Some researchers argue that the β-cell mass in T2D patients stays normal and remarks the functional abnormality of insulin secretion as the main problem of hyperglycemia. On the other hand, the scientific community discusses the reduction of the absolute β-cell mass, which is far more difficult to restore [34]. In this context, oxidative stress might inactivate key islet transcription factors, producing "stunned" β-cells, not responding to glucose [36–38]. Although it is difficult to measure the β-cell mass in vivo, there is a proposed positive correlation between high mass and high insulin sensitivity and secretion [34,39,40].

3.2. Thioredoxin-Interacting Protein (TXNIP) and Its Regulation of Pancreatic β-Cells

Thioredoxin-interacting protein (TXNIP) is an attractive aspect to focus on, as it has been suggested to be a major factor in the regulation of pancreatic β-cell dysfunction and death, representing key processes in the pathogenesis of T1D and T2D [19,41]. Therefore, TXNIP represents a very promising future target in the therapy for diabetes based on basic, preclinical and retrospective epidemiological analyses [41,42]. TXNIP inhibits thioredoxin (TRX) as a part of the intracellular antioxidant system, which manages different mechanisms in the β-cells, mainly the reduction of the antioxidant capacity and subsequent oxidative stress and apoptosis in the β-cells, resulting in reduced insulin production capacity (Figure 1) [43,44].

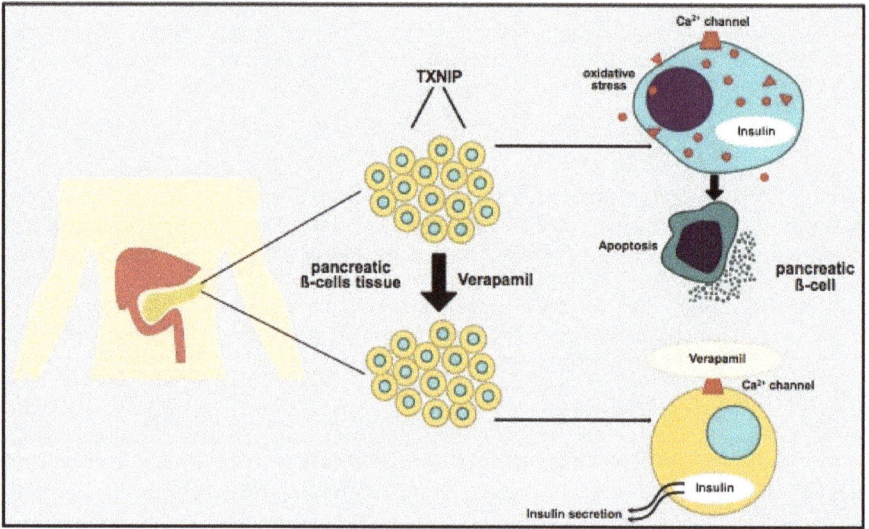

Figure 1. The role of pancreatic β-cells, oxidative stress and insulin secretion in T1D, [31]. Abbreviations: TXNIP, Thioredoxin interacting protein; Ca^{2+}, Calcium.

In detail, TXNIP regulates the glucose homeostasis as a signal complex, the TRX/TXNIP signal complex. This redoxisome represents the basis of TXNIP regulation as redox response. TXNIP has been shown to bind NOD-like receptor protein 3 (NLRP3) and activate the inflammasome [41]. TXNIP as a member of the ancestral α- Arrestin family binds to the Itchy E3 Ubiquitin Protein Ligase (ITCH) and enables the ubiquitination of the substrates. TXNIP in general is transcriptionally regulated by nuclear receptors (NR), such as glucocorticoid receptor (GR), vitamin D receptor (VDR), farnesoid X receptor (FXR) and peroxisome-proliferator activated receptor (PPARs) in a cell-specific manner [41]. These signal complex regulators are involved in the physiological regulation functions of TXNIP, for example in the regulation of glucose homeostasis, as pictured in Figure 2.

TXNIP has been shown to be activated by hyperglycemia and to be increased in diabetes, whereas TXNIP deletion seems to be associated with non-diabetes occurrence in general. In detail, TXNIP is one of the genes that is highly upregulated by hyperglycemia in murine and human β-cells. Therefore, in the case of β-cells the glucose sensor carbohydrate-response element-binding protein (ChREBP) directly binds to the promoter region of TXNIP and increases gene expression [41,45,46]. Furthermore, TXNIP inhibition has been proven for promoting insulin production and glucagon-like peptide 1 signaling via the microRBA regulation [42]. On the other hand, the glucose responsiveness of TXNIP is linked to the notable functions of induction of apoptosis as a reaction to hyperglycemic episodes [41,45,47]. This stress-induced upregulation of TXNIP can be noticed in the pancreatic islets during progression of diabetes in humans and mice [48,49]. Varying factors, such as glucocorticoids, lipids, inflammation/cytokines and oxidative stress, which influence and stimulate the TXNIP induction, are described in previous research [50–53].

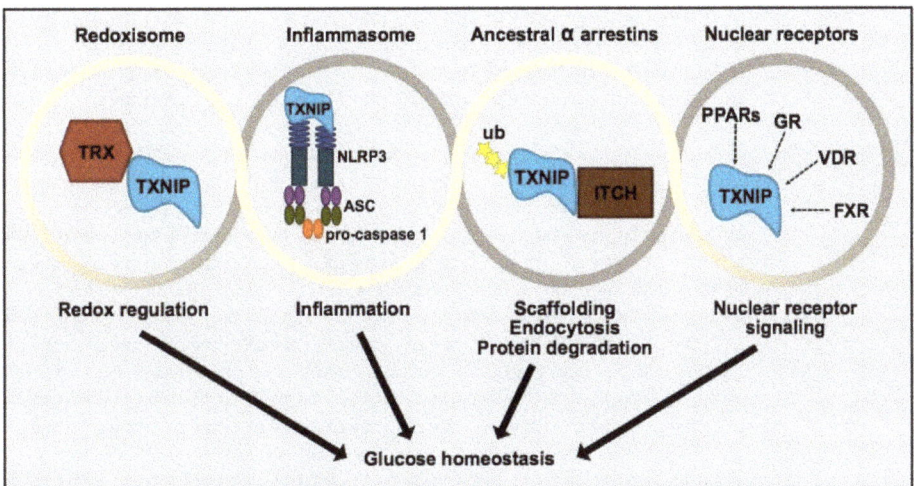

Figure 2. TXNIP signal complex regulating glucose homeostasis, [41]. Abbreviations: TRX, Thioredoxin; TXNIP, Thioredoxin interacting protein; NLRP3, NOD-like receptor protein 3; ITCH, Itchy E3 Ubiquitin Protein Ligase; PPARs, peroxisome-proliferator activated receptors; GR, glucocorticoid receptor; VDR, vitamin D receptor; FXR, farnesoid receptor.

In this context, there has been shown some scientific evidence that pancreatic β-cells as well as skeletal myocytes share common mechanisms of fuel sensing in order to cooperate and maintain glucose homeostasis in the whole-body system. Therefore, TXNIP has been recently shown to play a key role as a diabetogenic culprit disrupting the following both processes—on the one hand by activating the pancreatic isles by mobilizing insulin-containing vesicles and on the other hand by modulating the translocation of resident glucose transporters in the peripheries of the muscles [48,54]. The thioredoxin system plays an important role at a nodal point linking pathways of redox regulation, energy metabolism, antioxidant defense, and in the end cell growth and survival [44]. Hypoglycemic agents, carbohydrate-response-element-binding protein and cytosolic calcium levels regulate the β-cell TXNIP expression, and these different aspects contribute to regulation of whole-body glucose maintenance [42]. This vicious cycle may contribute to TXNIP triggered β-cell failure and overt diabetes [44].

Next to the mentioned TXNIP interactions, TXNIP is an α-Arrestin that acts as an adaptor for glucose transporter 1 (GLUT1), which plays upregulated—as a major glucose facilitator—an important role in the development of metabolic diseases, such as diabetes. TXNIP interacts with GLUT1 lipid nanodiscs in a 1:1 ratio and regulates the glucose uptake in response to intracellular as well as extracellular signals. TXNIP-GLUT1 interaction depends on TXNIP interaction with phosphatidylinositol 4,5-bisphosphate PI(4,5)P2 or PIP2 and TIXNP does not interact with GLUT5 [55].

In summary, the TRX/TXNIP signal complex has been shown to play an important role in the redox-related signal transduction in many different types of cells in various tissues. Additionally, TXNIP has several cellular functions, which largely rely on their scaffolding function as a member of the α-Arrestin family [41]. By both functions, i.e., the redox dependent and independent, TXNIP has emerged as master regulator for glucose homeostasis. Targeting TXNIP in diabetes seems to play an important role in the whole-body glucose metabolism regulation influenced by variable factors and circumstances and in the future might inaugurate new therapeutical potential in diabetes therapy.

3.3. Verapamil and Its Impact on Diabetes

The non-dihydropyridine CCB verapamil and its role in clinical routine as cardiac antiarrhythmic therapy and a blood-pressure-lowering drug was approved by the FDA in 1981 due to its advantageous pharmacodynamics for the treatment of angina, hypertension, supraventricular tachycardia and atrial fibrillation [21,22]. In recent years it has been considered as a promising novel approach in the therapy of TD1 and T2D [21]. The cardiac side effects and antidiabetic efficacy of R-form verapamil enantiomer (R-Vera) and S-form verapamil enantiomer (S-Vera) were evaluated in mouse models and R-Vera seems to represent an effective option in diabetes treatment by downregulating TXNIP and reducing β-cell apoptosis with an established safety profile and only weak adverse cardiac effects, such as negative inotropy [21]. While the rise of intracellular calcium concentration is known in general as the main trigger of exocytosis and subsequent insulin secretion, verapamil reduces by blocking calcium channels the intracellular calcium concentration and prevents long-term β-cell impairment, which is partly caused by chronic increased intracellular Ca^{2+} levels. This preventive mechanism contributes to preserved β-cell function by TXNIP downregulation, ameliorating less apoptosis in pancreatic β-cells and helping to preserve continuously endogenous insulin levels during glucose metabolism regulation [21].

In general, the three different subtypes of calcium channels, i.e., Ca_V 3.1, -3.2 and -3.3, are distributed over the whole body and have defined roles in cardiac regulation, vasculature tone regulation and the activation of the nervous system. The main effect of verapamil results in blocking of both L-Type and T-type channels with higher affinity for depolarized channels than for resting channels. The highest affinity, up to ten times higher, of verapamil is reported in depolarized L-type channels than in the resting channels [22]. The phenylalkylamine Br-verapamil binds in the central cavity of the pore on the intracellular side of the selectivity filter—blocking the ion-conducting pathway—and structure-based mutations of key amino-acid residues confirm the verapamil binding on both sides, as reported by Tang et al. [56]. These specific positive effects could be verified in several studies, as shown in mouse models resulting in improved β-cell survival and function, enhanced insulin secretion and reduced diabetes rate [19]. Next to these findings, several clinical observational studies, such as International Verapamil SR/Trandolapril (INVEST) and the Reasons for Geographic and Racial Differences in Stroke (REGARDS) study, confirmed decreased risk for newly diagnosed diabetes and lower fasting blood glucose levels in response to regular oral verapamil intake [25–27].

3.3.1. Verapamil Administration and β-Cell Mass in Mouse Model

In this regard TXNIP was identified as a target to halt the functional β-cell mass loss as described by Xu et al. in a mouse model [19]. Hyperglycemia and diabetes induce an upregulation of β-cell TXNIP expression, and TXNIP overexpression causes β-cell apoptosis. Although it has previously been shown that TXNIP is strongly dependent and induced by glucose, different proinflammatory cytokines, such as tumor necrosis factor α (TNF α), interleukin-1 β (IL-1 β) and interferon γ (IFNγ) each have distinct and partly opposing mechanisms and pathways on β-cell TXNIP expression [19,50].

Xu et al. could reveal positive effects due to inhibition of TXNIP expression, enhanced endogenous insulin levels as well as improved glucose homeostasis and sensitivity in the mouse model. These positive effects of TXNIP repression by orally administrated verapamil in a mouse model seem to be conditional by reduction of intracellular calcium levels, inhibition of calcineurin signaling and nuclear exclusion and decreased binding of carbohydrate response element-binding protein to the E-box repeat in the TXNIP promoter [19].

For the first time it was highlighted that oral medication of the CCB verapamil could effectively inhibit proapoptotic β-cell TXNIP expression, improve β-cell survival and function with weak adverse cardiac effects, and could represent a new therapeutic approach for the prevention and therapy of diabetes.

3.3.2. Clinical Implications in Type 1 Diabetes (T1D)

To translate these positive findings reported in a mouse model [19,50] into humans, Ovalle et al. performed a trial in order to assess the efficacy and safety of using oral verapamil in subjects with recent onset T1D in order to downregulate TXNIP and enhance the patients' endogenous β-cells mass and insulin production [18]. Therefore, in a double-blind, placebo-controlled Phase 2 trial, 32 participants were randomized to assess the efficacy and safety of orally administered verapamil in subjects with recent onset T1D in order to downregulate TXNIP, and to evaluate the maintenance of endogenous β-cell mass and insulin production. Furthermore, 26 participants were randomized to the two treatment groups, i.e., placebo control group versus oral medication with verapamil for 12 months. The initial dose of verapamil was 120 mg daily and was advanced to a maximum dose of 360 mg daily, if tolerated. The primary outcome measures assessed the functional β-cell mass by the area under the curve (AUC) from a two-hour mixed meal stimulated c-peptide after 12 months. As secondary outcome measures the changes from baseline in exogenous insulin requirements both within 12 weeks and 12 months, hypoglycemic events as well as the HbA1c values within 12 weeks and 12 months were defined. An improved endogenous β-cell activity, lower exogenous insulin requirements and lower hypoglycemic episodes were demonstrated in the verapamil group for at least 24 months and lost upon discontinuation [18,57]. These positive findings were shown and consistent to the previous results in preclinical diabetic mouse model studies and in isolated human islets [18,50]. Evaluating secondary endpoints, as the total daily dose of insulin (TDDI) to maintain glycemic control, a significant treatment difference of −43% in the verapamil group compared to the placebo group could be revealed within the first follow-up year, as well as non-significant lower HbA1c levels ($p = 0.083$) in the verapamil group. Moreover, an improved glycemic control with significant less hypoglycemic episodes in the verapamil group ($p = 0.0387$) as well as more time within the target range of 3.9–10.0 mmol/L assessed by a continuous glucose monitoring (CGM) system were reported within the verapamil group. Verapamil treatment did not affect fasting glucagon levels and no severe adverse events occurred in the verapamil group causing treatment discontinuation. These positive effects, especially the comparable glucagon levels in both groups, might be assumed by an improved insulin sensitivity due to verapamil administration resulting in an overall better glucose control. These aspects might contribute to lower exogenous insulin requirements, which in turn could reduce the hypoglycemic episodes [18]. These different mechanisms might result in an overall improved glucose control and stable glucagon levels in both groups might serve as a positive feedback control mechanism. Importantly, verapamil administration did not cause any severe episodes of hypotension, heart rate abnormalities or electrocardiogram (ECG) alterations. These results emphasize the potential translational implications and its impact on clinical care and encourage the scientific community for larger follow-up trials in order to develop novel therapeutical approaches [18,19].

The clinical implications of TXNIP targeting in T1D subjects seem to preserve additional therapeutic opportunities to decrease long term micro- and macrovascular complications, such as diabetic vascular dysfunction, diabetic retinopathy as well as diabetic nephropathy, and to decrease the rate of diabetes-related morbidity and mortality [58,59]. These positive effects are based on the established mode of verapamil, i.e., the blockade of L-type calcium channels resulting in a decrease of intracellular calcium level followed by an inhibition of TXNIP transcription [19]. In this context, tissue with a high expression level of L-type calcium channels, as the heart or the β-cells, consequently benefits from the TXNIP inhibition and positive effects have been shown in diabetic heart disease [60,61].

A recently published exploratory study of Xu et al. assessed the potential systemic changes in response to verapamil treatment by global proteomics analyzed by using liquid chromatography-tandem mass spectrometry (LC-MS) and revealed positive systemic and cellular effects of orally administered verapamil in TD1 subjects [57]. The initial trial was registered by clincicaltrials.gov (NCT02372253 2/20/2015) and previous research was published by Ovalle et al. 2018 [18]. The participants were randomized to oral verapamil (360 mg sustained-release daily) or placebo.

In this study, focusing on continuous use of verapamil, several positive effects, such as delayed T1D progression, promotion of endogenous β-cell function and consecutive lowered insulin requirements by continuous verapamil application were revealed. These positive effects were sustained for at least two years by regular application and were lost upon discontinuation. No further follow up after two years was performed in this exploratory trial. Therefore, the current studies point out crucial mechanistic and clinically beneficial effects of administered verapamil in T1D patients [57]. These positive effects of orally administered verapamil might be assumed by TXNIP inhibition causing β-cell protective and anti-diabetic effects. Analyzing chromogranin A (CHGA) serum levels as a potential therapeutic marker before and after treatment revealed a positive correlation with loss of β-cell function, reflected changes in verapamil treatment and discontinuation and persisted over a follow up time of at least two years. In summary, the results of this exploratory study suggested that a continuous orally administered verapamil treatment in T1D individuals may lower insulin requirements and decelerate disease progression for at least two years after diagnosis. These positive effects are associated with normalization of CHGA levels, and anti-oxidative effects, and immunomodulatory gene expression profile in pancreatic isles. The complex interaction is pictured in Figure 3. [57]. All these changes might contribute to the overall beneficial effects of verapamil use.

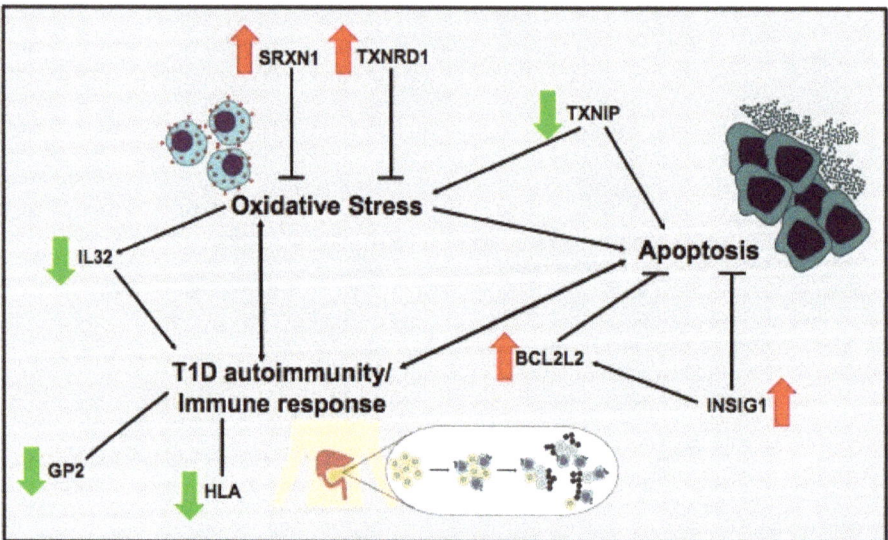

Figure 3. Systemic and cellular effects of verapamil treatment in subjects with type 1 diabetes, [57]. Abbreviations: TXNIP, Thioredoxin interacting protein; IL32, interleukin 32; BCL2L2, Bcl-2-like protein2; GP2, glycoprotein2; INSIG1, insulin-induced gene1; HLA, human leucocyte antigen; TXNRD1, Thioredoxin reductase; SRXN1, sulfiredoxin reductase; red arrow, represents upregulation by verapamil; green arrow, represents downregulation by verapamil.

These reported beneficial findings have to be confirmed in larger studies and might improve diabetes control in subjects with T1D in the future [18,57].

3.3.3. Clinical Implications in Type 2 Diabetes (T2D)

In a retrospective population-based cohort study from the Taiwan's National Health Insurance Research Database, regular oral verapamil use was associated with a decreased incidence of T2D in patients with unknown history of diabetes in comparison to a matched group of patients treated with other CCB with an adjusted hazard ratio 0.80 [6]. These positive findings are supported by the observational data analyses from the International Verapamil SR/Trandolapril (INVEST) studies, which revealed a lower risk for developing diabetes as well as the data derived from the study using the Reasons for Geographic and Racial Differences in Stroke (REGARDS) cohort, where lower fasting blood glucose levels were shown in patients using verapamil compared to subjects with diabetes without CCB [25–27]. The results of both mentioned observational studies highlight the positive effects of orally administered verapamil as a potentially preventive agent in T2D development. Next to these preventive aspects, positive results regarding the inhibition of gluconeogenesis are reported in T2D patients, which contributes to improved glucose homeostasis in T2D individuals [62].

Next to the reported studies, which have shown a lower incidence of T2D in verapamil-treated subjects, Malayeri et al. could reveal positive effects in T2D subjects in a randomized, double-blind, placebo-controlled trial [33]. In this study, verapamil administration showed a better glycemic control by means of decrease of HbA1c, decrease of TXNIP expression and increased glucagon-like peptide-1 receptor (GLP1R) mRNA providing increasing β-cell survival [33]. Additional findings by Carbovale et al. revealed significantly lowered plasma glucose levels in verapamil-treated subjects with T2D [63].

On this account, verapamil may serve as an effective oral adjunct therapy in combination with oral antidiabetic drugs in T2D patients in the future as it is safe, improves glycemic control, and might preserve β-cells function as demonstrated in T1D and T2D mouse models [21].

These previously described positive effects of orally administered verapamil, based on retrospective population-based and observational data analyses [6,25–27] as well as the presented data of a randomized, double-blind, placebo-controlled trial [33], could elucidate the positive effects of TXNIP regulation on glucose metabolism. Additionally, positive findings were revealed by Hong et al. in mouse models of T2D, who demonstrated for the first time new mechanistic insights and novel links between TXNIP and proinflammatory cytokines and microRNA signaling [50]. Furthermore, latest research results by Wu et al. revealed positive effects of verapamil use in type 2 diabetic rats on bone mass, microstructure as well as macro- and nano mechanical properties of the femur [64]. Taken together these several positive effects emphasize the important role of TXNIP and its effects on the pancreatic β-cell and TXNIP expression in T2D and underline through various systemic and cellular effects its potential as an adjunctive therapeutic approach.

4. Discussion

Since loss of functional β-cell mass is one of the key aspects of diabetes in general, different therapeutical approaches have been established in past decades in order to halt this process [20]. Chronic increased intracellular Ca^{2+} levels seem to contribute to impaired β-cell function and are associated with long term β-cell impairment. In this regard, excitotoxicity or overnutrition and the combination of both stresses seem to play an important role, as they might cause alterations in the β-cells transcriptome, mitochondrial energy metabolism, fatty acid β-oxidation, and mitochondrial biogenesis [65].

Next to the current physical activity recommendations of 150 min of moderate-intensity aerobic exercise per week resulting in optimized glycemic control in individuals with diabetes [66,67], additional early oral verapamil usage has been reported to improve insulin-stimulated glucose transport in skeletal muscle, resulting in optimized glycemic control and improved insulin sensitivity.

Next to the mentioned positive effects of orally administered verapamil on the β-cell preservation and the improved glycemic control [31,48], several overall beneficial effects observed with verapamil have been illustrated [57]. In summary, in our opinion these far reaching cellular and systemic regulatory effects seem to contribute to the positive assessment of verapamil, referring to its impact on diabetes. Next to the regulating effects on the thioredoxin system [57], in individuals with diabetes, who are predisposed to micro- and macrovascular complications during their lifetime, the management of autoimmune-related injury has to be focused. Verapamil promotes by regulation of the thioredoxin system several antioxidative, anti-apoptotic and immunomodulatory interactions in the human pancreatic islets [57]. Current scientific evidence suggests that TXNIP-targeting therapeutics, such as verapamil, seem to play an important role as central regulators of whole-body glucose homeostasis [41]; nevertheless, the basic molecular mechanisms of how TXNIP interacts with other proteins in different cellular tissues is not fully understood. In this context, up to now the interaction between TXNIP and glucagon is not completely understood, but Thielen et al. could identify a novel orally substituted quinazoline sulfonamide, SRI-37330, with an excellent safety profile and inhibition of TXNIP in human islets, inhibition of glucagon function and secretion, lowering hepatic glucose production and strong anti-diabetic effects in a mouse model of T1D [68]. These reported findings on SRI-37330 are consistent with previous observations on TXNIP targeting by blockage of the L-type calcium channels with verapamil. These positive effects for verapamil have been shown in mouse models [19,43], in a randomized controlled trial in individuals with T1D [18], as well as the association with reduced incidence of newly diagnosed T2D [6,25,26,42] and better overall glycemic control in subjects with diabetes [27]. By the lack of validated clinical approaches for detecting insulitis and β-cell decline in T1D preclinical models to diagnose eventual diabetes and to monitor the efficacy of therapeutical interventions, ultrasound imaging of the pancreatic perfusion dynamics revealed delayed diabetes development by orally administered verapamil [69]. These therapeutic strategies might provide a deployable future predictive marker for therapeutic prevention in asymptomatic T1D individuals [69].

Nevertheless, verapamil is a blood pressure medication and an anti-arrhythmic drug and its TXNIP capacity is linked to its function as L-type calcium channel blocker [68]. Therefore, in our opinion the daily administrated verapamil has to be limited to certain patient populations, especially those who tend to hypotension and left ventricular systolic dysfunction, suffer from hepatopathy or might be predisposed for potential polypharmacy drug interactions. These side effects might prohibit its regular clinical prescription.

Other important points that have to be mentioned are the lack of data referring to the long-term application of verapamil, specifically in its indication as a diabetes-modifying drug. The present exploratory studies reveal some far-reaching systemic and cellular effects of verapamil treatment in the context of T1D [57]. Next to the described preservation of β-cell function in the pancreatic tissue, unappreciated positive connections between immune system, regulation of proinflammatory cytokines, lowering of CHGA in response to verapamil use were revealed and might help to dampen the associated autoimmune processes in T1D [57]. In our opinion, these interesting aspects contribute to the positive overall effects of verapamil in diabetes. Nevertheless, the current scientific studies were limited to small numbers of subjects. In this context, the VER-A-T1D trial (VER-A-T1D; NCT04545151) as a multicenter, randomized, double-blind, placebo-controlled study will evaluate the effect of orally administered verapamil on the preservation of β-cell function as measured by stimulated c-peptide levels after 12 months. Furthermore, another multinational trial investigates the use of verapamil in children and adolescents with newly diagnosed T1D to assess hybrid closed loop therapy and verapamil for β-cell preservation in new onset T1D (CLVer; NCT04233034), which was initiated in July 2020 and will be completed in September 2022. Nevertheless, the outcomes of both initiated studies and the presented scientific research in general are limited to a small number of participants and a short follow-up time with a lack of long-term follow-up results. Future research and longer follow-up periods will be of great interest for the scientific community, such as safety profile and side effects, as well as their daily practicability regarding the regular continuous verapamil use as a new innovative therapeutical approach. In the end the previously described positive effects of oral adjunct verapamil administration in subjects with T1D have to be confirmed in larger studies.

5. Conclusions

In conclusion, daily orally administered CCB verapamil added early to standard therapy in diabetes, mainly T1D, might contribute to establishing an effective adjuvant T1D therapy. Inhibition of β-cells TXNIP expression seems to represent a new therapeutical approach for the future prevention and therapy of diabetes, while preserving and promoting the person's own endogenous β-cell function as well as optimizing overall glucose control by reducing exogenous insulin requirements and reducing hypoglycemic risk. Next to the mediated β-cell preservation, far-reaching positive systemic and cellular effects by daily orally administrated verapamil use seem to dampen the associated autoimmune processes in T1D. In patients with no history of diabetes mellitus, a decreased incidence of T2D could be revealed in observational data analyses compared to the usage of other CCB. This additional safe and effective novel approach might provide an adjunctive therapeutical treatment option in the future management of diabetes mellitus and has to be confirmed in further clinical investigation in larger patient cohorts.

Author Contributions: Conceptualization, P.Z. and F.A.; methodology, O.M.; software, P.Z.; validation, O.M.; formal analysis, O.M.; investigation, P.Z.; writing—original draft preparation, P.Z.; writing—review and editing, F.A., M.L.E., S.H., M.P.E. and O.M.; supervision, F.A.; project administration, O.M. All authors have read and agreed to the published version of the manuscript.

Funding: Funded by the Deutsche Forschungsgemeinschaft (DFG, German Research Foundation)—491183248.

Institutional Review Board Statement: Not applicable.

Informed Consent Statement: Not applicable.

Data Availability Statement: Not applicable.

Conflicts of Interest: M.L.E. received a KESS2/European Social Fund scholarship and travel grants from Novo Nordisk A/S and Sanofi-Aventis. F.A. received speaker honoraria from Eli Lilly, Merck Sharp & Dome, Boehringer Ingelheim, AstraZeneca and Amgen. O.M. has received lecture fees from Medtronic, Sanofi-Aventis and Novo Nordisk A/S, Novo Nordisk AT, Novo Nordisk UK, Medtronic AT, Sanofi-Aventis, research grants from Sêr Cymru II COFUND fellowship/European Union, Novo Nordisk A/S, Sanofi-Aventis, Dexcom Inc., and Novo Nordisk AT as well as material funding from Abbott Diabetes Care. P.Z. received speaker honoraria from Bayer, Daiichi Sankyō, Amarin Germany GmbH, and AstraZeneca GmbH. All other authors have no conflict of interest relevant to the article to declare.

References

1. Saeedi, P.; Petersohn, I.; Salpea, P.; Malanda, B.; Karuranga, S.; Unwin, N.; Colagiuri, S.; Guariguata, L.; Motala, A.A.; Ogurtsova, K.; et al. Global and regional diabetes prevalence estimates for 2019 and projections for 2030 and 2045: Results from the International Diabetes Federation Diabetes Atlas, 9th edition. *Diabetes Res. Clin. Pract.* **2019**, *157*, 107843. [CrossRef] [PubMed]
2. Boyko, E.J.; Magliano, D.G.; Karuranga, S.; Piemonte, L.; Riley, P.; Saeedi, P.; Sun, H. IDF Diabetes Atlas, 10 th Edition Committee. 2021. Available online: https://diabetesatlas.org/idfawp/resource-files/2021/07/IDF_Atlas_10th_Edition_2021.pdf (accessed on 19 June 2022).
3. Lu, J.; Xia, Q.; Zhou, Q. How to make insulin-producing pancreatic β cells for diabetes treatment. *Sci. China Life Sci.* **2017**, *60*, 239–248. [CrossRef] [PubMed]
4. Tuluc, P.; Theiner, T.; Jacobo-Piqueras, N.; Geisler, S. Role of High Voltage-Gated Ca^{2+} Channel Subunits in Pancreatic β-Cell Insulin Release. From Structure to Function. *Cells* **2021**, *10*, 2004. [CrossRef] [PubMed]
5. Campbell, J.E.; Newgard, C.B. Mechanisms controlling pancreatic islet cell function in insulin secretion. *Nat. Rev. Mol. Cell Biol.* **2021**, *22*, 142–158. [CrossRef]
6. Yin, T.; Kuo, S.-C.; Chang, Y.-Y.; Chen, Y.-T.; Wang, K.-W.K. Verapamil Use Is Associated With Reduction of Newly Diagnosed Diabetes Mellitus. *J. Clin. Endocrinol. Metab.* **2017**, *102*, 2604–2610. [CrossRef]

7. Rickels, M.R.; Evans-Molina, C.; Bahnson, H.T.; Ylescupidez, A.; Nadeau, K.J.; Hao, W.; Clements, M.A.; Sherr, J.L.; Pratley, R.E.; Hannon, T.S.; et al. High residual C-peptide likely contributes to glycemic control in type 1 diabetes. *J. Clin. Investig.* **2020**, *130*, 1850–1862. [CrossRef]
8. Carr, A.L.J.; Oram, R.A.; Marren, S.M.; McDonald, T.J.; Narendran, P.; Andrews, R.C. Measurement of Peak C-Peptide at Diagnosis Informs Glycemic Control but not Hypoglycemia in Adults With Type 1 Diabetes. *J. Endocr. Soc.* **2021**, *5*, bvab127. [CrossRef]
9. Zenz, S.; Mader, J.K.; Regittnig, W.; Brunner, M.; Korsatko, S.; Boulgaropoulos, B.; Magnes, C.; Raml, R.; Narath, S.H.; Eller, P.; et al. Impact of C-Peptide Status on the Response of Glucagon and Endogenous Glucose Production to Induced Hypoglycemia in T1DM. *J. Clin. Endocrinol. Metab.* **2018**, *103*, 1408–1417. [CrossRef]
10. Narendran, P.; Jackson, N.; Daley, A.; Thompson, D.; Stokes, K.; Greenfield, S.; Charlton, M.; Curran, M.; Solomon, T.; Nouwen, A.; et al. Exercise to preserve β-cell function in recent-onset Type 1 diabetes mellitus (EXTOD)a randomized controlled pilot trial. *Diabet. Med.* **2017**, *34*, 1521–1531. [CrossRef]
11. Chetan, M.R.; Charlton, M.H.; Thompson, C.; Dias, R.P.; Andrews, R.C.; Narendran, P. The Type 1 diabetes 'honeymoon' period is five times longer in men who exercise: A case-control study. *Diabet. Med.* **2019**, *36*, 127–128. [CrossRef]
12. Pastore, M.-R.; Bazzigaluppi, E.; Belloni, C.; Arcovio, C.; Bonifacio, E.; Bosi, E. Six Months of Gluten-Free Diet Do Not Influence Autoantibody Titers, but Improve Insulin Secretion in Subjects at High Risk for Type 1 Diabetes. *J. Clin. Endocrinol. Metab.* **2003**, *88*, 162–165. [CrossRef] [PubMed]
13. Weber, K.S.; Buyken, A.E.; Nowotny, B.; Strassburger, K.; Simon, M.-C.; Pacini, G.; Szendroedi, J.; Müssig, K.; Roden, M. The Impact of Dietary Factors on Glycemic Control, Insulin Sensitivity and Secretion in the First Years after Diagnosis of Diabetes. *Exp. Clin. Endocrinol. Diabetes* **2016**, *124*, 230–238. [CrossRef] [PubMed]
14. Bo, S.; Gentile, L.; Castiglione, A.; Prandi, V.; Canil, S.; Ghigo, E.; Ciccone, G. C-peptide and the risk for incident complications and mortality in type 2 diabetic patients: A retrospective cohort study after a 14-year follow-up. *Eur. J. Endocrinol.* **2012**, *167*, 173–180. [CrossRef] [PubMed]
15. Steffes, M.W.; Sibley, S.; Jackson, M.; Thomas, W. β-Cell Function and the Development of Diabetes-Related Complications in the Diabetes Control and Complications Trial. *Diabetes Care* **2003**, *26*, 832–836. [CrossRef] [PubMed]
16. Davis, A.K.; DuBose, S.N.; Haller, M.J.; Miller, K.M.; DiMeglio, L.A.; Bethin, K.E.; Goland, R.S.; Greenberg, E.M.; Liljenquist, D.R.; Ahmann, A.J.; et al. Prevalence of Detectable C-Peptide according to Age at Diagnosis and Duration of Type 1 Diabetes. *Diabetes Care* **2015**, *38*, 476–481. [CrossRef] [PubMed]
17. von Scholten, B.J.; Kreiner, F.F.; Gough, S.C.L.; von Herrath, M. Current and future therapies for type 1 diabetes. *Diabetologia* **2021**, *64*, 1037–1048. [CrossRef]
18. Ovalle, F.; Grimes, T.; Xu, G.; Patel, A.J.; Grayson, T.B.; Thielen, L.A.; Li, P.; Shalev, A. Verapamil and beta cell function in adults with recent-onset type 1 diabetes. *Nat. Med.* **2018**, *24*, 1108–1112. [CrossRef]
19. Xu, G.; Chen, J.; Jing, G.; Shalev, A. Preventing β-Cell Loss and Diabetes With Calcium Channel Blockers. *Diabetes* **2012**, *61*, 848–856. [CrossRef]
20. Pathak, V.; Pathak, N.M.; O'Neill, C.L.; Guduric-Fuchs, J.; Medina, R.J. Therapies for Type 1 Diabetes: Current Scenario and Future Perspectives. *Clin. Med. Insights Endocrinol. Diabetes* **2019**, *12*, 117955141984452. [CrossRef]
21. Chen, Y.-S.; Weng, S.-J.; Chang, S.-H.; Li, R.-Y.; Shane, G.-T.; Hsu, J.-P.; Yeh, S.-W.; Chang, A.-C.; Lee, M.-J. Evaluating the antidiabetic effects of R-verapamil in type 1 and type 2 diabetes mellitus mouse models. *PLoS ONE* **2021**, *16*, e0255405. [CrossRef]
22. Bergson, P.; Lipkind, G.; Lee, S.P.; Duban, M.-E.; Hanck, R.A. Verapamil Block of T-Type Calcium Channels. *Mol. Pharmacol.* **2011**, *79*, 411–419. [CrossRef] [PubMed]
23. Reynolds, N.A.; Wagstaff, A.J.; Keam, S.J. Trandolapril/Verapamil Sustained Release. *Drugs* **2005**, *65*, 1893–1914. [CrossRef] [PubMed]
24. Pratley, R.E.; Weyer, C. The role of impaired early insulin secretion in the pathogenesis of Type II diabetes mellitus. *Diabetologia* **2001**, *44*, 929–945. [CrossRef]
25. Cooper-DeHoff, R.; Cohen, J.D.; Bakris, G.L.; Messerli, F.H.; Erdine, S.; Hewkin, A.C.; Kupfer, S.; Pepine, C.J. Predictors of Development of Diabetes Mellitus in Patients With Coronary Artery Disease Taking Antihypertensive Medications (Findings from the INternational VErapamil SR-Trandolapril STudy [INVEST]). *Am. J. Cardiol.* **2006**, *98*, 890–894. [CrossRef] [PubMed]
26. Cooper-DeHoff, R.M.; Aranda, J.M., Jr.; Gaxiola, E.; Cangiano, J.L.; Garcia-Barreto, D.; Conti, C.R.; Hewkin, A.; Pepine, C.J. Blood pressure control and cardiovascular outcomes in high-risk Hispanic patients—Findings From the International Verapamil SR/Trandolapril Study (INVEST). *Am. Heart J.* **2006**, *151*, 1072–1079. [CrossRef] [PubMed]
27. Khodneva, Y.; Shalev, A.; Frank, S.J.; Carson, A.P.; Safford, M.M. Calcium channel blocker use is associated with lower fasting serum glucose among adults with diabetes from the REGARDS study. *Diabetes Res. Clin. Pract.* **2016**, *115*, 115–121. [CrossRef]
28. Kim, B.-Y.; Jung, C.-H.; Mok, J.-O.; Kang, S.-K.; Kim, C.-H. Association between serum C-peptide levels and chronic microvascular complications in Korean type 2 diabetic patients. *Geol. Rundsch.* **2011**, *49*, 9–15. [CrossRef]
29. Sari, R.; Balci, M.K. Relationship between C peptide and chronic complications in type-2 diabetes mellitus. *J. Natl. Med. Assoc.* **2005**, *97*, 1113–1118.
30. Juntti-Berggren, L.; Larsson, O.; Rorsman, P.; Ammala, C.; Bokvist, K.; Wahlander, K.; Nicotera, P.; Dypbukt, J.; Orrenius, S.; Hallberg, A.; et al. Increased activity of L-type Ca^{2+} channels exposed to serum from patients with type I diabetes. *Science* **1993**, *261*, 86–90. [CrossRef]
31. Lam, T.K.T.; Cherney, D.Z.I. Beta cell preservation in patients with type 1 diabetes. *Nat. Med.* **2018**, *24*, 1089–1090. [CrossRef]

32. Gilbert, E.R.; Liu, D. Regulation of Insulin Synthesis and Secretion and Pancreatic Beta-Cell Dysfunction in Diabetes. *Curr. Diabetes Rev.* **2012**, *9*, 25–53. [CrossRef]
33. Malayeri, A.; Zakerkish, M.; Ramesh, F.; Galehdari, H.; Hemmati, A.A.; Angali, K.A. The Effect of Verapamil on TXNIP Gene Expression, GLP1R mRNA, FBS, HbA1c, and Lipid Profile in T2DM Patients Receiving Metformin and Sitagliptin. *Diabetes Ther.* **2021**, *12*, 2701–2713. [CrossRef] [PubMed]
34. Weir, G.C.; Gaglia, J.; Bonner-Weir, S. Inadequate β-cell mass is essential for the pathogenesis of type 2 diabetes. *Lancet Diabetes Endocrinol.* **2020**, *8*, 249–256. [CrossRef]
35. Hara, M.; Fowler, J.; Bell, G.; Philipson, L. Resting beta-cells—A functional reserve? *Diabetes Metab.* **2016**, *42*, 157–161. [CrossRef]
36. Halban, P.A.; Polonsky, K.S.; Bowden, D.W.; Hawkins, M.A.; Ling, C.; Mather, K.J.; Powers, A.C.; Rhodes, C.J.; Sussel, L.; Weir, G.C. β-Cell Failure in Type 2 Diabetes: Postulated Mechanisms and Prospects for Prevention and Treatment. *Diabetes Care* **2014**, *37*, 1751–1758. [CrossRef] [PubMed]
37. Ferrannini, E. The Stunned β Cell: A Brief History. *Cell Metab.* **2010**, *11*, 349–352. [CrossRef] [PubMed]
38. Guo, S.; Dai, C.; Guo, M.; Taylor, B.; Harmon, J.S.; Sander, M.; Robertson, R.P.; Powers, A.C.; Stein, R. Inactivation of specific β cell transcription factors in type 2 diabetes. *J. Clin. Investig.* **2013**, *123*, 3305–3316. [CrossRef]
39. Ferrannini, E.; Natali, A.; Muscelli, E.; Nilsson, P.M.; Golay, A.; Laakso, M.; Beck-Nielsen, H.; Mari, A. Natural history and physiological determinants of changes in glucose tolerance in a non-diabetic population: The RISC Study. *Diabetologia* **2011**, *54*, 1507–1516. [CrossRef]
40. Ward, W.K.; Bolgiano, D.C.; McKnight, B.; Halter, J.B.; Porte, D. Diminished B cell secretory capacity in patients with noninsulin-dependent diabetes mellitus. *J. Clin. Investig.* **1984**, *74*, 1318–1328. [CrossRef]
41. Yoshihara, E. TXNIP/TBP-2: A Master Regulator for Glucose Homeostasis. *Antioxidants* **2020**, *9*, 765. [CrossRef]
42. Thielen, L.; Shalev, A. Diabetes pathogenic mechanisms and potential new therapies based upon a novel target called TXNIP. *Curr. Opin. Endocrinol. Diabetes Obes.* **2018**, *25*, 75–80. [CrossRef]
43. Chen, J.; Hui, S.T.; Couto, F.M.; Mungrue, I.; Davis, D.B.; Attie, A.D.; Lusis, A.J.; Davis, R.A.; Shalev, A. Thioredoxin-interacting protein deficiency induces Akt/Bcl-xL signaling and pancreatic beta-cell mass and protects against diabetes. *FASEB J.* **2008**, *22*, 3581–3594. [CrossRef] [PubMed]
44. Muoio, D.M. TXNIP Links Redox Circuitry to Glucose Control. *Cell Metab.* **2007**, *5*, 412–414. [CrossRef]
45. Minn, A.H.; Hafele, C.; Shalev, A. Thioredoxin-Interacting Protein Is Stimulated by Glucose through a Carbohydrate Response Element and Induces β-Cell Apoptosis. *Endocrinology* **2005**, *146*, 2397–2405. [CrossRef] [PubMed]
46. Shalev, A.; Pise-Masison, C.A.; Radonovich, M.; Hoffmann, S.C.; Hirshberg, B.; Brady, J.N.; Harlan, D.M. Oligonucleotide Microarray Analysis of Intact Human Pancreatic Islets: Identification of Glucose-Responsive Genes and a Highly Regulated TGFβ Signaling Pathway. *Endocrinology* **2002**, *143*, 3695–3698. [CrossRef]
47. Shalev, A. Lack of TXNIP protects β-cells against glucotoxicity. *Biochem. Soc. Trans.* **2008**, *36*, 963–965. [CrossRef]
48. Parikh, H.; Carlsson, E.; Chutkow, W.A.; Johansson, L.E.; Storgaard, H.; Poulsen, P.; Saxena, R.; Ladd, C.; Schulze, P.C.; Mazzini, M.J.; et al. TXNIP Regulates Peripheral Glucose Metabolism in Humans. *PLOS Med.* **2007**, *4*, e158. [CrossRef]
49. Yoshihara, E.; Fujimoto, S.; Inagaki, N.; Okawa, K.; Masaki, S.; Yodoi, J.; Masutani, H. Disruption of TBP-2 ameliorates insulin sensitivity and secretion without affecting obesity. *Nat. Commun.* **2010**, *1*, 127. [CrossRef]
50. Hong, K.; Xu, G.; Grayson, T.B.; Shalev, A. Cytokines Regulate β-Cell Thioredoxin-interacting Protein (TXNIP) via Distinct Mechanisms and Pathways. *J. Biol. Chem.* **2016**, *291*, 8428–8439. [CrossRef]
51. Karunakaran, U.; Moon, J.S.; Lee, H.W.; Won, K.C. CD36 initiated signaling mediates ceramide-induced TXNIP expression in pancreatic beta-cells. *Biochim. Biophys. Acta-Mol. Basis Dis.* **2015**, *1852*, 2414–2422. [CrossRef]
52. Reich, E.; Tamary, A.; Sionov, R.V.; Melloul, D. Involvement of thioredoxin-interacting protein (TXNIP) in glucocorticoid-mediated beta cell death. *Diabetologia* **2012**, *55*, 1048–1057. [CrossRef] [PubMed]
53. Wang, J.; Wang, J.; Wang, J.-J.; Zhang, W.-F.; Jiao, X.-Y. Role of autophagy in TXNIP overexpression-induced apoptosis of INS-1 islet cells. *Sheng Li Xue Bao Acta Physiol. Sin.* **2017**, *69*, 445–451.
54. Muoio, D.M.; Newgard, C.B. Obesity-Related Derangements in Metabolic Regulation. *Annu. Rev. Biochem.* **2006**, *75*, 367–401. [CrossRef] [PubMed]
55. Dykstra, H.; LaRose, C.; Fisk, C.; Waldhart, A.; Meng, X.; Zhao, G.; Wu, N. TXNIP interaction with GLUT1 depends on PI(4,5)P2. *Biochim. Biophys. Acta-Biomembr.* **2021**, *1863*, 183757. [CrossRef]
56. Tang, L.; El-Din, T.M.G.; Swanson, T.M.; Pryde, D.C.; Scheuer, T.; Zheng, L.; Catterall, W.A. Structural basis for inhibition of a voltage-gated Ca2+ channel by Ca^{2+} antagonist drugs. *Nature* **2016**, *537*, 117–121. [CrossRef]
57. Xu, G.; Grimes, T.D.; Grayson, T.B.; Chen, J.; Thielen, L.A.; Tse, H.M.; Li, P.; Kanke, M.; Lin, T.-T.; Schepmoes, A.A.; et al. Exploratory study reveals far reaching systemic and cellular effects of verapamil treatment in subjects with type 1 diabetes. *Nat. Commun.* **2022**, *13*, 1159. [CrossRef]
58. Wondafrash, D.Z.; Nire'A, A.T.; Tafere, G.G.; Desta, D.M.; Berhe, D.A.; Zewdie, K.A. Thioredoxin-Interacting Protein as a Novel Potential Therapeutic Target in Diabetes Mellitus and Its Underlying Complications. *Diabetes Metab. Syndr. Obes. Targets Ther.* **2020**, *13*, 43–51. [CrossRef]
59. Lido, P.; Romanello, D.; Tesauro, M.; Bei, A.; Perrone, M.A.; Palazzetti, D.; Noce, A.; di Lullo, L.; Calò, L.; Cice, G. Verapamil: Prevention and treatment of cardio-renal syndromes in diabetic hypertensive patients? *Eur. Rev. Med. Pharmacol. Sci.* **2022**, *26*, 1524–1534. [CrossRef]

60. Afzal, N.; Ganguly, P.K.; Dhalla, K.S.; Pierce, G.N.; Singal, P.K.; Dhalla, N.S. Beneficial Effects of Verapamil in Diabetic Cardiomyopathy. *Diabetes* **1988**, *37*, 936–942. [CrossRef]
61. Chen, J.; Cha-Molstad, H.; Szabo, A.; Shalev, A. Diabetes induces and calcium channel blockers prevent cardiac expression of proapoptotic thioredoxin-interacting protein. *Am. J. Physiol. Metab.* **2009**, *296*, E1133–E1139. [CrossRef]
62. Thrane, M.T.; Holst, J.J.; Busch-Sørensen, M.; Sjøstrand, H.; Sengelov, H.; Lyngsøe, J. Influence of short term verapamil treatment on glucose metabolism in patients with non-insulin dependent diabetes mellitus. *Eur. J. Clin. Pharmacol.* **1991**, *41*, 401–404. [CrossRef]
63. Carnovale, C.; Dassano, A.; Mosini, G.; Mazhar, F.; D'Addio, F.; Pozzi, M.; Radice, S.; Fiorina, P.; Clementi, E. The β-cell effect of verapamil-based treatment in patients with type 2 diabetes: A systematic review. *Geol. Rundsch.* **2020**, *57*, 117–131. [CrossRef] [PubMed]
64. Wu, X.; Gong, H.; Hu, X.; Shi, P.; Cen, H.; Li, C. Effect of verapamil on bone mass, microstructure and mechanical properties in type 2 diabetes mellitus rats. *BMC Musculoskelet. Disord.* **2022**, *23*, 363. [CrossRef] [PubMed]
65. Osipovich, A.B.; Stancill, J.S.; Cartailler, J.-P.; Dudek, K.D.; Magnuson, M.A. Excitotoxicity and Overnutrition Additively Impair Metabolic Function and Identity of Pancreatic β-Cells. *Diabetes* **2020**, *69*, 1476–1491. [CrossRef] [PubMed]
66. Colberg, S.R.; Sigal, R.J.; Yardley, J.E.; Riddell, M.C.; Dunstan, D.W.; Dempsey, P.C.; Horton, E.S.; Castorino, K.; Tate, D.F. Physical Activity/Exercise and Diabetes: A Position Statement of the American Diabetes Association. *Diabetes Care* **2016**, *39*, 2065–2079. [CrossRef]
67. Mendes, R.; Sousa, N.; Almeida, A.; Subtil, P.; Guedes-Marques, F.; Reis, V.; Themudo-Barata, J.L. Exercise prescription for patients with type 2 diabetes—a synthesis of international recommendations: Narrative review: Table 1. *Br. J. Sports Med.* **2016**, *50*, 1379–1381. [CrossRef]
68. Thielen, L.A.; Chen, J.; Jing, G.; Moukha-Chafiq, O.; Xu, G.; Jo, S.; Grayson, T.B.; Lu, B.; Li, P.; Augelli-Szafran, C.E.; et al. Identification of an Anti-diabetic, Orally Available Small Molecule that Regulates TXNIP Expression and Glucagon Action. *Cell Metab.* **2020**, *32*, 353–365.e8. [CrossRef]
69. Pham, V.T.; Ciccaglione, M.; Ramirez, D.G.; Benninger, R.K.P. Ultrasound Imaging of Pancreatic Perfusion Dynamics Predicts Therapeutic Prevention of Diabetes in Preclinical Models of Type 1 Diabetes. *Ultrasound Med. Biol.* **2022**, *48*, 1336–1347. [CrossRef]

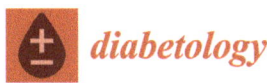

Review

Insulin in Frail, Older People with Type 2 Diabetes—Low Threshold for Therapy

Ahmed Abdelhafiz [1,*], Shail Bisht [1], Iva Kovacevic [1], Daniel Pennells [1] and Alan Sinclair [2,3]

1. Department of Geriatric Medicine, Rotherham General Hospital, Moorgate Road, Rotherham S60 2UD, UK; shail.bisht@nhs.net (S.B.); iva.kovacevic@nhs.net (I.K.); d.pennells@nhs.net (D.P.)
2. King's College, London WC2R 2LS, UK; sinclair.5@btinternet.com
3. Foundation for Diabetes Research in Older People (fDROP), Droitwich Spa WR9 0QH, UK
* Correspondence: ahmedhafiz@hotmail.com; Tel.: +44-01709427576

Abstract: The global prevalence of comorbid diabetes and frailty is increasing due to increasing life expectancy. Frailty appears to be a metabolically heterogeneous condition that may affect the clinical decision making on the most appropriate glycaemic target and the choice of the most suitable hypoglycaemic agent for each individual. The metabolic profile of frailty appears to span across a spectrum that starts at an anorexic malnourished (AM) frail phenotype on one end and a sarcopenic obese (SO) phenotype on the other. The AM phenotype is characterised by significant weight loss and less insulin resistance compared with the SO phenotype, which is characterised by significant obesity and increased insulin resistance. Therefore, due to weight loss, insulin therapy may be considered as an early option in the AM frail phenotype. Insulin-related weight gain and the anabolic properties of insulin may be an advantage to this anorexic phenotype. There is emerging evidence to support the idea that insulin may improve the muscle function of older people with diabetes, although this evidence still needs further confirmation in future large-scale prospective studies. Long acting insulin analogues have a lower risk of hypoglycaemia, comapred to intermediate acting insulins. Additionally their simple once daily regimen makes it more appropriate in frail older patients. Future research on the availability of new once-weekly insulin analogues is appealing. The goals of therapy are to achieve relaxed targets, avoid hypoglycaemia and to focus on the maintenance of quality of life in these vulnerable patients.

Keywords: older people; diabetes mellitus; management; insulin therapy; frailty; sarcopenia

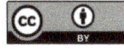

1. Introduction

The global prevalence of diabetes is increasing, particularly, in the older age groups. For example, 44% of people with diabetes are above the age of 65 years [1]. Frailty is an emerging new complication of diabetes and increasingly recognised in clinical guidelines for diabetes management [2–6]. Frailty is not a homogeneous concept and appears to have a spectrum of different metabolic phenotypes, which may influence the choice of the most suitable hypoglycaemic agents for an individual [6]. The metabolic spectrum of frailty starts by the anorexic malnourished (AM) phenotype with significant weight loss and less insulin resistance on one end, and the sarcopenic obese (SO) phenotype with excess weight and increased insulin resistance on the other end [6]. Based on our experience in managing older people with diabetes, we hypothesise that insulin therapy, especially the long-acting insulin analogues, may be a good option to be introduced early in the AM phenotype due to its anabolic effects and the possible positive benefits on muscle function and body weight. This manuscript reviews the potential positive effects of insulin on muscle function in older people (≥60 years of age) with diabetes, explores the hypoglycaemic safety of insulin analogues in this population and presents a literature-based recommendation for an early introduction of insulin in the AM frail phenotype.

2. Methods

We undertook a literature search of the following databases: Google Scholar, PubMed and Embase. Medical Subject Heading (MeSH) terms used were: diabetes mellitus, older people, old age, elderly, frailty, sarcopenia, muscle function, muscle strength, muscle mass, muscle quality, insulin, therapy, management, anabolic effects, quality of life and hypoglycaemia, individually and in combination. Articles were reviewed for relevance by abstract. A manual search of citations in the retrieved articles was performed in addition to the electronic literature search. The search for articles on the effect of insulin on skeletal muscle was limited to studies published over the last 10 years and reported clear outcomes. The search for articles on the safety of long-acting insulin analogues in older people was limited to studies published over the last 5 years. The inclusion criteria were: 1. Studies that reported the impact of insulin therapy on muscle mass, strength, quality or function, and 2. Studies that investigated the safety of long-acting insulin analogues in older people aged $\geq$60 years with diabetes. The exclusion criteria were: 1. Non-English language or non-human studies, 2. Studies with no clear outcome, 3. Studies that compared first- with second-generation long-acting insulin analogues and 4. Case reports, review articles, editorials, abstracts, conference proceedings or expert opinions. All articles derived from the search enquiry were independently examined by the authors and data were extracted from each study in a predesigned standardised information table that included author, study design, year of publication, country of origin, participants studied, aim of the study and the main findings. Any disagreements between authors were resolved by consensus.

3. Effects of Insulin on Skeletal Muscles

Although insulin has physiologic anabolic properties, data on the effects of insulin on skeletal muscle mass, strength or function are limited. Insulin may have the potential to improve muscle mass and increase body weight in frail, older people with diabetes, especially in the AM phenotype where insulin-associated weight gain could be seen as an advantage. Previous studies have shown that insulin can stimulate muscle protein synthesis and anabolism in younger individuals, but this anabolic effect is blunted in older people, which suggests that higher doses of insulin may be required to achieve this anabolic effect in older age groups [7,8]. Through our literature search and after the application of exclusion criteria, five studies investigated the effect of insulin on muscle function and were included in this manuscript. Although the evidence is limited, these studies have shown some emerging evidence that insulin may be associated with some positive effects on skeletal muscles of older people with diabetes. (Table 1) Tanaka et al., in their cross-sectional study of 191 older Japanese men, with a mean (SD) age of 60.2 (12.5) years, with type 2 diabetes mellitus, found endogenous insulin to be significantly and positively correlated with skeletal muscles mass of the upper and lower limbs [9]. Insulin levels were also significantly lower in subjects with sarcopenia compared to those without ($p < 0.05$) [9]. This may suggest that the reduction in endogenous insulin plays an important role in the pathogenesis of sarcopenia in older people with diabetes mellitus, and maintaining endogenous insulin secretion may be important to prevent sarcopenia. Although this study included a reasonably large sample size, it included only men and excluded patients on insulin therapy; therefore, it was not able to draw similar conclusions for women or investigate the effect of exogenous therapeutic insulin on skeletal muscles. Bouchi et al., in their retrospective analysis of 312 Japanese older patients with type 2 diabetes, with a mean (SD) age of 64 (11) years, showed the positive effect of insulin therapy on the skeletal muscle index. They also demonstrated an improvement of the decline in muscle mass in the lower extremities after one year of insulin treatment compared to those not on insulin [10]. They concluded that insulin treatment could attenuate the progression of sarcopenia in older people with type 2 diabetes. Compared to patients not on insulin therapy, those who received insulin had a significantly longer duration of diabetes (10 vs. 6 years, $p < 0.001$). It is speculated that, compared to patients who have had diabetes for a short duration, those with a long duration of diabetes exhibit lower endogenous insulin levels, resulting in impaired insulin signalling in skeletal muscles and lower muscle mass [11]. Therefore, the efficient supply of exogenous insulin could improve insulin signalling in the skeletal muscles, promote protein synthesis and protect against the loss of muscle mass among patients with a longer duration of diabetes [10]. Authors have also adjusted for change in muscle mass and HbA1c and found that the protective effects of insulin treatment on the decline in muscle mass may be independent of the improvement in glycaemic control. This is clinically relevant as muscle mass improvement may be achieved without tighter glycaemic control in older people with diabetes who are at an increased risk of hypoglycaemia. The cross-sectional analysis by Cui et al. found that insulin use was not significantly different among older people with combined diabetes and sarcopenia, and those with diabetes but no sarcopenia (68.4% vs. 74.5%, $p = 0.48$), respectively [12]. However, 36 out of 132 participants did not use exogenous insulin, and fasting insulin and HOMA-IR in the sarcopenia group were all significantly lower than those in the non-sarcopenia group ($p < 0.05$). In addition, the small sample size of this study (132 subjects) and the fact that the duration of diabetes in the sarcopenic and non-sarcopenic groups was similar, may have attenuated the significance effect between both groups. Recently, in the population-based KORA-Age study that included 118 older German people with type 2 diabetes, with a mean (SD) age of 74.6 (6.2) years, insulin therapy was associated with preserved muscle mass, but not muscle function parameters [13]. The strength of this study was the longitudinal design with a follow-up period of three years and the inclusion of relatively older participants with a longer duration of diabetes mellitus, with a mean (SD) duration of 10.1 (9.9) years, but it is limited by the small number of participants (only 20) treated with insulin. In addition, the discrepancy between the positive effects of insulin on muscle mass compared to its effects on muscle function needs future exploration. The most recent large prospective study conducted by Sugimoto et al., which included 588 Japanese older people with type 2 diabetes mellitus, with a mean age (SD) of 70.0 (8.0) years, found that insulin use significantly increased skeletal muscle mass index after one year of follow-up [14]. The strength of this study was the relatively large sample size, good number (25.9%) of participants on insulin treatment at baseline, its longitudinal design and the positive effect of insulin was independent of confounding factors. Although data from the above studies have their limitations, it appears that there is emerging evidence to suggest that insulin therapy may have some advantages on the skeletal muscle parameters of older people with diabetes.

Table 1. Recent studies exploring effects of insulin on skeletal muscle in older people with diabetes.

Study	Patients	Aim to	Main Findings
Tanaka K et al., cross-sectional, Japan, 2015 [9].	191 men with type 2 DM, mean (SD) age 60.2 (12.5) Y.	Examine association of muscle mass with endogenous insulin secretion.	A. Endogenous insulin significantly and positively correlated with muscle mass of arms and legs as well as RSMI ($p < 0.05$). B. Endogenous insulin significantly lower in subjects with compared to those without sarcopenia ($p < 0.05$).
Bouchi R et al., retrospective observational, Japan, 2017 [10].	312 patients with type 2 DM, mean (SD) age 64.0 (11.0) Y.	Examine impact of insulin treatment on muscle mass.	A. Insulin was protective against annual decline in SMI (standardized β 0.195; $p = 0.025$) adjusted for covariates. B. In a cohort matched by propensity scores, insulin significantly increased the 1-year change in SMI compared with non-insulin-treated group; mean (SE) 2.40 (0.98%) vs. −0.43 (0.98%), $p = 0.050$).
Cui M et al., cross-sectional, China, 2020 [12].	132 patients with type 2 DM, aged ≥65 Y.	Explore factors associated with sarcopenia.	A. Insulin use was not significantly different between patients with sarcopenia and those with no sarcopenia (68.4% vs. 74.5%, $p = 0.48$). B. Metformin was significantly less used in patients with compared to those with no sarcopenia (13.2% vs. 41.5%, $p = 0.002$).

Table 1. Cont.

Study	Patients	Aim to	Main Findings
Ferrari U et al., prospective, Germany, 2020 [13].	731 (118 type 2 DM) participants of KORA-Age study, mean (SD) age 74.6 (6.2) Y, F/UP 3 Y.	Investigate association of type 2 DM and insulin treatment with changes in muscle mass, muscle strength and physical performance.	A. DM associated with change in SMI (β −0.1 (95% CI −0.3 to −0.02) kg/m^2, p = 0.02), but not with a change in GS (β −0.9, 95% CI −1.9 to 0.04 kg) or TUG (β −0.1, 95% CI −0.7 to 0.5 s). B. Insulin therapy positively associated with change in SMI (β 0.6 (95% CI 0.3 to 0.9) kg/m^2, p = 0.001), but not in GS (β −1.6, 95% CI −4.1 to 0.8 kg) or TUG (β 1.6, 95% CI −0.2 to 3.4 s).
Sugimoto K et al., observational longitudinal, Japan, 2021 [14].	588 patients with type 2 DM, mean (SD) age 70.0 (8.0) Y, F/U 1Y.	Examine relationship between glycaemic control and effect of antidiabetic agents on sarcopenia.	After 382 (53) days of F/U: A. Frequency of sarcopenia non-significantly increased (7.8% vs. 6.3%, p = 0.12). B. Patients with ≥1% drop in HbA1c had significant increase in SMI (B = 0.113, p = 0.027), gait speed (B = 0.145, p = 0.002), but non-significant change in handgrip strength (B = −0.005, p = 0.914). C. Insulin use significantly increased SMI (B = 0.115, p = 0.022). D. Oral antidiabetic therapy has no effect on sarcopenia.

DM = Diabetes mellitus, SD = Standard deviation, Y = Year, RSMI = Relative skeletal muscle index, SMI = Skeletal muscle index, SE = Standard error, F/U = Follow-up, CI = Confidence interval, GS = Grip strength, TUG = Timed up and go.

4. Insulin Analogues Safety

Insulin analogues, such as insulin glargine, detemir and degludec, are structurally altered human insulins that mimic the pharmacokinetic properties of endogenous insulin more closely than intermediate-acting insulins. Because of the long duration of action and the less pronounced insulin peak, long-acting insulin analogues have less risk of hypoglycaemia especially nocturnal hypoglycaemia. The evidence of this benefit was conflicting in earlier clinical trials [15–22]. However, most of these earlier studies predominantly included patients under the age of 60 years, which caused it to be less powered in detecting the efficacy and safety of long-acting insulin analogues in older age groups who are at increased risk of hypoglycaemia and its severe consequences than younger people. Through our literature search and following the application of the exclusion criteria, five studies investigated the safety of long-acting insulin analogues in older people with diabetes and were included in this manuscript. The recent studies that included older people with type 2 diabetes have shown some benefits of the new long-acting insulin analogues, compared to the older human insulins (Table 2). Fujimoto et al. showed that twice-daily insulin degludec/insulin aspart to improve daily glucose level variability, morning and evening glucose control and quality of life (QOL) in 22 Japanese men, with a mean (SD) age of 68.0 (9.9) years, previously treated with premixed insulin [23]. However, there was no significant difference in the incidence of hypoglycaemia before and after insulin switching. The total and therapy-related QOL feeling scores favoured insulin degludec/insulin aspart; whereas social, physical and daily activities scores were not significantly different. The flexibility of injection timing and glycaemic control may explain the improvement in the total and therapy-related feeling subscores in the QOL questionnaire. However, this study was limited by the small sample size and the short duration of follow-up, which may suggest that the switch in the insulin regimen might not explain all the changes in the endpoints, and other factors, such as lifestyle changes and physicians' motivations, might have contributed to the results. Another limitation was that the incidence in hypoglycaemia may have not been accurate, because the frequency of this event was calculated based on self-measured blood glucose levels or patients' symptoms. Lipska et al., in their large retrospective observational study of 22,489 patients with type 2 diabetes, found that the initiation of a basal insulin analogue (glargine or detemir) was not associated with a reduced risk of hypoglycaemia-related emergency department (ED) visits or hospital admissions compared with NPH insulin. Glycaemic control was similar in both groups after one year of follow-up [24]. However, the population included in this study were relatively young, with a mean (SD) age of 60.2 (11.8) years. Previous studies using the national registries in Finland that included participants of similar ages to those presented in Lipska et al.'s study showed a significantly increased risk of hospitalisation related to severe hypoglycaemia with the use of NPH insulin compared with insulin detemir or glargine [25,26]. In addition, although Lipska et al.'s was a large study, only 1928 participants of the total 25,489 used insulin analogues, and despite matching on the propensity score quintiles, some differences between the two groups remained, suggesting that the study did not fully adjust for the confounding factors. Recently, Bradley et al. showed that the initiation of long-acting insulin analogues was associated with a lower risk of ED visits or hospitalisations for hypoglycaemia compared with NPH insulin in older patients (≥65 years) with type 2 diabetes in Medicare beneficiaries [27]. The strength of this study was the large sample size of 575,008 patients with type 2 diabetes, of an older age, with a mean (SD) of 74.9 (6.7) years, and the fact that a large proportion of patients were treated with insulin glargine (407,018 patients) or insulin detemir (141,588 patients). The hazard ratio (HR) for hypoglycaemia was 0.71, 95% confidence interval (CI) 0.63 to 0.80 for glargine vs. NPH insulin, and 0.72, 0.63 to 0.82 for detemir vs. NPH insulin. The older ages of the participants in this study compared to the study conducted by Lipska et al., suggest that age may have contributed to the disparity between the two studies [24]. In the post hoc analysis, Bradley et al. observed that in participants aged 65–68 years; the use of glargine or detemir was not associated with ED visits or hospitalisations for hypoglycaemia compared with NPH insulin [27]. However, in older participants (69–87 years of age), the use of long-acting analogues was associated with a reduced risk of hypoglycaemia compared with NPH insulin. Betônico et al. demonstrated better glycaemic control and fewer nocturnal hypoglycaemia in 34 patients, mean (SD) age 63.0 (7.0) years, using insulin glargine compared with 16 patients, with a mean (SD) age of 60.0 (8.7) years, using NPH insulin [28]. The importance of this study was that it included patients with chronic kidney disease (CKD) stages 3 and 4, which is more common in older people. CKD is associated with a slower insulin degradation, increasing its duration of action that might increase the risk of hypoglycaemia [29]. However, because the insulin analogue has no peak action, it showed less risk of hypoglycaemia in this population. This is clinically relevant as, with the progression of CKD, most hypoglycaemic medications need dose reductions, and the adjustment of these medications, in the face of renal impairment, may not be enough to keep diabetes under control, and therefore insulin is the most effective therapy in this situation [30]. Özçelik et al. showed that the switch from premixed and intensive insulin to twice daily degludec/aspart insulin was associated with a significant reduction in the daily insulin dose requirement and the incidence of hypoglycaemia [31]. The use of premixed and intensive insulin is a complex regimen and may not be an easy option for daily life in older people with diabetes; therefore, the switch to degludec/aspart insulin may be a less complex regimen, as demonstrated in this study and previous studies [32]. Figure 1 illustrates the advantage of the physiological, clinical and therapeutic properties of insulin in the AM frail phenotype.

Table 2. Recent studies exploring efficacy and safety of insulin analogues compared with human insulin.

Study	Patients	Aim to	Main Findings
Fujimoto K. et al., prospective, observational, Japan, 2018 [23].	22 patients with type 2 DM, mean (SD) age 68.0 (9.9) Y, treated with premixed insulin for 2 M, then IDegAsp for next 2 M.	Investigate changes in glucose variability and QOL during switch from premixed insulin to IDegAsp twice daily.	Switching to IDegAsp from premixed insulin: A. Improved daily glucose level variability, morning and evening glucose control and QOL. B. No change in day-to-day variability of morning fasting glucose levels.
Lipska KJ et al., retrospective observational, US, 2018 [24].	25,489 patients with type 2 DM initiated basal or NPH insulin, mean (SD) age 60.2 (11.8) Y. F/Up 1.7Y.	Compare rates of hypoglycaemia-related ED visits or hospitalisation associated with initiation of long-acting insulin analogues vs. NPH insulin.	A. In 1928 patients initiated on insulin analogue, there were 39 hypoglycaemia-related ED visits or hospital admissions (11.9 events, 95% CI 8.1 to 15.6/1000 person–years) compared with 354 events among 23,561 patients on NPH (8.8 events, 7.9 to 9.8/1000 person–years), $p = 0.07$). B. Adjusted HR 1.16, 95% CI, 0.71 to 1.78 for hypoglycaemia-related events with insulin analogue use. C. After one year, there was no significant difference in glycaemic control between both groups.
Bradley MC et al., retrospective, US, 2021 [27].	Medicare 575, 008 patients, mean (SD) age 74.9 (6.7) Y with type 2 DM, 407,018 initiated insulin glargine, 141,588 detemir, 26,402 NPH.	Examine risk of ED visits or hospitalisations due to hypoglycaemia in older community patients with type 2 DM who initiated long acting or NPH insulin.	A. Incidence rates for ED visits or hospitalisations for hypoglycaemia per 1000 person–years were 17.37 (95% CI 16.89 to17.84) for glargine and 26.64 (95% CI 26.01–27.3) for NPH. B. For detemir and NPH, incidence rates were 16.69 (15.92 to 17.51) and 25.04 (24.01 to 26.11), respectively. C. Glargine or detemir use associated with reduced risk of hypoglycaemia compared with NPH (HR for glargine vs. NPH 0.71, 95% CI 0.63 to 0.80, and detemir vs. NPH insulin 0.72, 0.63 to 0.82).
Betônico CC et al., prospective, randomized, 2-way, crossover, open-label, Brazil, 2019 [28].	34 patients with type 2 DM randomly assigned to glargine U100 {16 patients, mean (SD) age 63.0 (7.0) Y} or NPH {18 patients, mean (SD) age 60.0 (8.7) Y}.	Compare glycaemic response to glargine U100 or NPH in patients with type 2 DM and CKD stages 3 and 4.	A. After 24 weeks, mean HbA1c declined from 8.86% (72.7 mmol/mol) to 7.95% (62.8 mmol/mol) in glargine group, but increased from 8.21% (66.2 mmol/mol) to 8.44% (69.4 mmol/mol) in INPH group, $p = 0.029$. B. Incidence of nocturnal hypoglycaemia was 3 times lower with glargine (0.5 events/patient) than with INPH (1.5 events/patient; $p = 0.047$).
Ozcelik et al., prospective observational, Turkey, 2021 [30].	115 patients with type 2 DM, group 1, 55 on premixed insulin switched to IDegAsp; group 2, 60 on intensive insulin switched to bd IDegAsp, median (IQR) age 67.0 (62.0–69.0). Y.	Evaluate efficacy and safety of transition from premixed and intensive insulin to twice-daily insulin IDegAsp.	A. Mean (SD) rate hypoglycaemia 1.5 (0.85)/week before treatment switch in group 1 decreased to 0.03 (0.11)/week after IdegAsp ($p < 0.0001$). B. In group 2, episodes of hypoglycaemia were 0.93 (1.17)/week before treatment transition, decreased to 0.07 (0.25)/week after IDegAsp ($p < 0.0001$).

DM = Diabetes mellitus, SD = Standard deviation, Y = Year, M = Month, IDegAsp = Insulin degludec/aspart, QOL = Quality of life, NPH = Neutral protamine Hagedorn, F/U = Follow-up, ED = Emergency department, CI = Confidence interval, HR = Hazard ratio, CKD = Chronic kidney disease, IQR = Inter quartile range.

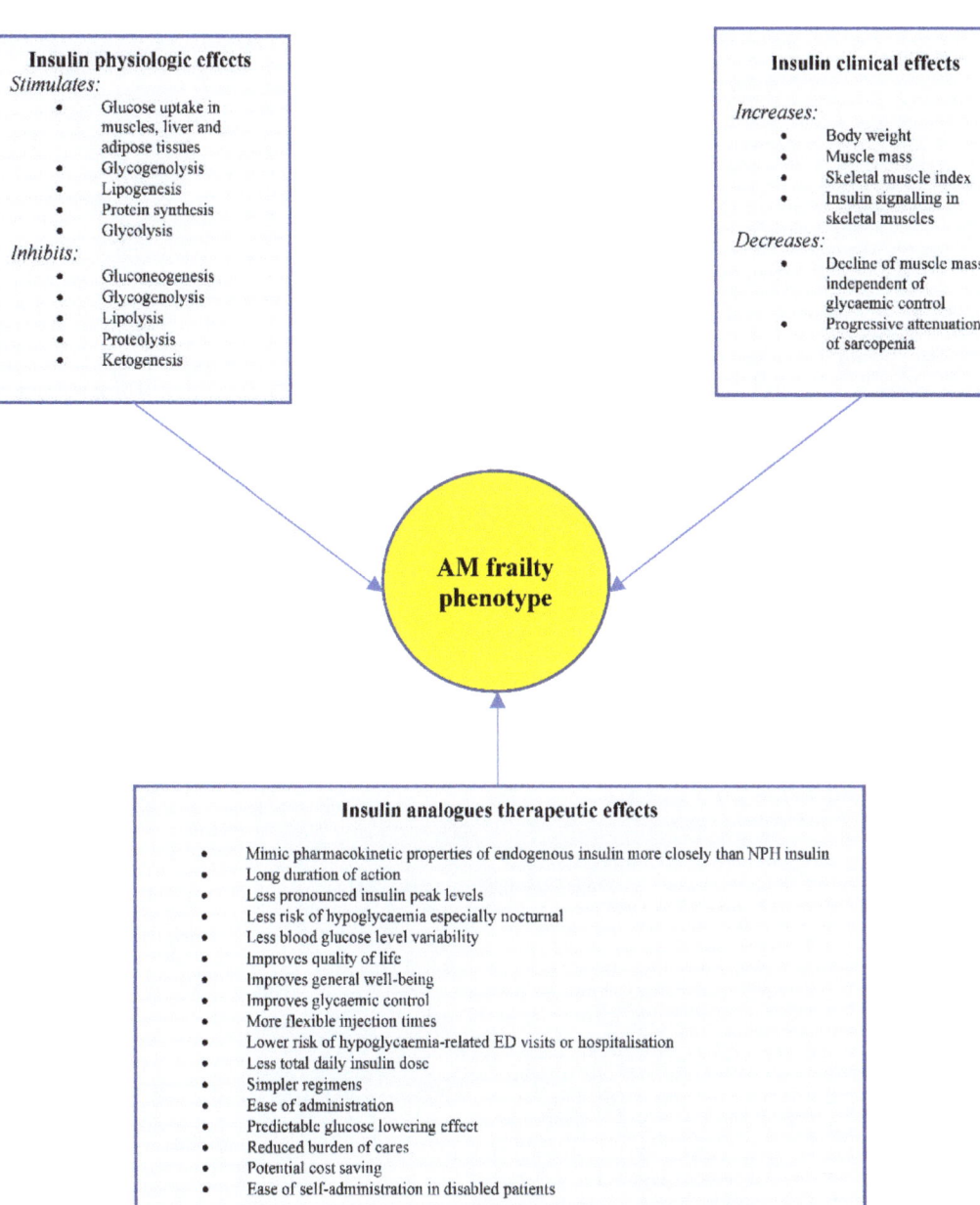

Figure 1. Advantage of the physiologic, clinical and therapeutic effects of insulin in the AM frailty phenotype. AM = Anorexic malnourished, ED = Emergency department.

5. Insulin—Low Threshold of Therapy

The potential effect on body weight should be considered when prescribing hypoglycaemic agents in frail older people with type 2 diabetes. For example, the use of weight limiting agents, such GLP-1RA and SGLT-2 inhibitors in the AM phenotype, are inappropriate due to the increased risk of further weight loss, dehydration, hypotension and increased risk of falls. Acarabose is associated with weight loss, significant gastrointestinal side effects and is less tolerated. Insulin secretagogues, such as sulfonylureas or glinides, although they have the advantage of desirable weight gain in the malnourished frail phenotype, are unsafe due to their high risk of hypoglycaemia. This population is also likely to have a high prevalence of dementia, which may be associated with erratic eating patterns, and the use of insulin secretagogues may significantly increase their risk of hypoglycaemia. Metformin may not be a suitable choice for many patients who have renal impairments. Additionally, pioglitazone is associated with the increased risk of lower-limb oedema, volume overload and exacerbation of congestive cardiac failure. Insulin has always been perceived as a last resort hypoglycaemic therapy after oral agents due to the associated side effects, such as the increased risk of hypoglycaemia, undesirable weight gain, inconvenience of frequent injections and the burden of blood glucose monitoring. However, in the AM phenotype of frailty, insulin may be a preferred early stage therapy. This phenotype is characterised by anorexia and significant weight loss. As a result, this phenotype has less insulin resistance and is likely to be more responsive to insulin therapy, in comparison to the SO phenotype that is characterised by increased insulin resistance [6]. Insulin-related weight gain is an advantage in this frailty phenotype. It may also have the potential to improve muscle mass and muscle function independent of glycaemic control. Therefore, in the milder form of the AM phenotype, such as people who are still compliant with oral therapy and nutrition, metformin, dipeptidyl peptidase-4 (DPP-4) inhibitors or glitazones can be used as first-line therapy, mainly due to their lower risk of hypoglycaemia. However, in patients with severe malnutrition and those less compliant with oral medications, insulin could be the first line of therapy. Insulin therapy has been shown to produce a sustained improvement in the well-being of older people [33]. Insulin-associated side effects, such as the inconvenience of frequent injections, blood glucose monitoring and the increased risk of hypoglycaemia, should be considered. The new insulin analogues appear as potentially favourable therapy in the AM frail phenotype due to the low risk of hypoglycaemia and the convenience of a once daily injection. In the SO phenotype, insulin therapy remains a last resort choice due to the significantly increased insulin resistance and undesirable weight gain in this phenotype. Metformin is the preferred first-line agent due to its cardiovascular benefits, weight-neutral effects and a potential positive effect on frailty [34,35]. GLP-1RA and SGLT-2 should be considered as a second-line, or first choice in patients not tolerant to metformin, due to their advantage of inducing significant weight loss and their cardio-renal protective effects [36]. Dipeptidyl peptidase-4 (DPP-4) is well tolerated with a low risk of hypoglycaemia or weight gain. Acarabose can be considered as an add-on therapy, if well tolerated. Although it can cause diarrhoea, it may have some cardiovascular benefits, low risk of hypoglycaemia and it promotes weight loss [37]. Insulin secretagogues and glitazones should be avoided in this frailty phenotype due to their increased risk of further weight gain (Figure 2).

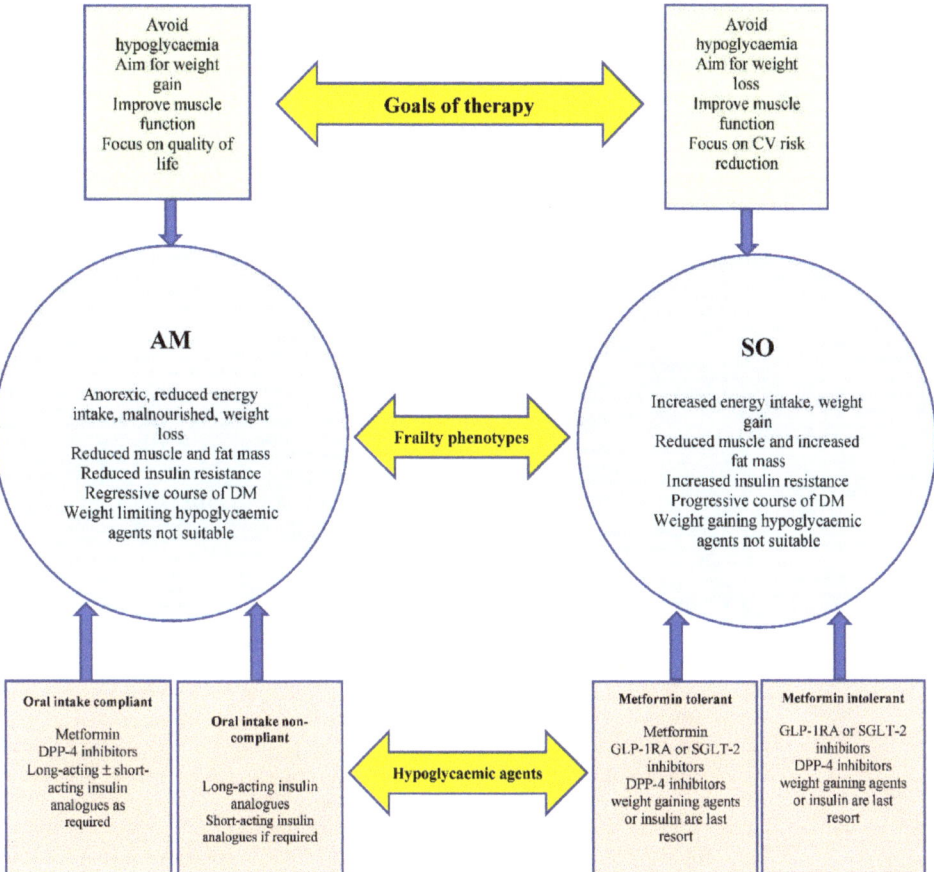

Figure 2. Two main metabolic frailty phenotypes' characteristics, hypoglycaemic agents and goals of therapy. Long-acting insulin analogues should be considered as an early option in AM frail patients with reduced and non-compliant oral intake. Weigh limiting agents should be considered as an early choice in the SO frailty phenotype. AM = Anorexic malnourished, SO = Sarcopenic obese.

6. Insulin Use in Frail, Older People with Diabetes

The decision to choose the type of insulin does not depend on the efficacy, but is largely based on other considerations, such as the risk of hypoglycaemia, impact on body weight, frequency of administration, cost and accessibility [38]. Barriers to the use of insulin, when clinically indicated, still exist at the physician, patient and healthcare system levels. These barriers include the complexity of an insulin regimen, lack of time and knowledge to appropriately prescribe insulin, anxiety about injections and monitoring, fear of hypoglycaemia and the lack of support [39,40]. These barriers may result in a significant delay in starting insulin in eligible patients [40,41]. The simplicity of the basal insulin analogues regimen may help to improve this clinical inertia. When choosing an insulin regimen for frail, older people with diabetes, the predictability of the glucose lowering effect, risk of hypoglycaemia, ease of administration and simplicity, as well as the flexibility of injection times, are important factors. Therefore, a single-dose regimen of a basal insulin analogue can play an important role in controlling hyperglycaemia in the AM frail, older patients. Multiple daily injections are too complex and not suitable or frail, older people, especially those with cognitive and physical dysfunctions. Long-acting, peakless insulin analogues have prolonged duration of action, present less blood glucose variability and should be administered only once daily to avoid the risk of hypoglycaemia. Although long-acting insulin analogues may have a higher acquisition cost than basal human insulins, their longer duration of action, predictability, less monitoring required and once-daily injection translate into a reduced burden of care and potential cost savings. The once-daily injection with the prolonged half-life of insulin analogues enables a flexible dosing regimen without compromising its efficacy and safety, and provides a breathing space and convenience for the administering healthcare workers and carers. With the single daily dose, self-administration may still be possible in patients who develop certain clinical conditions, such as arthritis, tremors or visual impairments. In addition, the reduced risk of nocturnal hypoglycaemia of the long-acting insulin analogues is an important value, as nocturnal hypoglycaemia is associated with the greatest reduction in quality of life and is a major barrier for hypoglycaemic therapy titration [42]. In older people with diabetes, hypoglycaemia may present less specific symptoms due to reduced autonomic responses in old age [43,44]. Therefore, educational diabetes programmes are important for patients and their carers. For example, in a study that delivered a diabetes educational programme to staff in care homes, staff knowledge improved and was retained after one year, and led to the improved quality of care for residents with diabetes [45]. It is also important to recognise that relaxed glycaemic targets are not an assurance of a lower risk of hypoglycaemia, as continuous glucose monitoring has unmasked frequent episodes of hypoglycaemia in older people with diabetes and high HbA1c levels [46].

7. Goals of Therapy

In the advanced AM frailty phenotypes who have limited life expectancy, glycaemic control with tight HbA1c should not be the focus of treatment. The goals of therapy should be aimed at achieving the best suitable blood glucose levels that control symptomatic hyperglycaemia and avoid side effects, especially hypoglycaemia, and focus on quality of life, rather than long-term HbA1c objectives. Hyperglycaemia increases the risk of frailty, probably through inducing mitochondrial dysfunction, microvascular damage, increased inflammation and oxidative stress [47]. On the other hand, hypoglycaemia increases the risk of frailty by inducing repeated minor subclinical cerebral injuries or recurrent falls and fractures that may, over time, lead to functional impairment [48]. Therefore, in frail patients with a reasonable life expectancy, the ideal short-term glycaemic control is to avoid the wide glycaemic excursions to prolong time spent in the normal glycaemic range. Zaslavsky et al. found a U-shaped relationship between blood glucose levels and the risk of incident frailty with blood glucose levels <8.9 mmol/L (<160 mg/dL) and >10.0 mmol/L (>180 mg/dL) to be associated with an increased risk of frailty ($p = 0.001$) [49]. The ideal HbA1c that reduces the risk of frailty/physical dysfunction or mortality in older people remains less clear. The U-shaped relationship reported by Zaslavsky et al. found the HbA1c of 7.6% (59.6 mmol/mol) to be associated with the least risk of frailty [49]. Other studies found HbA1c ≥ 8.0 (>63.9 mmol/mol) to be associated with a slow walking speed, and HbA1c >7.0% (53.0 mmol/mol) with functional disability [50,51]. Similarly, in a UK population-based cohort study of >25,000 older people (aged 80–89 years) with type 2 diabetes followed-up for a median of 2 years, a U-shaped relationship between HbA1c and mortality was observed [52]. The lowest mortality was found in older people with HbA1c of 7–7.4% (53–57 mmol/mol), compared with HbA1c of <6.0% (<42 mmol/mol) or ≥ 8.5% (≥ 69 mmol/mol). The results from the National Health and Nutrition Examination Surveys (NHANES) showed that, following a follow-up period of 8.9 years, HbA1c >8.0% (>63.9 mmol/mol) was associated with an increased risk of all-cause and cause-specific mortality in older people with diabetes [53]. Not only glycaemic targets, but also the choice of hypoglycaemic agent and the physical function of the individual, appear to have had an impact on the outcome. It was shown that a lower HbA1c (<7.0%) was associated with an increased mortality risk, compared with moderate levels (≥ 7.0% <8.5%) in patients using regimens that were associated with hypoglycaemia [54]. High levels of HbA1c were consistently associated with an elevated mortality risk in those regimens that had a lower risk of hypoglycaemia. These data suggest that the individualisation of glycaemic targets should consider the classes of glucose-lowering therapy, with less aggressive targets in patients treated with agents associated with a high risk of hypoglycaemia [54]. Similarly, a recent systematic review reported that better glycaemic control, HbA1c <7.0% (53.0 mmol/mol), and low glycaemic variability were associated with better maintenance of physical function. Higher HbA1c 8.0–8.9% (63.9–73.8 mmol/mol) was associated with a reduction in the composite outcome of death or functional decline in frail community-dwelling older people with diabetes who were in need for skilled assistance or classified as nursing-home-eligible [55]. These finding suggest that the greater the decline in function and the increase in frailty, the higher the targets should be.

8. Future Perspectives

Clinical guidelines still consider frail, older people with diabetes as one category, and therefore clinical practice does not characterise the metabolic profile of frailty and its impact on glycaemic control and choice of hypoglycaemic agents [56,57]. Recently, five different subtypes of patients with type 2 diabetes with different characteristics, insulin resistance, disease progression and risk of diabetes-related complications were identified [58]. Future clinical trials should consider the clear characterisation of older participants, rather than characterisation by age alone. Although we suggested that frail, older people with diabetes may have a wide spectrum of the metabolic profile, there is currently no research or evidence to support this view. Another limitation of this review was that the participants recruited to the studies included in this manuscript were of a relatively younger age, again, due to paucity of research in older age groups. Therefore, the metabolic spectrum of frailty and its effect on the choice of hypoglycaemic agents is another potential direction for future research. Little is known about the effects of hypoglycaemic agents on frailty, and future research is needed [59–64]. The anabolic properties of insulin and its effect on body muscle needs further exploration. The current scarce evidence suggests that insulin may have a positive effect on muscle function and attenuate the progression of sarcopenia in older people with diabetes, but this evidence is not yet substantial or evident in older age groups. In addition, frailty was not assessed in these studies. Therefore, future confirmation in large prospective studies is still required. The positive effect of insulin on muscle parameters appears to be independent of glycaemic control, which is an advantage in old age to achieve this beneficial outcome without inducing hypoglycaemia. Prospective studies that include muscle biopsies are also required to assess the effect of insulin therapy on muscle quality. The new insulin analogues appear as a potentially favourable therapy in the AM frail phenotype, as long as hypoglycaemia is avoided, but evidence is still required to explore its effect on muscle function and whether it can delay the progression of frailty to disability. The current research on the use of once-weekly insulin injections is an appealing convenience choice for frail, older people with diabetes, and may further encourage the early introduction of insulin in this vulnerable group of patients [65].

9. Conclusions

Frail, older people with diabetes appear to have a heterogeneous metabolic spectrum that clusters at an anorexic malnourished (AM) phenotype at one end and a sarcopenic obese (SO) phenotype at the other end. The use of oral hypoglycaemic medications in the AM phenotype may be limited by organ dysfunction and polypharmacy. In addition, the new agents of GLP-1RA and SGLT-2 inhibitors may not be suitable in this frailty phenotype due to their side effects of further weight loss, dehydration, hypotension and increased risk of falls. Therefore, insulin use may be considered as an early option in this group of vulnerable frail patients. The long-acting insulin analogues appear as safer options due to their low risk of hypoglycaemia and the convenience of single daily administration. The side effects of insulin-induced weight gain may be an advantage in this frailty phenotype. Insulin-related anabolic properties and its potential positive effect on muscle function is another advantage, although this important effect still needs further exploration in future large prospective studies. The goals of therapy in this frailty phenotype should maintain a relaxed glycaemic control, avoid hypoglycaemia as much as possible and focus on the maintenance of good quality of life.

10. Key Points

- Frailty and sarcopenia are newly emerged diabetes-related complications in older people with diabetes.
- Frailty appears to be metabolically heterogeneous with anorexic malnourished (AM) phenotypes at one end, and sarcopenic obese (SO) phenotypes at the other end of the spectrum.
- The AM phenotype is likely to be less tolerant to oral hypoglycaemic therapy due to multiple comorbidities and organ dysfunction.
- Insulin therapy, especially long-acting insulin analogues, are an early option in the AM phenotype.
- Insulin may have positive effects on muscle function in this frail phenotype, although future confirmation studies are required.

Author Contributions: Authors contributed equally to the writing of this manuscript. All authors have read and agreed to the published version of the manuscript.

Funding: This research received no external funding.

Data Availability Statement: Not applicable.

Conflicts of Interest: The authors declare no conflict of interest.

References

1. Sinclair, A.; Saeedi, P.; Kaundal, A.; Karuranga, S.; Malanda, B.; Williams, R. Diabetes and global ageing among 65–99-year-old adults: Findings from the International Diabetes Federation Diabetes Atlas, 9th edition. *Diabetes Res. Clin. Pract.* **2020**, *162*, 108078. [CrossRef] [PubMed]
2. Sinclair, A.J.; Abdelhafiz, A.H.; Rodríguez-Mañas, L. Frailty and sarcopenia-newly emerging and high impact complications of diabetes. *J. Diabetes Complicat.* **2017**, *31*, 1465–1473. [CrossRef] [PubMed]
3. Hanlon, P.; Fauré, I.; Corcoran, N.; Butterly, E.; Lewsey, J.; McAllister, D.; Mair, F.S. Frailty measurement, prevalence, incidence, and clinical implications in people with diabetes: A systematic review and study-level meta-analysis. *Lancet Health Longev.* **2020**, *1*, e106–e116. [CrossRef]
4. Sinclair, A.J.; Abdelhafiz, A.; Dunning, T.; Izquierdo, M.; Manas, L.R.; Bourdel-Marchasson, I.; Morley, J.E.; Munshi, M.; Woo, J.; Vellas, B. An International Position Statement on the Management of Frailty in Diabetes Mellitus: Summary of Recommendations 2017. *J. Frailty Aging* **2018**, *7*, 10–20. [CrossRef] [PubMed]
5. Leroith, D.; Biessels, G.J.; Braithwaite, S.S.; Casanueva, F.F.; Draznin, B.; Halter, J.B.; Hirsch, I.B.; McDonnell, M.; Molitch, M.E.; Murad, M.H.E.; et al. TReatment of diabetes in older adults: An endocrine society clinical practice guideline. *J. Clin. Endocrinol. Metab.* **2019**, *104*, 1520–1574. [CrossRef]
6. Abdelhafiz, A.H.; Emmerton, D.; Sinclair, A.J. Impact of frailty metabolic phenotypes on the management of older people with type 2 diabetes mellitus. *Geriatr. Gerontol. Int.* **2021**, *21*, 614–622. [CrossRef]
7. Abdulla, H.; Smith, K.; Atherton, P.J.; Idris, I. Role of insulin in the regulation of human skeletal muscle protein synthesis and breakdown: A systematic review and meta-analysis. *Diabetologia* **2016**, *59*, 44–55. [CrossRef]
8. Fujita, S.; Glynn, E.L.; Timmerman, K.L.; Rasmussen, B.B.; Volpi, E. Supraphysiological hyperinsulinaemia is necessary to stimulate skeletal muscle protein anabolism in older adults: Evidence of a true age-related insulin resistance of muscle protein metabolism. *Diabetologia* **2009**, *52*, 1889–1898. [CrossRef]
9. Tanaka, K.-I.; Kanazawa, I.; Sugimoto, T. Reduction in Endogenous Insulin Secretion is a Risk Factor of Sarcopenia in Men with Type 2 Diabetes Mellitus. *Calcif. Tissue Res.* **2015**, *97*, 385–390. [CrossRef]
10. Bouchi, R.; Fukuda, T.; Takeuchi, T.; Nakano, Y.; Murakami, M.; Minami, I.; Izumiyama, H.; Hashimoto, K.; Yoshimoto, T.; Ogawa, Y. Insulin Treatment Attenuates Decline of Muscle Mass in Japanese Patients with Type 2 Diabetes. *Calcif. Tissue Res.* **2017**, *101*, 1–8. [CrossRef]
11. Kalyani, R.R.; Tra, Y.; Yeh, H.C.; Egan, J.M.; Ferrucci, L.; Brancati, F.L. Quadriceps strength, quadriceps power, and gait speed in older U.S. adults with diabetes mellitus: Results from the National Health and Nutrition Examination Survey, 1999–2002. *J. Am. Geriatr. Soc.* **2013**, *61*, 769–775. [CrossRef] [PubMed]
12. Cui, M.; Gang, X.; Wang, G.; Xiao, X.; Li, Z.; Jiang, Z.; Wang, G. Associations between sarcopenia and clinical characteristics of patients with type 2 diabetes. *Medicine* **2020**, *99*, e18708. [CrossRef] [PubMed]

13. Ferrari, U.; Then, C.; Rottenkolber, M.; Selte, C.; Seissler, J.; Conzade, R.; Linkohr, B.; Peters, A.; Drey, M.; Thorand, B. Longitudinal association of type 2 diabetes and insulin therapy with muscle parameters in the KORA-Age study. *Acta Diabetol.* **2020**, *57*, 1057–1063. [CrossRef]
14. Sugimoto, K.; Ikegami, H.; Takata, Y.; Katsuya, T.; Fukuda, M.; Akasaka, H.; Tabara, Y.; Osawa, H.; Hiromine, Y.; Rakugi, H. Glycemic Control and Insulin Improve Muscle Mass and Gait Speed in Type 2 Diabetes: The MUSCLES-DM Study. *J. Am. Med. Dir. Assoc.* **2021**, *22*, 834–838.e1. [CrossRef] [PubMed]
15. Rosenstock, J.; Schwartz, S.L.; Clark, C.M., Jr.; Park, G.D.; Donley, D.W.; Edwards, M.B. Basal insulin therapy in type 2 diabetes: 28-week comparison of insulin glargine (HOE 901) and NPH insulin. *Diabetes Care* **2001**, *24*, 631–636. [CrossRef] [PubMed]
16. Riddle, M.C.; Rosenstock, J.; Gerich, J. Insulin Glargine 4002 Study Investigators. The treat-to-target trial: Randomized addition of glargine or human NPH insulin to oral therapy of type 2 diabetic patients. *Diabetes Care* **2003**, *26*, 3080–3086. [CrossRef]
17. Fritsche, A.; Schweitzer, M.A.; Häring, H.U.; 4001 Study Group. Glimepiride combined with morning insulin glargine, bedtime neutral protamine hagedorn insulin, or bedtime insulin glargine in patients with type 2 diabetes: A randomized, controlled trial. *Ann. Intern. Med.* **2003**, *138*, 952–959. [CrossRef]
18. Haak, T.; Tiengo, A.; Draeger, E.; Suntum, M.; Waldhausl, W. Lower within-subject variability of fasting blood glucose and reduced weight gain with insulin detemir compared to NPH insulin in patients with type 2 diabetes. *Diabetes Obes. Metab.* **2005**, *7*, 56–64. [CrossRef]
19. Hermansen, K.; Davies, M.; Derezinski, T.; Martinez Ravn, G.; Clauson, P.; Home, P. A 26-week, randomized, parallel, treat-to-target trial comparing insulin detemir with NPH insulin as add-on therapy to oral glucose-lowering drugs in insulin-naïve people with type 2 diabetes. *Diabetes Care* **2006**, *29*, 1269–1274. [CrossRef]
20. Eliaschewitz, F.G.; Calvo, C.; Valbuena, H.; Ruiz, M.; Aschner, P.; Villena, J.; Ramirez, L.A.; Jimenez, J. Therapy in Type 2 Diabetes: Insulin Glargine vs. NPH Insulin Both in Combination with Glimepiride. *Arch. Med. Res.* **2006**, *37*, 495–501. [CrossRef]
21. Horvath, K.; Jeitler, K.; Berghold, A.; Ebrahim, S.H.; Gratzer, T.W.; Plank, J.; Kaiser, T.; Pieber, T.R.; Siebenhofer, A. Long-acting insulin analogues versus NPH insulin (human isophane insulin) for type 2 diabetes mellitus. *Cochrane Database Syst. Rev.* **2007**, CD005613. [CrossRef] [PubMed]
22. Singh, S.R.; Ahmad, F.; Lal, A.; Yu, C.; Bai, Z.; Bennett, H. Efficacy and safety of insulin analogues for the management of diabetes mellitus: A meta-analysis. *CMAJ* **2009**, *180*, 385–397. [CrossRef] [PubMed]
23. Fujimoto, K.; Iwakura, T.; Aburaya, M.; Matsuoka, N. Twice-daily insulin degludec/insulin aspart effectively improved morning and evening glucose levels and quality of life in patients previously treated with premixed insulin: An observational study. *Diabetol. Metab. Syndr.* **2018**, *10*, 64. [CrossRef] [PubMed]
24. Lipska, K.J.; Parker, M.M.; Moffet, H.H.; Huang, E.S.; Karter, A.J. Association of Initiation of Basal Insulin Analogs vs Neutral Protamine Hagedorn Insulin with Hypoglycemia-Related Emergency Department Visits or Hospital Admissions and with Glycemic Control in Patients With Type 2 Diabetes. *JAMA* **2018**, *320*, 53–62. [CrossRef] [PubMed]
25. Haukka, J.; Hoti, F.; Erästö, P.; Saukkonen, T.; Mäkimattila, S.; Korhonen, P. Evaluation of the incidence and risk of hypoglycemic coma associated with selection of basal insulin in the treatment of diabetes: A Finnish register linkage study. *Pharmacoepidemiol. Drug Saf.* **2013**, *22*, 1326–1335. [CrossRef]
26. Strandberg, A.Y.; Khanfir, H.; Mäkimattila, S.; Saukkonen, T.; Strandberg, T.; Hoti, F. Insulins NPH, glargine, and detemir, and risk of severe hypoglycemia among working-age adults. *Ann. Med.* **2017**, *49*, 357–364. [CrossRef]
27. Bradley, M.C.; Chillarige, Y.; Lee, H.; Wu, X.; Parulekar, S.; Muthuri, S.; Wernecke, M.; MaCurdy, T.E.; Kelman, J.A.; Graham, D.J. Severe Hypoglycemia Risk with Long-Acting Insulin Analogs vs Neutral Protamine Hagedorn Insulin. *JAMA Intern. Med.* **2021**, *181*, 598. [CrossRef]
28. Betônico, C.C.; Titan, S.M.O.; Lira, A.; Pelaes, T.S.; Correa-Giannella, M.L.C.; Nery, M.; Queiroz, M. Insulin Glargine U100 Improved Glycemic Control and Reduced Nocturnal Hypoglycemia in Patients with Type 2 Diabetes Mellitus and Chronic Kidney Disease Stages 3 and 4. *Clin. Ther.* **2019**, *41*, 2008–2020. [CrossRef]
29. Alsahli, M.; Gerich, J.E. Hypoglycemia in Patients with Diabetes and Renal Disease. *J. Clin. Med.* **2015**, *4*, 948–964. [CrossRef]
30. Pecoits-Filho, R.; Abensur, H.; Betônico, C.C.R.; Machado, A.D.; Parente, E.B.; Queiroz, M.; Salles, J.E.N.; Titan, S.; Vencio, S. Interactions between kidney disease and diabetes: Dangerous liaisons. *Diabetol. Metab. Syndr.* **2016**, *8*, 50. [CrossRef]
31. Özçelik, S.; Çelik, M.; Vural, A.; Aydın, B.; Özçelik, M.; Gozu, M. Outcomes of transition from premixed and intensive insulin therapies to insulin aspart/degludec co-formulation in type 2 diabetes mellitus: A real-world experience. *Arch. Med. Sci.* **2021**, *17*, 1–8. [CrossRef] [PubMed]
32. Rodbard, H.W.; Cariou, B.; Pieber, T.R.; Endahl, L.A.; Zacho, J.; Cooper, J.G. Treatment intensification with an insulin degludec (IDeg)/insulin aspart (IAsp) co-formulation twice daily compared with basal IDeg and prandial IAsp in type 2 diabetes: A randomized, controlled phase III trial. *Diabetes Obes. Metab.* **2016**, *18*, 274–280. [CrossRef] [PubMed]
33. Reza, M.; Taylor, C.; Towse, K.; Ward, J.; Hendra, T. Insulin improves well-being for selected elderly type 2 diabetic subjects. *Diabetes Res. Clin. Pract.* **2002**, *55*, 201–207. [CrossRef]
34. Maruthur, N.M.; Tseng, E.; Hutfless, S.; Wilson, L.M.; Suarez-Cuervo, C.; Berger, Z.; Chu, Y.; Iyoha, E.; Segal, J.B.; Bolen, S. Diabetes Medications as Monotherapy or Metformin-Based Combination Therapy for Type 2 Diabetes. A Systematic Review and Meta-analysis. *Ann. Intern. Med.* **2016**, *164*, 740–751. [CrossRef] [PubMed]

35. Crowley, M.J.; Diamantidis, C.J.; McDuffie, J.R.; Cameron, C.B.; Stanifer, J.W.; Mock, C.K.; Wang, X.; Tang, S.; Nagi, A.; Kosinski, A.S.; et al. Clinical Outcomes of Metformin Use in Populations with Chronic Kidney Disease, Congestive Heart Failure, or Chronic Liver Disease: A Systematic Review. *Ann. Intern. Med.* **2017**, *166*, 191–200. [CrossRef] [PubMed]
36. Abdelhafiz, A.H.; Sinclair, A.J. Cardio-renal protection in older people with diabetes with frailty and medical comorbidities—A focus on the new hypoglycaemic therapy. *J. Diabetes Complicat.* **2020**, *34*, 107639. [CrossRef]
37. Chang, Y.C.; Chuang, L.M.; Lin, J.W.; Chen, S.T.; Lai, M.S.; Chang, C.H. Cardiovascular risks associated with second-line oral antidiabetic agents added to metformin in patients with Type 2 diabetes: A nationwide cohort study. *Diabet. Med.* **2015**, *32*, 1460–1469. [CrossRef]
38. Doyle-Delgado, K.; Chamberlain, J.J.; Shubrook, J.H.; Skolnik, N.; Trujillo, K. Pharmacologic Approaches to glycemic treatment of type 2 diabetes: Synopsis of the 2020 American diabetes Association's standards of medical care in diabetes clinical guideline. *Ann. Intern. Med.* **2020**, *173*, 813e21. [CrossRef]
39. Blonde, L.; Aschner, P.; Bailey, C.; Ji, L.; Leiter, L.A.; Matthaei, S.; Global Partnership for Effective Diabetes Management. Matthaei S on behalf of the Global Partnership for Effective Diabetes Management. Gaps and barriers in the control of blood glucose in people with type 2 diabetes. *Diabetes Vasc. Dis. Res.* **2017**, *14*, 172e83. [CrossRef]
40. Reach, G.; Pechtner, V.; Gentilella, R.; Corcos, A.; Ceriello, A. Clinical inertia and its impact on treatment intensification in people with type 2 diabetes mellitus. *Diabetes Metab.* **2017**, *43*, 501–511. [CrossRef]
41. Khunti, K.; Gomes, M.B.; Pocock, S.; Shestakova, M.V.; Pintat, S.; Fenici, P.; Hammar, N.; Medina, J. Therapeutic inertia in the treatment of hyperglycaemia in patients with type 2 diabetes: A systematic Review. *Diabetes Obes. Metabol.* **2018**, *20*, 427e37. [CrossRef]
42. Edelman, S.V.; Blose, J.S. The Impact of Nocturnal Hypoglycemia on Clinical and Cost-Related Issues in Patients with Type 1 and Type 2 Diabetes. *Diabetes Educ.* **2014**, *40*, 269–279. [CrossRef] [PubMed]
43. Jaap, A.; Jones, G.; McCrimmon, R.; Deary, I.J.; Frier, B.M. Perceived symptoms of hypoglycemia in elderly type 2 diabetic patients treated with insulin. *Diabet Med.* **1998**, *15*, 398–401. [CrossRef]
44. Goto, A.; Arah, O.; Goto, M.; Terauchi, Y.; Noda, M. Severe hypoglycaemia and cardiovascular disease: Systematic review and meta-analysis with bias analysis. *BMJ* **2013**, *347*, f4533. [CrossRef] [PubMed]
45. Deakin, T.A.; Littley, M.D. Diabetes care in residential homes: Staff training makes a difference. *J. Hum. Nutr. Dietet.* **2001**, *14*, 443–447. [CrossRef]
46. Munshi, M.N.; Slyne, C.; Segal, A.R.; Saul, N.; Lyons, C.; Weinger, K. Liberating A1C goals in older adults may not protect against the risk of hypoglycemia. *J. Diabetes Complicat.* **2017**, *31*, 1197–1199. [CrossRef]
47. Stout, M.B.; Justice, J.N.; Nicklas, B.J.; Kirkland, J.L. Physiological Aging: Links Among Adipose Tissue Dysfunction, Diabetes, and Frailty. *Physiology* **2017**, *32*, 9–19. [CrossRef]
48. Abdelhafiz, A.H.; Rodríguez-Mānas, L.; Morley, J.E.; Sinclair, A.J. Hypoglycemia in older people-a less well recognized risk factor for frailty. *Aging Dis.* **2015**, *10*, 156–167. [CrossRef]
49. Zaslavsky, O.; Walker, R.L.; Crane, P.K.; Gray, S.L.; Larson, E.B. Glucose levels and risk of frailty. *J. Gerontol. A Biol. Sci. Med. Sci.* **2016**, *71*, 1223–1229. [CrossRef]
50. Yoon, J.W.; Ha, Y.-C.; Kim, K.M.; Moon, J.H.; Choi, S.H.; Lim, S.; Park, Y.J.; Lim, J.-Y.; Kim, K.W.; Park, K.S.; et al. Hyperglycemia Is Associated with Impaired Muscle Quality in Older Men with Diabetes: The Korean Longitudinal Study on Health and Aging. *Diabetes Metab. J.* **2016**, *40*, 140–146. [CrossRef]
51. Godino, J.G.; Appel, L.J.; Gross, A.L.; Schrack, J.A.; Parrinello, C.M.; Kalyani, R.R.; Windham, B.G.; Pankow, J.S.; Kritchevsky, S.B.; Bandeen-Roche, K.; et al. Diabetes, hyperglycemia, and the burden of functional disability among older adults in a community-based study. *J. Diabetes* **2017**, *9*, 76–84. [CrossRef] [PubMed]
52. Hamada, S.; Gulliford, M.C. Mortality in individuals aged 80 and older with type 2 diabetes mellitus in relation to glycosylated hemoglobin, blood pressure, and total cholesterol. *J. Am. Geriatr. Soc.* **2016**, *64*, 1425–1431. [CrossRef] [PubMed]
53. Palta, P.; Huang, E.S.; Kalyani, R.R.; Golden, S.H.; Yeh, H.-C. Hemoglobin A1c and Mortality in Older Adults With and Without Diabetes: Results From the National Health and Nutrition Examination Surveys (1988–2011). *Diabetes Care* **2017**, *40*, 453–460. [CrossRef] [PubMed]
54. Currie, C.J.; Holden, S.E.; Jenkins-Jones, S.; Morgan, C.L.; Voss, B.; Rajpathak, S.N.; Alemayehu, B.; Peters, J.R.; Engel, S.S. Impact of differing glucose-lowering regimens on the pattern of association between glucose control and survival. *Diabetes Obes. Metab.* **2018**, *20*, 821–830. [CrossRef]
55. Bollig, C.; Torbahn, G.; Bauer, J.; Brefka, S.; Dallmeier, D.; Denkinger, M.; Eidam, A.; Klöppel, S.; Zeyfang, A.; Voigt-Radloff, S.; et al. Evidence gap on antihyperglycemic pharmacotherapy in frail older adults: A systematic review. Evidenzmangel für die antihyperglykämische Pharmakotherapie gebrechlicher älterer Patienten: Ein systematisches Review. *Z. Gerontol. Geriatr.* **2021**, *54*, 278–284. [CrossRef]
56. Ambrož, M.; de Vries, S.T.; Hoogenberg, K.; Denig, P. Trends in HbA$_{1c}$ thresholds for initiation of hypoglycemic agents: Impact of changed recommendations for older and frail patients. *Pharmacoepidemiol. Drug Saf.* **2021**, *30*, 37–44. [CrossRef]
57. Mangé, A.-S.; Pagès, A.; Sourdet, S.; Cestac, P.; McCambridge, C. Diabetes and Frail Older Patients: Glycemic Control and Prescription Profile in Real Life. *Pharmacy* **2021**, *9*, 115. [CrossRef]

58. Ahlqvist, E.; Storm, P.; Käräjämäki, A.; Martinell, M.; Dorkhan, M.; Carlsson, A.; Vikman, P.; Prasad, R.; Aly, D.M.; Almgren, P.; et al. Novel subgroups of adult-onset diabetes and their association with outcomes: A data-driven cluster analysis of six variables. *Lancet Diabetes Endocrinol.* **2018**, *6*, 361–369. [CrossRef]
59. Shea, M.K.; Nicklas, B.J.; Marsh, A.P.; Houston, D.; Miller, G.D.; Isom, S.; Miller, M.E.; Carr, J.; Lyles, M.F.; Harris, T.B.; et al. The Effect of Pioglitazone and Resistance Training on Body Composition in Older Men and Women Undergoing Hypocaloric Weight Loss. *Obesity* **2011**, *19*, 1636–1646. [CrossRef]
60. Marsh, A.P.; Shea, M.K.; Locke, R.M.V.; Miller, M.E.; Isom, S.; Miller, G.D.; Nicklas, B.J.; Lyles, M.F.; Carr, J.J.; Kritchevsky, S.B. Resistance Training and Pioglitazone Lead to Improvements in Muscle Power During Voluntary Weight Loss in Older Adults. *J. Gerontol. Ser. A* **2013**, *68*, 828–836. [CrossRef]
61. Rajaobelina, K.; Helmer, C.; Vélayoudom-Céphise, F.-L.; Nov, S.; Farges, B.; Pupier, E.; Blanco, L.; Hugo, M.; Gin, H.; Rigalleau, V. Progression of skin autofluorescence of AGEs over 4 years in patients with type 1 diabetes. *Diabetes Metab. Res. Rev.* **2017**, *33*, e2917. [CrossRef] [PubMed]
62. Rizzo, M.R.; Barbieri, M.; Fava, I.; Desiderio, M.; Coppola, C.; Marfella, R.; Paolisso, G. Sarcopenia in Elderly Diabetic Patients: Role of Dipeptidyl Peptidase 4 Inhibitors. *J. Am. Med. Dir. Assoc.* **2016**, *17*, 896–901. [CrossRef] [PubMed]
63. Perna, S.; Guido, D.; Bologna, C.; Solerte, S.B.; Guerriero, F.; Isu, A.; Rondanelli, M. Liraglutide and obesity in elderly: Efficacy in fat loss and safety in order to prevent sarcopenia. A perspective case series study. *Aging Clin. Exp. Res.* **2016**, *28*, 1251–1257. [CrossRef] [PubMed]
64. Yajima, T.; Yajima, K.; Takahashi, H.; Yasuda, K. The effect of dulaglutide on body composition in type 2 diabetes mellitus patients on hemodialysis. *J. Diabetes Complicat.* **2018**, *32*, 759–763. [CrossRef] [PubMed]
65. Bajaj, H.S.; Bergenstal, R.M.; Christoffersen, A.; Davies, M.J.; Gowda, A.; Isendahl, J.; Lingvay, I.; Senior, P.A.; Silver, R.J.; Trevisan, R.; et al. Switching to Once-Weekly Insulin Icodec Versus Once-Daily Insulin Glargine U100 in Type 2 Diabetes Inadequately Controlled on Daily Basal Insulin: A Phase 2 Randomized Controlled Trial. *Diabetes Care* **2021**, *44*, 1586–1594. [CrossRef]

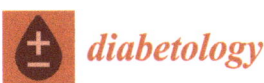

Opinion

Lipodystrophies from Insulin Injection: An Update of the Italian Consensus Statement of AMD-OSDI Study Group on Injection Technique

Sandro Gentile [1,2,*], Ersilia Satta [1], Giuseppina Guarino [1,2] and Felice Strollo [3] on behalf of the AMD-OSDI Study Group on Injection Technique

1. Nefrocenter Research, 84013 Cava dè Tirreni, Italy
2. Department of Internal Medicine, Campania University "Luigi Vanvitelli", 80138 Naples, Italy
3. Endocrinology and Diabetes Department, IRCCS, San Raffaele Pisana, 00163 Rome, Italy
* Correspondence: s.getile1949@gmail.com

Abstract: The causes and metabolic consequences of lipohypertrophy (LH) from incorrect insulin injection techniques have been well-known for a long time and are the subject of countless publications. However, only some researchers propose structured research modalities for LH and programs to teach patients how to prevent them and minimize their effects, thus contributing to complete rehabilitation. Experts and scientific societies have produced consensus documents and recommendations to spread the culture of LH and its complications among clinicians. However, they should go deeper into LH detection methods. This short article analyzes the recent literature on the best way to explore and find more or less evident LH lesions by using a structured and validated clinical methodology to benefit the many clinicians without access to technological equipment such as ultrasonography. This text also aims to bring awareness that since the last published recommendations on injection techniques, new needles for insulin injection, more technologically advanced and suitable for specific populations, have come to market but still need a thorough evaluation.

Keywords: diabetes; insulin; lipodystrophy; injection technique; clinical detection; recommendations; rehabilitation

1. Introduction

From the onset of insulin in the last century, it was immediately apparent that the daily injections necessary to administer it involved local skin complications such as subcutaneous lipoatrophy (LA) [1] due to impurities of the first insulin preparations and to related immune-allergic reactions [2]. Today, technology makes it possible to inject extremely pure insulin preparations without the devastating atrophying effects of the early insulin era. However, today, a further variant of insulin injection lipodystrophy (LD), the skin lipohypertrophy (LH), is present in numerous patients on multi-injection therapy [3]. From a purely descriptive point of view, therefore, with the term "lipodystrophies" we mean both forms of skin atrophy (LA) and hypertrophy (LH). The former lesions are now rare and represent less than 5% of all LDs. At the same time, the latter is much more frequent, being the main local complication of insulin injections [2]. LH is due to the anabolic action of insulin and in addition to the systematic puncture of narrow areas of the skin (usually an extension comparable with that of a credit card), reusing the same needle several times, injecting cold insulin, and using too long and thick needles [2,4,5].

The phenomenon of LH due to incorrect injection technique is well-present in the literature. Its diffusion concerns just under 50% of all subjects in multi-injection therapy with insulin [6–8], but with wide variations in frequency, linked to the research method, too often approximate, and the lack of healthcare provider experience or structured identification method [9–12]. In reality, this is a gap in scientific research. Indeed, when going through leading literature banks (e.g., Scopus and PubMed), we find numerous scientific articles describing case histories with and without LH and clinical cases of subjects with LD without giving due relevance to the identification method [13,14]. A sure cornerstone of literature concerns the comparison between manual and ultrasound research of LH, which undoubtedly decrees the diagnostic superiority of ultrasonography over manual [15]. However, due to the high number of patients self-injecting insulin, the equipment and dedicated personnel costs, and the time required for each examination, ultrasonography remains confined to the scientific field. Indeed, ultrasonography is unsuitable for widespread clinical use, especially in specific care settings such as outpatients or economically disadvantaged and developing countries [16]. Nevertheless, some handy yet evidence-based methodological indications at the clinical level may be helpful (Table 1) [13,14,16–18].

Table 1. Methodological indications on how to manually search for skin LH.

	CORRECT LH SEARCH SEQUENCE
1	Have the patient indicate all skin areas where he or she injects the insulin and examine all of them
2	Conduct the exam in a well-lit environment, preferably with natural light
3	Examine the patient supine without clothing and then in a standing position
4	Rotate the standing patient to take advantage of the incidence of light bringing out LH profile and elevation
5	Ask the patient to get muscles relaxed during the examination
6	Perform superficial palpation of the injection sites, passing the examining hand over and over again, looking for nodules or pasty areas of greater consistency than the surrounding skin
7	Repeat the palpation as described above, with more force to sense any deeper LH
8	Perform the pinching maneuver, taking a flap of skin between the index finger and thumb, to evaluate the thickness of the skin fold and compare it with nearby areas that are not affected by the injections: the LH is recognizable by a greater thickness of the fold
9	The set of previous findings allows us to describe an area of skin containing an LH
10	The LHs can be small or several centimeters large, protruding on the skin or flat; their recognition by sight alone risks not identify clear palpable LHs
11	Show identified LHs to the patient, explain why they form, what metabolic consequences they entail, and why the need to correctly perform the insulin injection
12	Give precise and motivated indications on how to correctly inject insulin (injection site rotation, no reuse of the same needle, insulin at room temperature, use of short and thin needles as recommended)
13	Skin examination (e.g., acanthosis nigricans, insulin injection or insertion sites, lipodystrophy) is a component of the comprehensive diabetes medical evaluation at initial and annual visits, besides every follow-up

If errors in insulin injection technique cause LH, recommendations on correct injection techniques are critical for current treatment and rehabilitation in case of marked LH-related glucose variability. In Italy, an intercompany study group of AMD (Italian Medical Association of Diabetologists) and OSDI (Italian Association of Nurses on Diabetes) [19] published recommendations on optimal insulin injection techniques in 2016, and similar recommendations were published shortly after, resulting from the conclusions of an international meeting of a panel of experts from 52 countries, held in Rome in 2015 [20].

Those conclusions are substantially similar and confirm the need for:

1. A preventive search for LH to avoid injecting insulin into them;
2. Constant injection site rotation ensuring a distance of at least 1 cm between two successive injections and utilization of the entire surface of injection areas identified in the abdomen, external and rear sides of the arms, upper external side of the thighs and buttocks;
3. Single use of each pen needle (1 needle = 1 injection);
4. Choice of 32 G × 4 mm needles even in overweight and obese subjects;
5. Proper insulin storage;
6. Ice-cold insulin avoidance;
7. No skin massage after the injection;
8. No injection through clothing;
9. Thorough hand and skin hygiene;
10. No pinch maneuver or acute angle needle inclination at the time of injection.

In 2017, the Italian AMD-OSDI study group updated the recommendations on injection techniques, also considering pregnant women and insulin pump (CSII) users. Their document suggested lateral areas of the abdomen in the first months and advised against using the whole abdominal area in the following months in pregnant women. For CSII users, it recommended an effective needle insertion site rotation and the choice of needles guided by the specialist care team [21]. ADA Standards of Medical Care in Diabetes—2022 accurately echoed the conclusions of such documents [17]. In particular, this document refers to the 2016 recommendations [20] and suggests skin examination as an inescapable component of the comprehensive diabetes medical evaluation at initial, follow-up, and annual visits. Furthermore, the ADA document considers the 4 mm and 32 G needles proposed in the 2016 document as the reference needle for obese subjects in the absence of evidence for subsequent shorter and thinner needles.

Indeed, 4 mm/33 G and 3.5 mm/34 G needles came to the market after the 2016 consensus was published. Two studies evaluated small cohorts of insulin-treated subjects for their non-inferiority to 4 mm/33 G and 3.5 mm/34 G in terms of (i) patient satisfaction, (ii) pain sensation at treatment start, (iii) bruising, (iv) insulin leakage, (v) variations in fructosamine, and (vi) fasting and post-meal glucose levels [22,23]. In essence, the effects of the two needle types are substantially overlapping, with only a slightly increased effort perceived by patients at pressing the button that is used to have insulin flowing through the needle due to reduced gauge (G). ADA experts did not consider these papers, probably due to the few cases they examined. However, 3.5 mm needles could be helpful in selected populations. The latter might include young children, skinny adults, pregnant women, and hemodialyzed subjects who are often malnourished and underweight and quickly develop LH [24]. These subjects could successfully use ultra-short needles to avoid the risk of intramuscular injections related to their ultra-thin subcutaneous adipose tissue.

However, using excessively thin needles requires an extra effort to press the pen button when injecting insulin, thus eventually causing trouble to older people with hand problems. Indeed, the elderly's hands are often home to arthrosis, arthritis, carpal tunnel syndrome, or, especially in North-European men, thickening of the palmar aponeurosis (Dupuytren's disease). Such abnormalities are easily diagnosed through an accurate physical examination and by asking the patient to write down a short sentence or to perform the tabletop test (i.e., placing fingers flat on a table). They prevent patients from pressing the pen button long enough to complete the full insulin dose injection and keep it pressed ten more seconds after that, as expected to avoid any drug leakage.

A further, too often disregarded issue is the need to add details in electronic medical records concerning LH presence, site, size, texture, and degree of projection on the skin surface, if so ever. Such a habit could let patients and healthcare providers follow up on LH changes and monitor the effectiveness of educational efforts over time by comparing progressive lesion improvement with metabolic parameters, including glucose time-in-range and variability, which are well-known risk factors for chronic diabetes complications worsening (Figure 1 and Table 2).

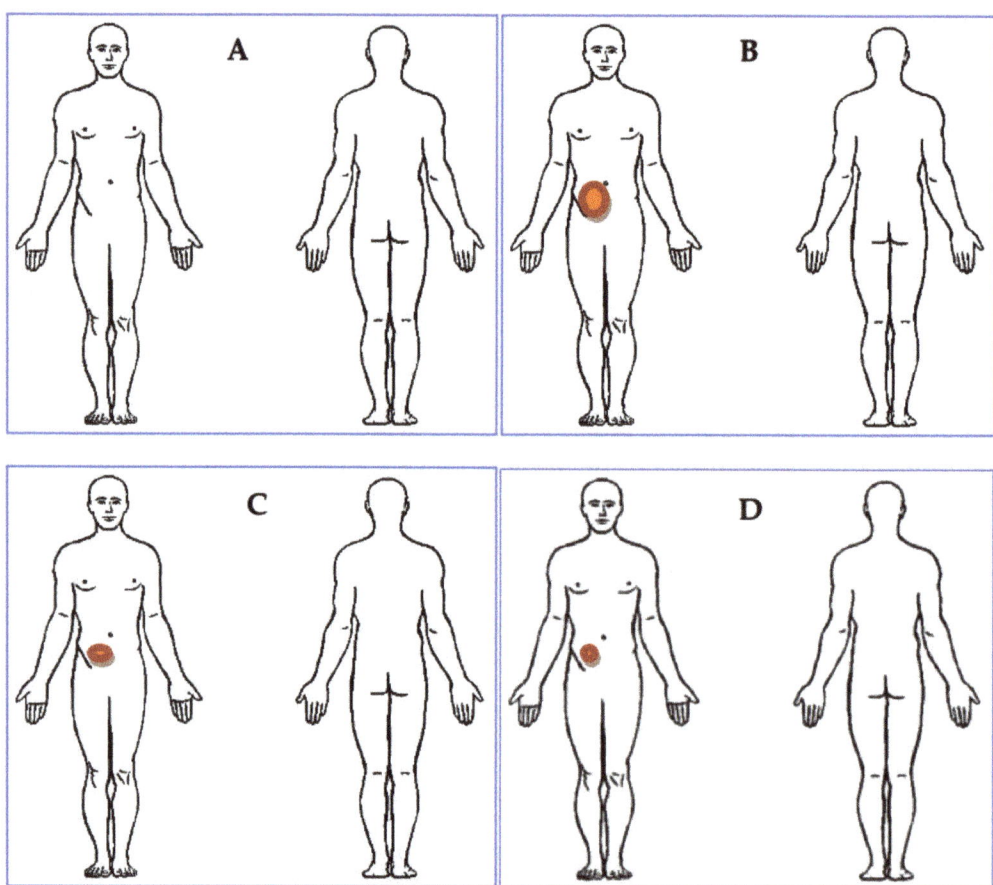

Figure 1. Body image suitable for LH site and size recording over time. Panel (**A**): no LH is present. Panel (**B**): a large abdominal LH is present. Panels (**C**,**D**): the LH size progressively decreases during follow-up.

Table 2. LH features recording grid. Tick the box accordingly.

LH Features	Right Arm	Left Arm	Right Thigh	Left Thigh	Right Hemi-Abdomen	Left Hemi-Abdomen	Right Buttock	Left Buttock
Present								
>4 cm								
<4 cm								
Protruding								
Flat								
Hard-elastic								
Soft								

Another handy and practical tool allowing the clinician to efficiently monitor lesions could be a digital checklist of actions to be taken for LH detection and follow-up. It should be included in each patient's medical record with a popup alert periodically encouraging the clinician to verify injection site conditions. A similar recording method could also help take note of educational activities performed and the patient's ability to accordingly act. For instance, healthcare providers should preliminarily check whether or not an individual patient can perpendicularly insert the needle in the pen so that the inner side of the needle does not bend and correctly penetrates the insulin reservoir rubber cap, which is a prerequisite for easy and reliable fluid flow into the skin at the time of injection.

Diabetes-related clinical records should include a detailed checklist devoted to all actions needed to identify LH in insulin-treated patients, as follows:

- Are you sure the explanations you gave to your patient when prescribing insulin were exhaustive and sufficiently clear to let him/her understand how to correctly perform injections?
- Did you explain to him/her how the insulin pen works?
- Did you show him/her how to insert the needle on top of the pen?
- Did you show him/her how to hold the pen at the time of injection?
- Did you provide him/her a chart or cartoon displaying clear indications of the best injection site selection?
- Did you give him/her clear information concerning the importance of selecting the correct needle length and inserting it onto the skin surface at a correct angle?
- Did you tell him/her how to store insulin and avoid ice-cold insulin injections?
- Did you tell him/her that too long needles pose him/her a risk of reaching the muscle tissue below the subcutaneous layer in the case of thin areas, and intramuscular injections make insulin absorption faster, thus often causing unexpected hypoglycemia?
- Did you take enough time to show him/her the best way to perform injection site rotation within separate skin areas?
- Did you explain to him/her the appropriate distance to keep among injection sites?
- Did you stress the importance of pressing the pen button for at least 10 s before taking the pen out of the skin enough?
- Did you repeatedly mention that disposable needles are to be used only once and then discarded?
- Did you remind him/her that, when repeatedly using the same injection site, he/she might give rise to skin nodules causing insulin absorption abnormalities with consequent large blood glucose variability, poor diabetes control, and ever-increasing insulin?
- Did you explain to him/her, especially when insulin-treated for a long time, that it is necessary to self-palpate the skin area in search of nodules and to avoid them if present?
- Did you make sure that, besides understanding all the information pills provided, he/she has taken the habit of correctly putting into practice the teachings you have told and shown so far?

It is easy to check all the abovementioned education elements by simply asking the patient to perform one or more injections in the presence of the diabetes team members and correct any errors in execution.

All insulin-treated subjects should undergo education sessions, including extensive retraining, regularly and at least annually [4,8,18], without forgetting to verify acquired habits in terms of the correct sequence of actions required to appropriately handle, store, and inject insulin.

Indeed, only regularly occurring meetings meant to verify the correct sequence of insulin injection-related actions may yield reliable long-term therapeutic results, thus preventing the worthlessness of the relentless ongoing technological advances in pen and needle engineering and progress in pharmacology/biotechnology in pursuit of progressively more "physiologic" and pure insulin preparations. All the above reflect practical economic considerations but are also better for health and are especially meant to improve the patient's quality of life as much as possible. Indeed, a steadily correct injection habit not only avoids the ever-increasing costs of insulin spoiled by intranodular trapping but also improves glucose control and dramatically reduces hypoglycemic events [4,8,18]. Our daily experience has been supported by experimental data so far. It provides us with a solid motivation to go on with what initially was a vast educational effort and gradually became routine. Indeed, now we feel fully rewarded by our patient's satisfaction with his/her easily perceived better quality of life. Should such a miracle happen, insulin-treated subjects would no more exchange their serene awareness of a present free of sudden, unexpected, and frightening hypoglycemic events and a future free of complications with a painless injection performed into an almost insensitive, denervated lipodystrophic nodule.

At present, while waiting for such a dream to come true in most diabetes wards worldwide, it is of utmost importance that healthcare teams verify that patients perform self-palpation efficiently enough to detect LHs and, after that, always choose healthy skin sites when injecting the drug, considering the possible "unintentional" choice of painless lesioned areas.

In conclusion, we underline the need for (i) a more careful, systematic, and structured search for cutaneous LH related to injection technique errors; (ii) care teams systematically searching for LH and teaching patients how to recognize and avoid LH while injecting insulin; (iii) updated guidelines and recommendations on correct injection techniques in the light of recent advances in insulin needle technology; and (iv) education of patients ignoring those documents and only trying to avoid discomfort at the time of injection [25,26]. Given the unstoppable growth of the population with diabetes—also due to the increase in the number of post-COVID-19 cases [27]—all what mentioned above is necessary and urgent to prevent the most potent available drug from being nullified and to avoid chronic diabetes complications by improving treatment effectiveness in people on multiple injection regimens. One hundred years have passed since the introduction of insulin into therapy, and some questions spontaneously arise: will all this be enough? Will it take another 100 years to solve the problems of insulin-induced LH [28]?

Finally, an additional interesting element to consider is the LH-inducing potential of non-insulin-containing anti-hyperglycemic drug preparations, if so ever. Indeed, such a theme deserves attention, in our view, because no investigators systematically explored it so far, and, what is even more intriguing, such injections would lack insulin's anabolic effects, which have been listed for years among typical LH contributing factors. To the best of our knowledge, only one paper related to that issue was published by our group some years ago, dealing with a formulation containing a once-weekly long-acting exenatide, i.e., a glucagon-like peptide-1 receptor agonist (GLP-1RA), repeatedly injected into the same skin site, as reflected by Figure 2 [29].

Possible LH-inducing effects of mixed basal insulin-GLP-1RAs also warrant investigation. Therefore, the scientific community is responsible for fostering awareness of the negative long-term consequences of careless injection habits to improve knowledge in the field and perform adequate, effective prevention and treatment measures.

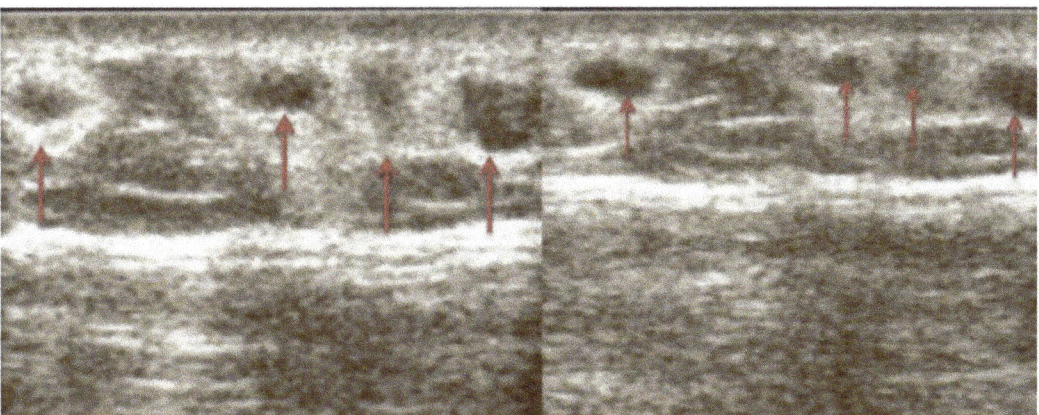

Figure 2. Ultrasound image of multiple nodules found 8 weeks after repeated subcutaneous injections. Formulation performed within a small skin area within the arm. Nodules displayed hypoechoic patterns with hyperechoic borders ([29], modified).

2. Summary Points

1. Lipohypertrophy (LH) due to incorrect injection technique is widespread, underdiagnosed, and mainly ignored by clinicians.
2. We have national and international recommendations on correct injection techniques, but LH is, nevertheless, ubiquitous.
3. A call to action is needed to implement the culture of LH and its complications.
4. Recommendations must take into account advances in technology, and new research is needed to prove the usefulness of the new devices.
5. It is necessary to implement structured clinical diagnostic paths for the identification of LH, especially in care settings without ultrasonography, an unsuitable and expensive method for population and screening studies.

Author Contributions: F.S., G.G., E.S. and S.G. equally contributed to the conception and drafting of this paper. All named authors meet the International Committee of Medical Journal Editors (ICMJE) criteria for authorship for this article, take responsibility for the integrity of the work as a whole. All authors have read and agreed to the published version of the manuscript.

Funding: This research received no external funding. None of the authors has received funds or any form of direct or indirect financing for this article or has incompatibility with the contents of the text.

Institutional Review Board Statement: The IRB from the Naples "Vanvitelli" University approved the study on 16 July 2022 under n. 11619/bis.

Informed Consent Statement: The manuscript does not directly use human or animal data for which it does not respond to this need and, therefore, does not even require an authorization procedure.

Data Availability Statement: Data are contained within the article.

Acknowledgments: We are indebted to Paola Murano, General Manager of the Nefrocenter Research Network, for the effective and continuous, spontaneously offered support toward carrying out the paper. Special thanks go to the members of AMD-OSDI Study Group (available on www.aemmedi.it, accessed on 3 February 2023).

Conflicts of Interest: The authors declare no conflict of interest.

References

1. Gentile, S.; Guarino, G.; Satta, E.; Romano, C.; Strollo, F. Why 100-years after the discovery of insulin and the appearance of insulin-induced lipodystrophy: Are we still struggling with this nasty complication? *Diabetes Res. Open. J.* **2022**, *8*, 23–29. [CrossRef]
2. Blanco, M.; Hernández, M.T.; Strauss, K.W.; Amaya, M. Prevalence and risk factors of lipohypertrophy in insulin-injecting patients with diabetes. *Diabetes Metab.* **2013**, *39*, 445–453. [CrossRef]
3. Gentile, S.; Strollo, F.; De Rosa, N. Injection-Related Local Side Effects in the Treatment of Diabetes Mellitus: A Methodological Approach and Possible Solutions. Consensus Statement of AMD-OSDI Study Group on Injection Technique. In e-Book Diabetes Complications. 2016. Available online: https://www.semanticscholar.org/paper/Gr-upSM-Injection-Related-Local-Side-Effects-in-the-Sandro-Felice/d29d49e463d1dbe98bde0089177870f2080bc46c (accessed on 3 February 2023).
4. Gentile, S.; Guarino, G.; Della Corte, T.; Marino, G.; Satta, E.; Pasquarella, M.; Romano, C.; Alfrone, C.; Strollo, F.; AMD-OSDI Study Group on Injection Technique, Nefrocenter Research and Nyx Start-Up. Role of structured education in reducing lypodistrophy and its metabolic complications in insulin-treated people with type 2 diabetes: A randomized multicenter case-control study. *Diabetes Ther.* **2021**, *12*, 1379–1398. [CrossRef] [PubMed]
5. Shen, M.; Shi, Y.; Zheng, S.; Fan, H.; Xu, J.; Yang, T. A systematic survey of physicians' insights into lipohypertrophy. *Front. Public Health* **2021**, *9*, 738179. [CrossRef] [PubMed]
6. Lin, Y.; Lin, L.; Wang, W.; Hong, J.; Zeng, H. Insulin-related lipohypertrophy: Ultrasound characteristics, risk factors, and impact of glucose fluctuations. *Endocrine* **2022**, *75*, 768–775. [CrossRef] [PubMed]
7. Deng, N.; Zhang, X.; Zhao, F.; Wang, Y.; He, H. Prevalence of lipohypertrophy in insulin-treated diabetes patients: A systematic review and meta-analysis. *J. Diabetes Investig.* **2017**, *9*, 536–543. [CrossRef]
8. Gentile, S.; Guarino, G.; Della Corte, T.; Marino, G.; Satta, E.; Pasquarella, M.; Romano, C.; Alfrone, C.; Giordano, L.; Loiacono, F.; et al. The Durability of an Intensive, Structured Education-Based Rehabilitation Protocol for Best Insulin Injection Practice: The ISTERP-2 Study. *Diabetes Ther.* **2021**, *12*, 2557–2569. [CrossRef]
9. Gentile, S.; Guarino, G.; Marino, G.; Strollo, F. Risk factors for severe hypoglycemia in people with insulin-treated diabetes: Are we sure we took into account all variables involved? *Nutr. Metab. Cardiovasc. Dis.* **2017**, *27*, 415–416. [CrossRef]
10. Gentile, S.; Satta, E.; Guarino, G.; Romano, G.; Maffettone, A.; Heinke, E.E.; Donnarumma, E.; Castellano, R.; Izzo, S.; Manzo, I.; et al. A Journey Through Guidelines, Consensus, Curriculum of Educators and Clinical Practice on Insulin-Induced Skin Lipohypertrophy: From the Earth to the Moons. *Med. Res. Arch.* **2022**, *10*. [CrossRef]
11. Gentile, S.; Strollo, F.; Guarino, G. Why are so huge differences reported in the occurrence rate of skin lipohypertrophy? Does it depend on method defects or on lack of interest? *Diabetes Metab. Syndr.* **2019**, *13*, 682–686. [CrossRef]
12. Strollo, F.; Satta, E.; Gentile, S. Insulin Injection-Related Skin Lipodystrophies: Blemish or Pathology? *Diabetology* **2022**, *3*, 615–619. [CrossRef]
13. Gentile, S.; Guarino, G.; Giancaterini, A.; Guida, P.; Strollo, F.; AMD-OSDI Italian Injection Technique Study Group. A suitable palpation technique allows to identify skin lipohypertrophic lesions in insulin-treated people with diabetes. *Springerplus* **2016**, *5*, 563. [CrossRef]
14. Gentile, S.; Strollo, F.; Guarino, G.; Giancaterini, A.; Ames, P.R.J.; Speese, K.; Guida, P.; Strauss, K. Factors hindering correct identification of unapparent lipohypertrophy. *J. Diabetes Metab. Disord. Control* **2016**, *3*, 42–47. [CrossRef]
15. Kapeluto, J.E.; Paty, B.W.; Chang, S.D.; Meneilly, G.S. Ultrasound detection of insulin-induced lipohypertrophy in Type 1 and Type 2 diabetes. *Diabet. Med.* **2018**, *35*, 1383–1390. [CrossRef] [PubMed]
16. Gentile, S.; Guarino, G.; Corte, T.D.; Marino, G.; Fusco, A.; Corigliano, G.; Colarusso, S.; Piscopo, M.; Improta, M.R.; Corigliano, M.; et al. Insulin-induced skin lipohypertrophy in Type 2 diabetes: A multicenter regional survey in Southern Italy. *Diabetes Ther.* **2020**, *11*, 2001–2017. [CrossRef]
17. American Diabetes Association Professional Practice Committee. 9. Pharmacologic approaches to glycemic treatment: Standards of Medical Care in Diabetes—2022. *Diabetes Care* **2022**, *45* (Suppl. 1), S125–S143. [CrossRef]
18. Gentile, S.; Guarino, G.; Della Corte, T.; Marino, G.; Satta, E.; Pasquarella, M.; Romano, C.; Alfrone, C.; Giordano, L.; Loiacono, F.; et al. AMD-OSDI Study Group on Injection Techniques, and ANIAD. The Economic Burden of Insulin Injection-Induced Lipohypertopy. Role of Education: The ISTERP-3 Study. *Adv. Ther.* **2022**, *39*, 2192–2207; Erratum in *Adv. Ther.* **2022**, *39*, 3058. [CrossRef]
19. Gentile, S.; Grassi, G.; Armentano, V.; Botta, A.; Cucco, L.; De Riu, S.; De Rosa, N.; Garrapa, G.; Gentile, L.; Giancaterini, A.; et al. AMD-OSDI consensus on injection techniques for people with diabetes mellitus. *Med. Clin. Rev.* **2016**, *2*, 3. [CrossRef]
20. Frid, A.H.; Kreugel, G.; Grassi, G.; Halimi, S.; Hicks, D.; Hirsch, L.J.; Smith, M.J.; Wellhoener, R.; Bode, B.W.; Hirsch, I.B.; et al. New insulin delivery recommendations. *Mayo Clin. Proc.* **2016**, *91*, 1231–1255. [CrossRef]
21. Consensus Document on the Italian Transposition of Forum for Injection Technique and Therapy Expert Recommendations 2015. Update and Integrations by the AMD-Osdi Inter-Corporate Group on Injective Techniques. 16 May 2017. Available online: https://aemmedi.it/wp-content/uploads/2016/09/FITTER2017.pdf (accessed on 13 February 2023).
22. Valentini, M.; Scardapane, M.; Bondanini, F.; Bossi, A.; Colatrella, A.; Girelli, A.; Ciucci, A.; Leotta, S.; Minotti, E.; Pasotti, F.; et al. Efficacy, safety and acceptability of the new pen needle 33G × 4 mm. AGO 01 study. *Curr. Med. Res. Opin.* **2015**, *31*, 487–492. [CrossRef]

23. De Berardis, G.; Scardapane, M.; Lucisano, G.; Abbruzzese, S.; Bossi, A.C.; Cipponeri, E.; D'Angelo, P.; Fontana, L.; Lancione, R.; Marelli, G.; et al. Efficacy, safety and acceptability of the new pen needle 34 G × 3.5 mm: A crossover randomized non-inferiority trial; AGO 02 study. *Curr. Med. Res. Opin.* **2018**, *34*, 1699–1704. [CrossRef]
24. Gentile, S.; Strollo, F.; Satta, E.; Della Corte, T.; Romano, C.; Guarino, G.; Nefrocenter Research Study Group: Nephrologists, Diabetologists, Nurses. Insulin-Related Lipohypertrophy in Hemodialyzed Diabetic People: A Multicenter Observational Study and a Methodological Approach. *Diabetes Ther.* **2019**, *10*, 1423–1433. [CrossRef] [PubMed]
25. Aronson, R. The role of comfort and discomfort in insulin therapy. *Diabetes Technol. Ther.* **2012**, *14*, 741–747. [CrossRef] [PubMed]
26. Bergenstal, R.M.; Strock, E.S.; Peremislov, D.; Gibney, M.A.; Parvu, V.; Hirsch, L.J. Safety and efficacy of insulin therapy delivered via a 4mm pen needle in obese patients with diabetes. *Mayo Clin. Proc.* **2015**, *90*, 329–338. [CrossRef] [PubMed]
27. Rubino, F.; Amiel, S.A.; Zimmet, P.; Alberti, G.; Bornstein, S.; Eckel, R.H.; Mingrone, G.; Boehm, B.; Cooper, M.E.; Del Prato, S.; et al. New-Onset Diabetes in COVID-19. *N. Engl. J. Med.* **2020**, *383*, 789–790. [CrossRef]
28. Di Bartolo, P.; Eckel, R.H.; Strollo, S.; Gentile, S. Hundred-year experience with insulin and lipohypertrophy: An unresolved issue. *Diabetes Res. Clin. Pract.* **2021**, *178*, 108924. [CrossRef]
29. Gentile, S.; Strollo, F. Subcutaneous Nodules during Treatment with an Exenatide Long-Acting Once-Weekly Formulation: An Ultrasound Evaluation. *Divers. Equal. Health Care* **2016**, *13*, 313–318.

Disclaimer/Publisher's Note: The statements, opinions and data contained in all publications are solely those of the individual author(s) and contributor(s) and not of MDPI and/or the editor(s). MDPI and/or the editor(s) disclaim responsibility for any injury to people or property resulting from any ideas, methods, instructions or products referred to in the content.

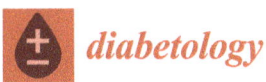

Study Protocol

Multicenter, Open Label, Randomized Controlled Superiority Trial for Availability to Reduce Nocturnal Urination Frequency: Study Protocol for a TOP-STAR Study

Hanako Nakajima [1], Hiroshi Okada [1], Akinori Kogure [2], Takafumi Osaka [3], Takeshi Tsutsumi [4], Toru Tanaka [5], Goji Hasegawa [6], Shinichi Mogami [7], Kazuteru Mitsuhashi [8], Noriyuki Kitagawa [9], Yoshitaka Hashimoto [10], Miho Yano [11], Muhei Tanaka [12], Akane Kitamura [13], Michiyo Ishii [14], Naoto Nakamura [15], Akio Kishi [16], Emi Ushigome [1], Masahide Hamaguchi [1,*] and Michiaki Fukui [1]

[1] Department of Endocrinology and Metabolism, Graduate School of Medical Science, Kyoto Prefectural University of Medicine, Kyoto 602-8566, Japan
[2] Department of Diabetes and Metabolic Medicine, Kyoto City Hospital, Kyoto 604-8845, Japan
[3] Department of Endocrinology and Diabetology, Ayabe City Hospital, Ayabe 623-0011, Japan
[4] Department of Endocrinology and Metabolism, Kyoto Yamashiro General Medical Center, Kizugawa 619-0214, Japan
[5] Department of Diabetes and Endocrinology, Japanese Red Cross Kyoto Daiichi Hospital, Kyoto 605-0981, Japan
[6] Division of Metabolism, Nephrology and Rheumatology, Japanese Red Cross Kyoto Daini Hospital, Kyoto 602-8026, Japan
[7] Department of Diabetes and Metabolism, Osaka General Hospital of West Japan Railway Company, Osaka 545-0053, Japan
[8] Department of Diabetes and Internal Medicine, Fukuchiyama City Hospital, Fukuchiyama 620-8505, Japan
[9] Department of Diabetology, Kameoka Municipal Hospital, Kameoka 621-0826, Japan
[10] Department of Diabetes and Endocrinology, Matsushita Memorial Hospital, Moriguchi 570-8540, Japan
[11] Department of Diabetology, Nishijin Hospital, Kyoto 602-8319, Japan
[12] Department of Endocrinology, Metabolism, and Diabetes, Saiseikai Suita Hospital, Osaka 564-0013, Japan
[13] Department of Diabetology, Nagitsuji Hospital, Kyoto 607-8163, Japan
[14] Department of Internal Medicine, Otsu City Hospital, Otsu 520-0804, Japan
[15] Division of Diabetes, Saiseikai Kyoto Hospital, Kyoto 617-8617, Japan
[16] Department of Diabetes, Kyoto Okamoto Memorial Hospital, Kyoto 613-0034, Japan
* Correspondence: mhama@koto.kpu-m.ac.jp; Tel.: +81-75-251-5505

Abstract: Nocturia is a common disease in patients with type 2 diabetes mellitus that can reduce the quality of life. Sodium glucose co-transporter 2 (SGLT2) inhibitors increase the urine volume and are often discontinued when polyuria occurs, although tofogliflozin, which has a short half-life in the blood, may improve nocturia by managing hyperglycemia and hypertension, without aggravating nocturia. As excessive sodium intake worsens nocturia and increases urine volume, sodium restriction is also effective in managing nocturia. This multicenter, open-label, randomized parallel-group trial will examine 80 patients with type 2 diabetes who experienced nocturia. After the baseline examination, the patients are randomly stratified into two groups and receive tofogliflozin treatment with or without sodium restriction for 12 weeks. The primary outcome is nocturia frequency at 12 weeks. The secondary outcomes are the frequency of daytime urine, changes in urine volume, and changes in home blood pressure.

Keywords: type 2 diabetes; sodium glucose co-transporter 2 (SGLT2) inhibitors; nocturia; sodium intake

1. Introduction

1.1. Background and Rationale

Nocturia is a condition of waking up at night to urinate one or more times during the night [1]. The frequency of nocturia in Japan increases with age, reaching 83.8% in men and

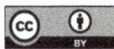

76.6% in women in their 60s [2]. Nocturia is caused by several factors, including nocturnal polyuria, cystourethral disturbance, sleep disturbance, and cardiovascular disease, and either one or a combination of these factors may be involved. In addition to age, diabetes mellitus, hypertension, stroke, heart disease, and obesity have been associated with nocturia [3–8]. Approximately 40% of patients with diabetes arise more than twice at night to void [9]. In our KAMOGAWA-DM cohort study [10], according to a questionnaire survey on the frequency of nocturia conducted in 396 patients, 80% had nocturia more than once, while 40% had nocturia more than twice. Nocturia is a common condition in patients with diabetes.

In addition, Hashimoto et al. [11] reported that sleep disorders were a major cause of poorer quality of life (QOL) in Japanese patients with type 2 diabetes (T2D), and more than half of them were frequently awakened by the urge to void. Nocturia is a risk factor for fractures and decreases the survival rate [12].

Sodium glucose co-transporter 2 (SGLT2) inhibitors can improve glycemic control, glycemic variability, and fat loss, as well as prevent heart and renal failure [13,14]. However, concerns have been raised regarding the adverse events of SGLT2 inhibitors, not only dehydration and urinary tract infection, but also polyuria [15]. In fact, frequent uri-nation and polyuria have been the primary reasons for the discontinuation of SGLT2 inhibitor treatment [16].

One SGLT2 inhibitor, tofogliflozin, which has a short half-life, promotes urinary glu-cose excretion during daytime without worsening nocturia [17] and may improve hyper-glycemia and hypertension. As sodium retention exacerbates nocturia by causing non-dipping nocturnal hypertension, SGLT2 inhibitors with a short half-life could im-prove nocturia by increasing the daytime excretion of sodium [18].

Therefore, to correct and prevent the worsening of nocturia, not only medication but also restriction of dietary salt intake should be considered. Reduction in sodium intake can decrease the frequency of nocturia, nocturnal urine volume, and nocturnal polyuria index; patients with nocturia accompanied by nocturnal polyuria should control their sodium intake.

The observational study in Japan, nocturia volume, the frequency of nocturia, and nocturnal polyuria index were evaluated after 12 weeks of dietary guidance in patients who experienced one episode of nocturia, exceeding the maximum daily salt intake (8 g for men and 7 g for women). This study reported that nocturia frequency, urine volume, and nocturnal polyuria index improved in the group of participants who had been successful in restricting salt intake [19,20].

As mentioned above, various factors constitute nocturia, such as nocturnal hypergly-cemia, excessive salt intake, and nocturnal hypertension; in particular, non-dipper-type nocturnal hypertension and heart failure are the risk factors for nocturia [21–23].

Nocturia should be managed with both medication and salt intake restriction in order to correct and prevent the exacerbation of nocturia; however, no study has evaluated the effect of a combination of salt intake restriction and SGLT2 inhibitor treatment on nocturia. It would be significant to examine the effect of tofogliflozin, an SGLT2 inhibitor with the shortest half-life, on nocturia in patients with T2D, and whether tofogliflozin treatment could be effective in combination with sodium restriction.

1.2. Objectives

1.2.1. Primary Objectives

The primary aim of this study is to evaluate the effect of tofogliflozin on nocturia in patients with T2D and to examine the efficacy of tofogliflozin with or without dietary sodium restriction on nocturia at 12 weeks after interventions.

1.2.2. Secondary Objectives

The secondary aim of this study is to assess below items at 12 weeks after interventions.

1. Frequency of urination during the day
2. Change in ratio of urinary volume at night to 24 h
3. Change in urine volume at night

4. Change in urine volume during the day
5. Change in total urinary sodium excretion and other urinalysis
6. Change in the results of blood tests
7. Change in home blood pressure at night
8. Change in body composition test
9. Change in questionnaire score (The Diabetes Treatment Satisfaction Questionnaire, status version, DTSQs score; Diabetes Diet-Related Quality of Life Revised, DDRQOL-R; Brief-type Self-administered Diet History Questionnaire, BDHQ; Core Lower Urinary Tract Symptoms score, CLSS)
10. Incidence of adverse events and diseases

2. Methods

2.1. Trial Design

This is a multicenter, open-label, randomized parallel group trial [Efficacy of dual therapy of TOfogliflozin and dietary instruction of sodium restriction in T2D patients with nocturia: A multicenter open-label randomized controlled superiority trial of the availability to reduce nocturnal urination frequency (TOP-STAR Study)] (Figure 1). Eighty patients with T2D and nocturia will be included in the study and randomly stratified into two groups.

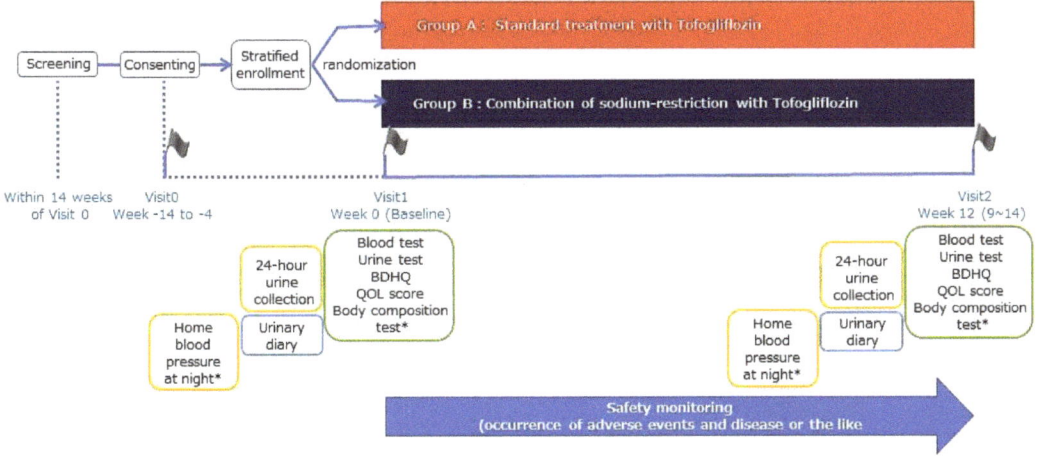

Figure 1. Study design of TOP-STAR study.

2.2. Eligibility Criteria, Recruitment, and Sample Size

Inclusion and exclusion criteria were established according to the study objectives and to ensure participant safety (Table 1).

This study will be conducted in 18 research institutions. In the previous study [20], the frequency of nocturia improved from 2.3 ± 0.9 times per day at baseline to 1.4 ± 1.0 times per day after 12 weeks in the group of participants who were successful in restricting salt intake. In the group of participants who were not successful in restricting salt intake, the frequency of nocturia did not improve (from 2.3 ± 1.1 days at baseline to 2.7 ± 1.1 days after 12 weeks). In this study, the frequency of nocturia was 2.3 ± 1.0 days in both groups at baseline, it remained unchanged (2.3 ± 1.0 days) in the tofogliflozin monotherapy group, and it was 1.3 ± 1.0 days in the combination group that received sodium restriction guidance after 12 weeks. Under these conditions and at a significance level of 5% in both groups, 10,000 tests were required to determine the differences in nocturia frequency between the groups after 12 weeks as shown in the results of Poisson regression analysis using data assuming a Poisson distribution. Therefore, the minimum number of patients required for this study was 36 patients per group. In addition, assuming a dropout rate of 10% during the study period, the target number of participants to be enrolled in this study was 40 patients per group or 80 patients in two groups.

Table 1. Inclusion and exclusion criteria.

Inclusion criteria	
Patients with all of the following criteria will be considered	
1	Patients with type 2 diabetes
2	Patients with nocturia more than once
3	Male and female between the ages of 20 and 90 at the time of obtaining consent
4	Patients who provide their consent in a written form
Exclusion criteria	
Patients who meet any of the following criteria are not eligible to the study	
1	Patients who use SGLT2 inhibitor at least 3 months prior to giving their content
2	Patients who have already been instructed by a nutritionist of sodium-restriction
3	Patients with an estimated sodium intake of less than 6 g/day by urinalysis at the time of obtaining consent
4	Patients for whom tofogliflozin is contraindicated
5	Patients whose HbA1c is 10.5% or higher within 3 months
6	Patients with eGFR less than 15 mL/min/1.73 m^2 or serum creatinine higher than 3.5 mg/dL or with hemodialysis
7	Patients with low blood pressure (less than 100/60 mmHg)
8	Patients with unstable hypertension
9	Patients with activities of daily living (ADL) of PS2 or higher
10	Patients with heart failure classified as New York Heart Association (NYHA) category III or IV
11	Patients being pregnant or planning to become pregnant.
12	Patients suffering from cancer. However, the treatment has been completed and/or the cancer has not recurred and/or is becoming apparent
13	Patients with anemia (Hb is 10 g/dL or less) caused by primary diseases other than diabetic nephropathy
14	Patients with hypoalbuminemia (serum albumin is 3.5 g/dL or less) caused by primary diseases other than diabetic nephropathy
15	Patients with nephrotic syndrome (less than 3.0 g/dL of serum albumin and more than 3.5 g/day of urinary protein) due to primary disease except diabetic nephropathy
16	Patients judged to be non-adherent by the attending physician
17	Patients who require substitute to obtain consent
18	Patients deemed inappropriate by the attending physician

2.3. Interventions

2.3.1. Random Grouping and Intervention Description

The participants are randomly assigned in different groups [Group A: standard treatment group]. Randomisation will be provided by a computer-generated program at the EviPRO Holdings Inc. (Tokyo, Japan). The study participants are administered with tofogliflozin 20 mg orally once a day before or after breakfast. The duration of tofogliflozin administration is 12 weeks (9–14 weeks) [Group B: group with dietary sodium restriction]. In addition to the oral administration of 20 mg of tofogliflozin once a day before or after breakfast, a nutritionist provides instructions on sodium restriction. The duration of tofogliflozin treatment is 12 weeks (9–14 weeks). SGLT2 inhibitor treatment is initiated on day 0 of the observation period. The study participants are requested to visit the research institutions at weeks 0 and 12, in addition to the date of obtaining consent.

2.3.2. Details of Instruction on Sodium Restriction

The nutritionist provided dietary instructions, with a target sodium intake of 6 g/day. In addition, for both groups, the target weight and amount of energy and protein in the diet were based on the nutritional guidelines that the patients received.

2.3.3. Details of Other Dietary Instruction

In both groups, the patients are instructed to stay properly hydrated to prevent dehydration (avoid excessive drinking or excessive water conservation).

Energy level: 25–35 kcal/kg/day for physical activity multiplied by the target weight.

Protein restriction: 0.8–1.0 g/kg/day (stage 3 diabetic nephropathy) and 0.6–0.8 g/kg/day (stage 4 diabetic nephropathy).

2.3.4. Observation Items

A baseline examination will be conducted prior to the intervention. The observations and schedules are presented in Tables 2 and 3. Generally, research participants will visit the research institution and undergo blood and urine tests at every visit.

Table 2. Observation items.

1. Eligibility information	
Observation point	At consenting and enrollment
Observation item	Inclusion criteria, exclusion criteria, gender, age, date of giving consent
2. Background information	
Observation point	At consenting, enrollment, or week 0
Observation item	Gender, age, height, weight, body mass index, duration of diabetes, presence of comorbidities (presence/absence of macrovascular/microvascular complications, renal disease, hepatic disease, hypertension, dyslipidemia), and history of illness (history of cardio-cerebrovascular disease)
3. Medication information	
Observation point	Week 0 and week 12
Observation item	Medications for diabetes, daily dosage, and other concomitant medication
4. Blood tests (fasting)	
Observation point	Week 0 and week 12
Observation item	Red blood cell count, white blood cell count, hematocrit, hemoglobin, estimated plasma volume, blood platelet count, hepatic enzymes (AST, ALT, serum albumin, LDH, gamma-GTP, ALP), UA, BUN, Cre, eGFR, T-Chol, HDL, LDL, TG, serum Na/K/Cl, HbA1c (or glycoalbumin), and plasma glucose
5. Special blood tests (fasting, using residual sample of "6 blood tests")	
Observation point	Week 0 and week 12
Observation item	Total ketone body, beta-hydroxybutyric acid, acetoacetic acid, and plasma metabolome[++]
6. Urine tests (total)	
Observation point	Week 0 and week 12
Observation item	Specific gravity, pH, protein, glucose, ketone body, occult blood, bilirubin, urobilinogen, u-mAlb, U-Cre, and U-Na/K/Cl
7. Body composition test (optional test)	
Observation point	Week 0 and week 12
Observation item	Skeletal muscle mass, skeletal muscle mass to total body weight ratio, and fat mass

Table 2. *Cont.*

8. QOL score (questionnaire to whom the participants directly answer)	
Observation point	Week 0 and week 12
Observation item	• The Diabetes Treatment Satisfaction Questionnaire, status version (DTSQs) score. DTSQs are questionnaires used for measuring the patients' satisfaction to treatments specific for diabetes mellitus, are implemented worldwide, and consists of 8 questions. • Diabetes Diet-Related Quality of Life Revised (DDRQOL-R) This questionnaire consists of nine items. It is used to determine the diabetic patients' level of satisfaction regarding their diet and quality of life in relation to the changes in their dietary habits. • Brief-type Self-administered Diet History Questionnaire (BDHQ) A questionnaire designed to quantitatively and precisely examine the status of nutrients and food intake. • Core Lower Urinary Tract Symptoms score (CLSS). It is a 10-item questionnaire developed in Japan to investigate significant urinary tract symptoms.
9. Other items that the participants should measure on their own: Urinary diary	
Observation point	Week 0: conducted within 7 days after obtaining consent until the observation period week 0. Urine volume will be measured for 3 days; week 12: conducted within 7 days before observation point week 12. Urine volume will be measured for 3 days.
Observation item	Time of going to bed, time of waking up, time of urination, frequency of urination, volume of urine, and alcohol consumption The study participants store urine using a measuring cup.
10. 24 h urine collection test	
Observation point	Week 0 (24 h before the observation point) and week 12 (24 h before the observation point)
Observation item	Time of going to bed, time of waking up, volume of urine, volume of urine at night, plasma glucose, urinary creatinine excretion for 24 h, and urinary sodium excretion for 24 h The study participants store urine using a measuring cup and dispense a small portion of this urine into a spit.
11. Home blood pressure at night	
Observation point	Week 0 (5 days before observation point. Urine volume will be measured 3 times a day for 3 days), week 12 (conducted within 7 days before observation point week 12, 3 times each day) Conducted in a period that is different from the urinary diary period
Observation item	Home blood pressure at night: The participants measure their blood pressure three times at night using an upper arm blood pressure monitor (Omron HEM-9601T) (automatic measurement). The participants record the results in their diaries.
12. Adherence to research medication regimen and sodium restriction	
Observation point	Week 12
Observation item	The research physician conducts an interview to collect data regarding the patient's medication status and adherence with sodium restriction, and record the collected data in the CRF.

Additionally, nocturnal home blood pressure measurements will be taken three times a day for five days. Next, the urinary frequency will be recorded for 7 days, and urine volume will be measured using a measuring cup for 3 days. In addition to the blood and urine tests, scores on the Japanese version of the Diabetes Treatment Satisfaction Questionnaire, status version (DTSQs) score, Diabetes Diet-Related Quality of Life Revised (DDRQOL-R), Brief-type Self-administered Diet History Questionnaire (BDHQ), and Core Lower Urinary Tract Symptoms score (CLSS) will be assessed using a patient questionnaire. DTSQs are questionnaires used for measuring the patients' satisfaction to treatments specific for diabetes mellitus, are implemented worldwide, and consists of 8 questions [24]. DDRQOL-R consists of nine items. It is used to determine the diabetic patients' level of satisfaction regarding their diet and quality of life in relation to the changes in their dietary habits [25]. BDHQ designed to quantitatively and precisely examine the status of nutrients and food intake [26]. CLSS is a 10-item questionnaire developed in Japan to investigate significant urinary tract symptoms [27].

Table 3. Observation schedule.

Observation Items	Enrollment	Baseline Week 0 *1	Week 12 (Week 9–14) or at Discontinuation *2
Obtaining consent	○		
① Eligibility information	○		
② Background information		○	
③ Medication information		○	○
④ Blood tests		○	○
⑤ Special blood tests		○	○
⑥ Urine tests		○	○
⑦ Body composition		▲	▲
⑧ Questionnaire		○	○
⑨ Urination log		○	○
⑩ 24 h urine collection		○	○
⑪ Nocturnal home blood pressure		▲	▲
⑫ Compliance with drug regimen/Compliance with sodium restriction			○
⑬ Adverse event and disease or the like		←○→	

○ Item is required to be observed at indicated observation. ▲ Item is optionally observed at indicated observation period/observation point. *1 The observation points at week 0 could be conducted on the same day as enrollment. However, it must be conducted prior to the initiation of the intervention and prior to the instruction on sodium restriction. *2 In the event of discontinuation, collect as much information as possible up to this point.

2.4. Criteria for Discontinuing or Modifying Allocated Interventions

2.4.1. Criteria and Coping Strategies for Study Discontinuation

If the investigator judges that it is difficult to continue the clinical trial for any of the following reasons, the investigator will immediately take necessary measures such as discontinuing the administration of the study drug. Patients' data will be used as data of a "study discontinuation case." The investigator will note the date, when the study started, the reason for withdrawal, and the process on the card and on the case report form (CRF). At the time of discontinuation, the necessary tests will be conducted. The efficacy and safety the procedure will be assessed at this point. Moreover, investigators will evaluate the efficacy and safety of the treatment, following up on the endpoints and analyzing the safety of the medical treatment received.

2.4.2. Criteria for Discontinuation of Study in Each Participant

(1) A study participant voluntarily withdraws from the study or withdraws her or his consent.

(2) Discontinuation of the study is required due to the occurrence of adverse events and diseases.

(3) The continuous use of the study agent worsens the primary disease or causes complications.

(4) Patients have remarkably poor adherence with medication or sodium intake restrictions (the medication rate is estimated to be less than 60% or higher than 120% of the expected dosage).

(5) The study participant is found pregnant.

(6) A serious deviation from the research protocol occurs, which is judged to have a significant impact on the research results.

(7) The investigators have decided that the discontinuation of the study is appropriate due to other reasons.

2.4.3. Criteria for Discontinuation of Study

(1) When continuation of the study is difficult for any of the following reasons, the principal investigator will determine whether the study could be continued or not. When it is determined that continuation is inappropriate, the principal investigator shall inform the principal investigators of all collaborating institutions of the reasons for the discontinuation and how to deal with the participants, and have them take the necessary actions. The principal investigator shall inform the accreditation review committee in written form of the discontinuation of the study.

(1-1) Significant information regarding the efficacy, safety and quality of the study agent was obtained.

(1-2) Participant recruitment and the planned number of study participants were difficult to achieve.

(1-3) Protocol modification was instructed but was not executed.

(2) When discontinuing a study, the investigator should immediately discontinue the study and report the decision to the president of his/her institution. The principal investigator must also take appropriate action promptly and notify the participant of the decision to discontinue the study.

2.4.4. Coping with Adverse Events

SGLT2 inhibitors can cause dehydration, urinary tract infections, normoglycemic ketoacidosis, and polyuria, and we carefully explain the possibility of these side effects at the recruitment of previous study. If a study participant suffers an adverse event during the study which may or may not be attributable to the SGLT2 inhibitor, the investigator will promptly take appropriate medical treatment. Investigators should report the adverse event to the responsible investigator and director of the institution and document the necessary information on the medical carte and CRF according to the study protocol. If it is necessary to interrupt the administration of study drug or medical treatment due to an adverse event, the study participant should be briefed on how to manage serious adverse events [SAEs].

2.5. Deviation from the Protocol

The investigator shall document in the carte and CRF any deviation or modification from the study protocol that is necessary to avoid immediate risk to study participants or for other compelling medical reasons, and the details and reasons for such deviation or modification shall be stated in the Carte and CRF. Study participants will be followed up throughout the study. If the investigator is unable to follow the protocol exactly, he/she should continue to collect sufficient information for the study. Data handling will be determined by the data handling committee in a blinded situation.

2.6. Management of Incompatibility

Incompatibility refers to non-compliance with legal regulations or operational protocols, fabrication and falsification of test data. The management of incompatibility shall be performed as follows:

1. When the responsible investigator becomes aware of the incompatibility of present study, the responsible investigator must immediately report this fact to the principal investigator.
2. When the investigator becomes aware of the non-conformity of the study, the investigator immediately reports this fact to the responsible investigator.
3. When there are serious incompatibilities, the investigator must immediately ask the accreditation review committee members for their opinions.

2.7. Strategies to Improve Adherence to Interventions

2.7.1. Management of the Study Agent

No placebo will be used in this study. Both groups will use commercially available, approved drugs for the study. Additionally, this is an open-label study. Therefore, specific management of the study agent is not conducted, and the study agent is managed in the same manner as general drugs.

2.7.2. Outcomes

The investigators collect and enter the results of the examinations list in Table 2 in the CRF and send the CRF to the data center. Adverse events are considered as safety endpoints throughout the study. The items measured by the study participants themselves are recorded in specific documents and sent to the data center by the investigators.

2.8. Data Collection and Management

2.8.1. Plans for Assessment and Collection of Outcomes

Original Documents

The research institution preserves and manages the following information as original source documents, and responds to monitoring, audits, and certifying review committees' requests.

1. Original documents for all data items (medical data, nurse records, drug records, laboratory data, subject logbooks, CRFs, QOL questionnaires, etc.).
2. Records of informed consent indicating the patient's agreement to the study participation.

2.8.2. Documents to Be Served as Source Documents

In addition to the original source documents, the research institution preserves and controls the information described below as source documents and provides them to the monitoring, accreditation review committees, and audit.

1. Withdrawal of consent form.
2. Medication adherence information.
3. Adverse event and disease information.

2.8.3. Data Management and Confidentiality

Central registry numbers will be used to identify study participants. When electronic data on subjects are transferred, the consent of the data management must be obtained. If data are transferred from an unsecured electronic network, encryption of the data must be performed at the source. If the data center needs to provide participant data to other research institutions, approval from the principal investigator and data management is required. Plan for collection, laboratory evaluation, and preservation of biospecimens for genetic or molecular analysis for the study/future use.

All involved individuals in this study are required to protect the personal information of the study participants. We will conduct this study in compliance with the Personal Information Protection Act and other applicable laws and regulations. Study participant's unique information (medical record number, initials) will be securely contained within the research institution, and information that would allow someone external to the research organization to recognize the study participant (name, phone number, address, etc.) will not be included in the CRF or registry database.

The researcher will use the correspondence table to identify the research participant (anonymization) and will maintain it privately. Correspondence sheets will be securely stored and appropriately managed by the researcher for the retention period specified by the Clinical Trials Act (until the day after five years have elapsed from the date of study completion) or the retention period specified by each research institute, whichever is later. Anonymized data acquired for analysis will be preserved for any future secondary research, such as meta-analyses. Prior approval from the Ethics Review Committee is required before anonymized data will be used for further research.

Specific blood test samples will be assayed in laboratories made available by each research organization and will be disposed of after data acquisition under the responsibility and procedures of the respective companies.

2.9. Patient and Public Involvement Statement

Patients will not be included in the research design, selection of the study questions, or measurement of the results. No participants will be included in the analysis or publication of the results. Patients will receive a brief summary of the study results written in Japanese after the completion of the study.

2.10. Statistical Methods

2.10.1. Analysis of the Primary Endpoint

The primary and secondary endpoints are analyzed using the full analysis set and, if necessary, using the per-protocol set (PPS). The safety endpoints are analyzed in the safety analysis population. The two-sided significance level of the analysis was set at 5%. The person in charge of the statistical analysis is responsible for preparing a separate statistical analysis plan and specifying the details of the statistical method, including data handling. A statistical analysis plan is prepared prior to data fixation. If changes were made to the original analysis plan, the statistical analysis plan should be revised with a revision history, and the changes should be recorded.

The primary endpoint is the frequency of nocturia at 12 weeks, and the difference between groups is evaluated to determine its statistical significance. Poisson regression analysis (generalized linear model assuming a Poisson distribution) is performed with group as the fixed effect and the allocation adjustment factors and days of nocturnal voiding at baseline as covariates to test the following null hypothesis: that the days of nocturnal voiding in the two groups are equal. The summary statistics (number of cases, minimum, median, and maximum, mean, standard deviation) are calculated for each time point and each group.

2.10.2. Analysis of the Secondary Endpoints

With regard to the primary endpoint, the frequency of urination during the day is assessed for statistical significance using Poisson regression analysis with group as the fixed effect and the allocation adjustment factor and baseline value as covariates. For the other change endpoints, group differences are evaluated using analysis of covariance with the group as the fixed effect and allocation adjustment factors and baseline values as covariates. In addition, the summary statistics of the measurements and changes at each time point for each endpoint are calculated for each group. The incidence of adverse events and diseases are analyzed as part of the safety endpoints.

2.10.3. Methods for Additional Analyses (e.g., Subgroup Analyses)

For the primary and secondary endpoints, the combined salt intake restriction guidance group (tofogliflozin plus salt intake restriction guidance group) is subdivided into a successful salt reduction group and an unsuccessful salt reduction group, and the three groups are compared with the standard treatment group (tofogliflozin group). The details are described in a separate statistical analysis section.

Methods used for analyzing the protocol nonadherence and any statistical methods used for handle missing data

Data on protocol non-compliance will not be part of the per-protocol population analysis, but will be part of the full analysis.

2.11. Ethics and Dissemination

2.11.1. Data Handling Committee

The data handling committee will be responsible for processing all data, both missing data and data departing from the protocol, in a blinded manner prior to statistical analysis. The committee consist of the principal investigator, responsible officer, and a biomedical statistics expert.

2.11.2. Composition of the Data Monitoring Committee, Its Role, and Reporting Structure

Third-party institution (Evipro Holdings Corporation) will conduct the monitoring according to the standard operating procedures for monitoring. The responsible investigator will regularly monitor the persons in charge of data quality and investigate whether the study is being conducted in compliance with the research protocol, ethical guidelines for medicine, and the Clinical Trials Act, as well as the progress of the study by taking appropriate measures to ensure compliance with the protocol. Monitoring personnel is tasked to provide a monitoring report and submit it periodically to the principal investigator. The adverse events and diseases are monitored and promptly reported to ensure the safety of the study participants.

2.12. Adverse Event Reporting and Harms

2.12.1. Reporting of Adverse Events

Adverse events outside of SAEs will be reported by noting them on the CRF associated with those occurrences and sending it to the data center. The data center shall summarize the appropriate report and inform the responsible investigator and receive instructions on how to handle the event. The investigational drug manufacturer/distributor (Kowa Company, Ltd., Aichi Japan) will also be notified.

2.12.2. Frequency and Plans for Auditing Trial Conduct

EviPRO Holdings, a third-party institution, will conduct the audits. Audits will be performed according to the protocol and Standard Operating Procedures to ensure compliance with the study protocol. The results of the audit will be reported by the auditor to the investigator, other investigator.

2.12.3. Dissemination Plans

Results of the study will be reported in peer-reviewed international journals.

3. Discussion

This study was designed based on the hypothesis that SGLT2 inhibitors, which are anti-diabetic drugs with cardioprotective and renal protective effects, may relieve nocturia not only by improving hyperglycemia and hypertension, but also by increasing daytime sodium excretion, with a focus on managing polyuria and nocturia, which are common complaints of patients with type 2 diabetes. In addition, comparing the efficacy of SGLT2 inhibitors alone with that of salt restriction combined with SGLT2 inhibitors is meaningful as it will enable the researchers to examine the efficacy and superiority of each treatment for nocturia. In addition, the long-term intention of this study is to improve health quality of life through the improvement of nocturia, hoping that this will lead to an improvement in the overall health of the patients.

In this pilot study, the frequency of nocturia is the primary endpoint, while the frequency of urination during the day and change in urine volume as secondary endpoints, which provides insight into the effect of SGLT2 inhibitors and sodium restriction on urination frequency and volume. This finding will be essential for developing future randomized trials.

In previous observational studies, the frequency of nocturia, urine volume, and nocturnal polyuria index improved in patients who successfully restricted salt intake, but nocturia did not improve in patients with unsuccessfully restricted salt intake by nearly 70% of the time. SGLT2 inhibitors are effective in preventing the progression of macrovascular disease and diabetic complications, and their use is expected to increase in the future. However, SGLT2 inhibitors have some disadvantages, such as nocturia; hence, we hope that this study will expand the possibilities of SGLT2 inhibitors. In previous observational studies, the frequency of nocturia, urine volume, and nocturnal polyuria index improved in patients who successfully restricted salt intake, but nocturia did not improve in patients with unsuccessfully restricted salt intake by nearly 70% of the time. SGLT2 inhibitors are effective in preventing the progression of macrovascular disease and diabetic complications, and their use is expected to increase in the future. However, SGLT2 inhibitors have some disadvantages, such as nocturia; hence, we hope that this study will expand the possibilities of SGLT2 inhibitors.

Author Contributions: H.N. led the drafting of the manuscript; H.O., M.H. and M.F. reviewed the manuscript and study design and contributed to the final draft. The other authors recruited the participants and contributed to the final draft. All authors have read and agreed to the published version of the manuscript.

Funding: The author(s) disclosed receipt of the following financial support for the research, authorship, and/or publication of this article: The TOP-STAR study, including the article processing charge, is funded by Kowa Co., Ltd. The grant number is not applicable. No drugs will be donated or funded by the sponsor. The funding bodies had no role in the study design, data collection and analysis, decision to publish, or preparation of the manuscript.

Institutional Review Board Statement: This study was registered with the Japan Clinical Trial Registry (jRCTs051210212) and was approved by the ethics committees of the Kyoto Prefectural University of Medicine (CRB5200001). The TOP-STAR study is to be conducted in accordance with the Declaration of Helsinki.

Informed Consent Statement: Written informed consent has been obtained from all the participants.

Data Availability Statement: Data will not be publicly available.

Acknowledgments: We would like to thank all the clinical staff for their assistance with the execution of the clinical trial and EviPRO Holdings. Inc. for their technical assistance in the launch and execution of this trial.

Conflicts of Interest: H.O. received personal fees from MSD K.K., Mitsubishi Tanabe Pharma Corporation, Sumitomo Dainippon Pharma Co., Ltd., Novo Nordisk Pharma Ltd., Daiichi Sankyo Co., Ltd., Eli Lilly Japan K.K., Kyowa Hakko Kirin Company Ltd., Kissei Pharmaceutical Co., Ltd., Takeda Pharmaceutical Co., Ltd., Kowa Pharmaceutical Co., Ltd., Ono Pharmaceutical Co., Ltd. and Sanofi K.K. M.H. received personal fees from Ono Pharma Co. Ltd., AstraZeneca K.K., Oishi Kenko Inc., Yamada Bee Farm, Sumitomo Dainippon Pharma Co., Ltd., Eli Lilly, Japan, Daiichi Sankyo Co. Ltd., Mitsubishi Tanabe Pharma Corp., Sanofi K.K. and Kowa Pharma Co. Ltd., outside the submitted work. M.F. received personal fees from Oishi Kenko inc., Yamada Bee Farm, Sanofi K.K., Terumo Corp., Nippon Chemiphar Co., Ltd., Johnson & Johnson K.K. Medical Co., Abbott Japan Co. Ltd., Kissei Pharma Co., Ltd., Sumitomo Dainippon Pharma Co. Ltd., Mitsubishi Tanabe Pharma Corp., Daiichi Sankyo Co. Ltd., Sanofi K.K., Astellas Pharma Inc., MSD K.K., Kyowa Kirin Co. Ltd., Taisho Pharma Co., Ltd., Kowa Pharma Co. Ltd., Mochida Pharma Co. Ltd., Novo Nordisk Pharma Ltd., Ono Pharma Co. Ltd., Sanwa Kagaku Kenkyusho Co. Ltd., Eli Lilly Japan K.K., Takeda Pharma Co. Ltd., Bayer Yakuhin, Ltd., AstraZeneca K.K., Nippon Boehringer Ingelheim Co., Ltd., Teijin Pharma Ltd., Medtronic Japan Co. Ltd., Arkray Inc. and Nipro Corp. outside the submitted work. The other authors have nothing to disclose.

References

1. Abrams, P.; Cardozo, L.; Fall, M.; Griffiths, D.; Rosier, P.; Ulmsten, U.; van Kerrebroeck, P.; Victor, A.; Wein, A. The standardisation of terminology of lower urinary tract function: Report from the standardisation sub-committee of the international continence society. *Am. J. Obstet. Gynecol.* **2002**, *187*, 116–126. [CrossRef] [PubMed]
2. Aoki, Y.; Yokoyama, O. Pathogenesis and management of nocturia in the elderly. *Jpn. J. Geriatr.* **2013**, *50*, 434–439. (In Japanese)
3. Yoshimura, K.; Terada, N.; Matsui, Y.; Terai, A.; Kinukawa, N.; Arai, Y. Prevalence of and risk factors for nocturia: Analysis of a health screening program. *Int. J. Urol.* **2004**, *11*, 282–287. [CrossRef] [PubMed]

4. Wang, Y.; Hu, H.; Xu, K.; Zhang, X.; Wang, X.; Na, Y.; Kang, X. Prevalence, risk factors, and symptom bother of nocturia: A population-based survey in China. *World J. Urol.* **2015**, *33*, 677–683. [CrossRef] [PubMed]
5. Wen, L.; Wen, Y.B.; Wang, Z.M.; Wen, J.G.; Li, Z.Z.; Shang, X.P.; Liu, Z.S.; Jia, L.H.; Qin, G.J.; Heesakkers, J.; et al. Risk Factors of Nocturia (Two or More Voids Per Night) in Chinese People Older Than 40 Years. *Neurourol. Urodyn.* **2015**, *570*, 566–570. [CrossRef] [PubMed]
6. Madhu, C.; Coyne, K.; Hashim, H.; Chapple, C.; Milsom, I.; Kopp, Z. Nocturia: Risk factors and associated comorbidities; findings from the EpiLUTS study. *Int. J. Clin. Pr.* **2015**, *69*, 1508–1516. [CrossRef]
7. Chow, P.M.; Liu, S.P.; Chuang, Y.C.; Lee, K.S.; Yoo, T.K.; Liao, L.; Wang, J.; Liu, M.; Sumarsono, B.; Jong, J.J. The prevalence and risk factors of nocturia in China, South Korea, and Taiwan: Results from a cross-sectional, population-based study International Index of Erectile Function. *World J. Urol.* **2018**, *36*, 1853–1862. [CrossRef]
8. Hirayama, A.; Torimoto, K.; Mastusita, C.; Okamoto, N.; Morikawa, M.; Tanaka, N.; Yoshida, K.; Fujimoto, K.; Hirao, Y.; Kurumatani, N. Evaluation of Factors Influencing the Natural History of Nocturia in Elderly Subjects: Results of the Fujiwara-kyo Study. *J. Urol.* **2013**, *189*, 980–986. [CrossRef]
9. Furukawa, S. Smoking and prevalence of nocturia in Japanese patients with type 2 diabetes mellitus: A post-hoc analysis of The Dogo Study. *Neurourol. Urodyn.* **2017**, *36*, 1336–1341. [CrossRef]
10. Kawano, R.; Takahashi, F.; Hashimoto, Y.; Okamura, T.; Miki, A.; Kaji, A.; Sakai, R.; Kitagawa, N.; Senmaru, T.; Majima, S.; et al. Short energy intake is associated with muscle mass loss in older patients with type 2 diabetes: A prospective study of the KAMOGAWA-DM cohort. *Clin. Nutr.* **2021**, *40*, 1613–1620. [CrossRef]
11. Hashimoto, Y.; Sakai, R.; Ikeda, K.; Fukui, M. Association between sleep disorder and quality of life in patients with type 2 diabetes: A cross-sectional study. *BMC Endocr. Disord.* **2020**, *4*, 98. [CrossRef] [PubMed]
12. Nakagawa, H.; Niu, K.; Hozawa, A.; Ikeda, Y.; Kaiho, Y.; Ohmori-Matsuda, K.; Nakaya, N.; Kuriyama, S.; Ebihara, S.; Nagatomi, R.; et al. Impact of Nocturia on Bone Fracture and Mortality in Older Individuals: A Japanese Longitudinal Cohort Study. *J. Urol.* **2010**, *184*, 1413–1418. [CrossRef] [PubMed]
13. Perkovic, V.; Jardine, M.J.; Neal, B. Canagliflozin and Renal Outcomes in Type 2 Diabetes and Nephropathy. *N. Engl. J. Med.* **2019**, *380*, 2295–2306. [CrossRef] [PubMed]
14. McMurray, J.J.; Solomon, S.D.; Inzucchi, S.E.; Køber, L.; Kosiborod, M.N.; Martinez, F.A.; Ponikowski, P.; Sabatine, M.C.; Anand, I.S.; Bělohlávek, J.; et al. Dapagliflozin in Patients with Heart Failure and Reduced Ejection Fraction. *N. Engl. J. Med.* **2019**, *381*, 1995–2008. [CrossRef]
15. The Japan Diabetes Society. Recommendations for the Appropriate Use of SGLT2 Inhibitors. Available online: http://www.fa.kyorin.co.jp/jds/uploads/recommendation_SGLT2.pdf (accessed on 22 February 2022). (In Japanese).
16. Takegoshi, S.; Miyata, Y.; Ogata, N.; Saito, T. Availability and efficacy of 20-mg tofogliflozin administered every other day to type 2 diabetic patients. *Prog. Med.* **2015**, *35*, 1077–1088. (In Japanese)
17. Takeishi, S.; Tsuboi, H.; Takekoshi, S. Comparison of tofogliflozin 20 mg and ipragliflozin 50 mg used together with insulin glargine 300 U/ml using continuous glucose monitoring (CGM): A randomized crossover study. *Endocr. J.* **2017**, *64*, 995–1005. [CrossRef] [PubMed]
18. Kawasoe, S.; Maruguchi, Y.; Kajiya, S.; Uenomachi, H.; Miyata, M.; Kawase, M.; Kubozono, T.; Ohishi, M. Mechanism of the blood pressure-lowering effect of sodium-glucose cotransporter 2 inhibitors in obese patients with type 2 diabetes. *BMC Pharmacol. Toxicol.* **2017**, *18*, 23. [CrossRef]
19. Matsuo, T.; Miyata, Y.; Sakai, H. Effect of salt intake reduction on nocturia in patients with excessive salt intake. *Neurourol. Urodyn.* **2019**, *38*, 927–933. [CrossRef]
20. Ushigome, E.; Oyabu, C.; Iwai, K.; Kitagawa, N.; Kitae, A.; Kimura, T.; Yokota, I.; Ushigome, H.; Hamaguchi, M.; Asano, M.; et al. Effects of dietary salt restriction on home blood pressure in diabetic patients with excessive salt intake: A pilot study. *J. Clin. Biochem. Nutr.* **2019**, *65*, 252–257. [CrossRef]
21. Matsuo, T.; Miyata, Y.; Sakai, H. Daily salt intake is an independent risk factor for pollakiuria and nocturia. *Int. J. Urol.* **2017**, *24*, 384–389. [CrossRef]
22. Matsumoto, T.; Tabara, Y.; Murase, K.; Setoh, K.; Kawaguchi, T.; Nagashima, S.; Kosugi, S.; Nakayama, T.; Wakamura, T.; Hirai, T.; et al. Nocturia and increase in nocturnal blood pressure: The Nagahama study. *J. Hypertens.* **2018**, *36*, 2185–2192. [CrossRef] [PubMed]
23. Okumura, K.; Obayashi, K.; Tai, Y.; Yamagami, Y.; Negoro, H.; Kataoka, H.; Kurumatani, N.; Saeki, K. Association between NT-proBNP and nocturia among community-dwelling elderly males and females: A cross-sectional analysis of the HEIJO-KYO study. *Neurourol. Urodyn.* **2021**, *40*, 112–119. [CrossRef]
24. Ishii, H. The Japanese version of the Diabetes Treatment Satisfaction Questionnaire (DTSQ): Translation and clinical evaluation. *J. Clin. Exp. Med.* **2000**, *192*, 809–814.
25. Sato, E.; Ochiai, R.; Shibayama, T.; Nishigaki, M.; Abe, Y.; Sawa, T.; Suzukamo, Y.; Kazuma, K. Reliability and validity of revised and short form versions of diabetes diet-related quality of life scale. *Diabetol. Int.* **2017**, *8*, 181–192. [CrossRef] [PubMed]

26. Kobayashi, S.; Honda, S.; Murakami, K.; Sasaki, S.; Okubo, H.; Hirota, N.; Notsu, A.; Fukui, M.; Date, C. Both comprehensive and brief self-administered diet history questionnaires satisfactorily rank nutrient intakes in Japanese adults. *J. Epidemiol.* **2012**, *22*, 151–159. [CrossRef]
27. Homma, Y.; Yoshida, M.; Yamanishi, T.; Gotoh, M. Core lowerurinary tract symptom (CLSS) questionnaire: A reliable tool in the overall assessment of lower urinary tract symptoms. *Int. J. Urol.* **2008**, *15*, 816–820. [CrossRef]

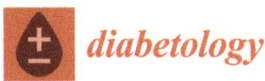

Commentary

Insulin Injection-Related Skin Lipodystrophies: Blemish or Pathology?

Felice Strollo [1], Ersilia Satta [2] and Sandro Gentile [2,3,*]

[1] Endocrinology and Diabetes, IRCCS San Raffaele Pisana, I-00163 Rome, Italy
[2] Nefrocenter Research & Nyx Start-Up, I-80030 Naples, Italy
[3] Department of Internal Medicine, Luigi Vanvitelli University of Campania, I-50138 Naples, Italy
* Correspondence: s.gentile1949@gmail.com

Abstract: The number of adult individuals with insulin-treated diabetes mellitus (DM) is steadily increasing worldwide. The main local complications of insulin injection are lipohypertrophies (LHs), i.e., subcutaneous nodules consisting of aggregates of macro-adipocytes and fibrin. These nodules result from errors repeatedly made by patients while injecting insulin. Despite being very common, LH lesions/nodules due to incorrect insulin injection techniques are often flat and hardly visible and thus require thorough deep palpation examination and ultrasonography (US) for detection. Identifying LHs is crucial, especially in elderly and frail subjects, because they may eventually result in poor diabetes control due to associated unpredictable insulin release patterns. Raising awareness of the adequate detection of LHs and their clinical consequences is crucial and urgent. A call to action is required on this topic at all levels of undergraduate and postgraduate education.

Keywords: diabetes; insulin; injection technique; lipohypertrophy

1. Introduction

Lipohypertrophy (LH) at insulin injection sites is a typical complication in insulin-requiring type 2-diabetic people resulting from the localized accumulation of subcutaneous fat [1,2]. Unfortunately, it occurs frequently, affecting 47% (range 5–70%) of patients on insulin [1,3]. However, LH can be prevented by overcoming severe educational defects that cause the patient to progressively acquire bad injection habits, including the choice of restricted skin areas, the repeated utilization of a single needle, or ice-cold preparations.

2. What May Happen to People with LHs

LHs do not only represent skin imperfections. Indeed, they often have severe metabolic consequences due to scattering insulin absorption and, inevitably, high blood glucose oscillations [4,5]. A few years ago, we published the case of a woman who had a prominent LH on her abdomen and, wishing to wear a bikini, steadily and vigorously massaged her unsightly abdominal lump with the most disparate cosmetic creams. As a result, she woke up in the emergency room of a hospital after a severe hypoglycemic event—which she did not remember—caused by the sudden release of the insulin trapped in the LH nodule [6].

3. A Case of Monster LH

In another case, we described the presence of two abdominal tangerine-like symmetrical bumps with a central hyperchromic navel, which, on ultrasound examination, turned out to be LHs with a gelatinous/fluid content. When analyzed, the latter had a 13 times higher insulin concentration than in the blood. These lesions only disappeared after three years of correct injection behavior and regularly occurring educational training. However, despite the size of the scarring umbilications having decreased, the dyschromia still subsided [7] (see Figure 1).

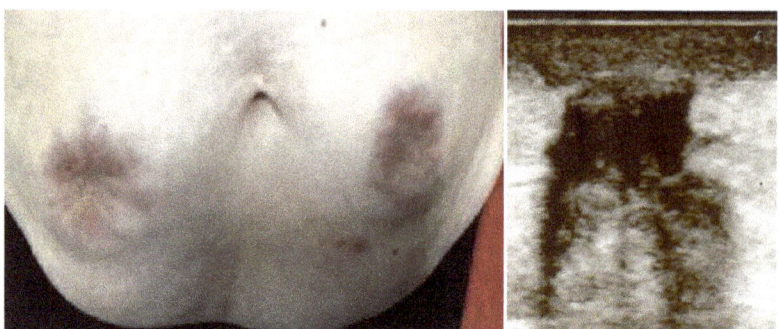

Figure 1. Two major LH swellings were evident at the two sides of the navel markedly protruding from the cutaneous plane (**left** panel). The central areas of both LH lesions were easily identified by sight and touch as umbilicated, hyperchromic, and clefted. In the (**right** panel), ultrasound scans of lipo-hypertrophic area are also provided: the thickening of the dermis is clearly visible together with the central, colliquative area.

4. Practical Considerations

Why do patients stubbornly inject insulin into lipodystrophic nodules? The answer is complex and largely depends on educational deficiencies when starting insulin therapy, which are aggravated by the lack of required periodic injection site inspections by diabetes teams, as previously described by our team in [7]. However, another reason behind it is the painlessness of mistreated and thus denervated skin tissue hosting LHs. Indeed, about half of patients on insulin self-injecting the drug four times a day, i.e., 1460 times per year, unconsciously or secretly accept risking high blood sugar levels by avoiding frequent painful injections [8].

5. Why Do People with Diabetes Forget the Lessons over Time?

The answer is not simple, but one can resort to a fundamental principle of therapeutic education, borrowing the axiom "knowing is not the same thing as knowing how to do". Evidence for this stems from a Charlie Brown strip where the famous cartoon character—drawn by Charles Monroe Schulz in the 1950s—informed Lucy of having taught Snoopy to whistle. When she objected that Snoopy could not whistle yet, he retorted that he had only said he had taught him, not that Snoopy had learned! In addition to this, we cannot rule out the role for comfortable movements, especially for older adults with joint difficulties, a certain degree of habit, and, for some, the tendency for depression and poor self-care, which are typical traits of chronic diseases with a longstanding asymptomatic phase such as diabetes. Finally, we should remember how difficult it is to change consolidated habits involving errors and bad clinical practice [1,8].

6. What Are the Consequences of Injection Technique Errors?

First, an unpredictable absorption of the preparation injected into the LH alters the expected synchronism between the post-meal rise in blood sugar and the immediate insulin action [4,5]. The direct consequence of such a phenomenon is considerable variability in circulating glucose levels, which is a recognized severe cardiovascular risk factor [9]. Secondly, such variability entails poor glycemic control and, even worse, repeated dangerous hypoglycemic episodes in the absence of eating errors, missed meals, vomiting, diarrhea, and insulin dose calculation errors The abovementioned LH consequences also burden patients with a poor quality of life and the national health system with excess medical and social expenditure [10]. The skin undergoes fundamental structural changes with aging, potentially increasing the risk for LHs. Therefore, LH side effects are hazardous in elderly individuals because of their inner frailty, frequently associated comorbidities, and possible hypoglycemia-related acute cardiovascular events [11].

When undergoing a severe episode of hypoglycemia, the patient can become unconscious and thus requires the intervention of family members, caregivers, or anyone else making emergency calls to the GP or first-aid services. This event might end in hospitalization, with the patient's and caregiver's absence from the workplace.

The above entails an apparent increase in costs quantifiable through the national tariff for health services and would not occur if adequate educational training was provided [9].

Indeed, our recent data document tenfold higher hypoglycemic event-related costs in patients with LH than without LH, and over eightfold lower costs—therefore, approaching those of patients injecting insulin correctly—after adequate systematic, multimodal, and repeated educational training [7,8,10].

Moreover, when injected into healthy skin instead of LH nodules, required insulin doses decrease by 20–25%. Despite being twenty times lower than those due to less unpredictable hypoglycemic events, the resulting savings are of great value when projected on large populations and compared to the annual costs of insulin, especially in the case of new rapid or basal analogs [1,2,9].

7. What Can We Do to Prevent Lipohypertrophies?

Indeed, the picture is not comforting. Suffice it to say that a recent survey conducted in China and other countries on health professionals (doctors and nurses) mercilessly documents that over 50% of patients have poor knowledge about LHs, associated metabolic consequences, and, even worse, how to avoid or counteract this type of complication [12–18].

In Italy, the situation is similar. Indeed, the occurrence of LH in at least 45% of insulin patients documents the similar level of our treatment system's inefficiency.

Unfortunately, apart from a few willing people who are stubbornly engaged in therapeutic education, including that involving correct injection techniques, LH is most often forgotten or ignored, thus becoming a "non-problem".

8. A Proposal for the Future

Considering that three to four million persons in Italy have diabetes, and about 40–50% of them will sooner or later require insulin, correct insulin injection techniques should have a more prominent place in undergraduate, postgraduate, and specialization courses. Specifically, doctors and nurses should follow dedicated training procedures on proper injection techniques. Outpatient general medicine practices and diabetes wards should also become involved in practical education paths, including primarily structured LH identification methods (Figure 2) [3]. In our youthful memories, none of this existed, and it was the experience in the field that sometimes compensated this absence. Another practical solution to the problem may also come from insulin manufacturers, who could include in pens and vial packages dedicated visuals and detailed descriptions on how to inject and use insulin correctly.

The relaxed, even condescending attitude towards LHs has to change, and we count on our most resourceful readers to make this happen as fast as possible.

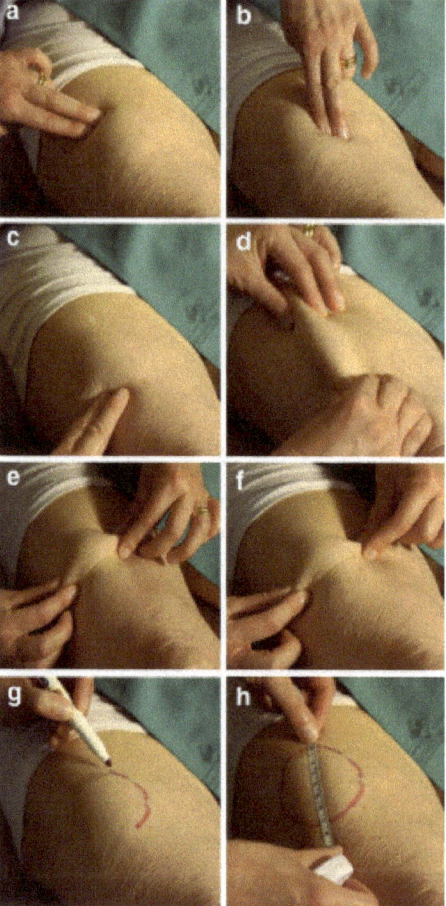

Figure 2. LH identification technique. The figure shows how to identify a lesion after a thorough inspection of the area by performing repeated vertical and horizontal fingertip movements over and around it (**a–c**), pinching it (**d–f**), and marking it (**g**), as well as how to finally measure it (**h**).

9. Key Summary Points

1. Improper Insulin injection causes skin lipohypertrophic lesions (LHs), which are often flat and barely visible, thus requiring thorough deep palpation examination and ultrasonography (US) for identification;
2. The detection of LHs is crucial to prevent poor diabetes control due to unpredictable insulin-release patterns;
3. The skin undergoes fundamental structural changes with aging, potentially increasing the risk of developing LHs;
4. Too many healthcare professionals (doctors and nurses) know little or nothing about lipohypertrophy and its associated metabolic consequences and, worse, they do not know how to avoid or counteract this type of complication;
5. The data from the literature suggest the need (i) to take specific actions to prevent and control the high risk of acute hypoglycemia-related cardiovascular events, especially in older subjects, and (ii) to identify specific, better-targeted, practical, and structured educational programs suited to older patients.

Author Contributions: S.G., E.S. and F.S. ideated and wrote this text and shared responsibilities jointly. All authors have read and agreed to the published version of the manuscript.

Funding: The authors received no funding for this manuscript.

Institutional Review Board Statement: The IRB from the Naples "Vanvitelli" University approved the study on 16 July 2022 under the n. 11619.

Informed Consent Statement: Not applicable.

Data Availability Statement: Data is contained within the article.

Conflicts of Interest: The authors declare no conflict of interest.

References

1. Gentile, S.; Guarino, G.; Della Corte, T.; Marino, G.; Satta, E.; Pasquarella, M.; Romano, C.; Alfrone, C.; Strollo, F. Role of Structured Education in Reducing Lypodistrophy and its Metabolic Complications in Insulin-Treated People with Type 2 Diabetes: A Randomized Multicenter Case–Control Study. *Diabetes Ther.* **2021**, *12*, 1379–1398. [CrossRef] [PubMed]
2. Blanco, M.; Hernández, M.; Strauss, K.; Amaya, M. Prevalence and risk factors of lipohypertrophy in insulin-injecting patients with diabetes. *Diabetes Metab.* **2013**, *39*, 445–453. [CrossRef] [PubMed]
3. Gentile, S.; Guarino, G.; Giancaterini, A.; Guida, P.; Strollo, F.; AMD-OSDI Italian Injection Technique Study Group. A suitable palpation technique allows to identify skin lipohypertrophic lesions in insulin-treated people with diabetes. *SpringerPlus* **2016**, *5*, 1–7. [CrossRef] [PubMed]
4. Gentile, S.; Agrusta, M.; Guarino, G.; Carbone, L.; Cavallaro, V.; Carucci, I.; Strollo, F. Metabolic consequences of incorrect insulin administration techniques in aging subjects with diabetes. *Geol. Rundsch.* **2010**, *48*, 121–125. [CrossRef] [PubMed]
5. Famulla, S.; Hövelmann, U.; Fischer, A.; Coester, H.-V.; Hermanski, L.; Kaltheuner, M.; Kaltheuner, L.; Heinemann, L.; Heise, T.; Hirsch, L. Insulin Injection Into Lipohypertrophic Tissue: Blunted and More Variable Insulin Absorption and Action and Impaired Postprandial Glucose Control. *Diabetes Care* **2016**, *39*, 1486–1492. [CrossRef] [PubMed]
6. Improta, M.; Strollo, F.; Gentile, S.; AMD-OSDI Study Group on Injection Technique. Lessons learned from an unusual case of severe hypoglycemia. *Diabetes Metab. Syndr. Clin. Res. Rev.* **2019**, *13*, 1237–1239. [CrossRef] [PubMed]
7. Gentile, S.; Guarino, G.; Strollo, F. How to treat improper insulin injection-related lipohypertrophy: A 3-year follow-up of a monster case and an update on treatment. *Diabetes Res. Clin. Pract.* **2020**, *171*, 108534. [CrossRef] [PubMed]
8. Gentile, S.; Guarino, G.; Della Corte, T.; Marino, G.; Satta, E.; Pasquarella, M.; Romano, C.; Alfrone, C.; Giordano, L.; Loiacono, F.; et al. The Durability of an Intensive, Structured Education-Based Rehabilitation Protocol for Best Insulin Injection Practice: The ISTERP-2 Study. *Diabetes Ther.* **2021**, *12*, 2557–2569. [CrossRef] [PubMed]
9. Nusca, A.; Tuccinardi, D.; Albano, M.; Cavallaro, C.; Ricottini, E.; Manfrini, S.; Pozzilli, P.; Di Sciascio, G. Glycemic variability in the development of cardiovascular complications in diabetes. *Diabetes/Metabolism Res. Rev.* **2018**, *34*, e3047. [CrossRef] [PubMed]
10. Gentile, S.; Strollo, F. Cost saving effects of a short-term educational intervention entailing lower hypoglycaemic event rates in people with type 1 diabetes and lipo-hypertrophy. *Diabetes Res. Clin. Pr.* **2018**, *143*, 320–321. [CrossRef] [PubMed]
11. Gentile, S.; Guarino, G.; Della Corte, T.; Marino, G.; Fusco, A.; Corigliano, G.; Colarusso, S.; Piscopo, M.; Improta, M.R.; Corigliano, M.; et al. Lipohypertrophy in Elderly Insulin-Treated Patients With Type 2 Diabetes. *Diabetes Ther.* **2020**, *12*, 107–119. [CrossRef] [PubMed]
12. Wu, X.; Zhao, F.; Zhang, M.; Yuan, L.; Zheng, Y.; Huang, J.; Li, Y.; Li, C. Insulin Injection Knowledge, Attitudes, and Practices of Nurses in China: A Cross-Sectional Nationwide Study. *Diabetes Ther.* **2021**, *12*, 2451–2469. [CrossRef] [PubMed]
13. Adhikari, S.; Poudel, R.S.; Rajbanshi, L.; Shrestha, S. Assessment of Insulin Injection Practice of Nurses Working in a Tertiary Healthcare Center of Nepal. *Nurs. Res. Pract.* **2018**, *2018*, 1–6. [CrossRef] [PubMed]
14. Mushta, A.M. Study of insulin injection technique amongst the nursing staff. *Pak. J. Med. Sci.* **2006**, *22*, 310–312.
15. Yacoub, M.; Demeh, W.; Darawad, M.; Barr, J.; Saleh, A.; Saleh, M. An assessment of diabetes-related knowledge among registered nurses working in hospitals in Jordan. *Int. Nurs. Rev.* **2014**, *61*, 255–262. [CrossRef] [PubMed]
16. Theofanidis, D. In-Hospital Administration of Insulin by Nurses in Northern Greece: An Observational Study. *Diabetes Spectr.* **2017**, *30*, 175–181. [CrossRef] [PubMed]
17. Robb, A.; Reid, B.; A Laird, E. Insulin knowledge and practice: A survey of district nurses in Northern Ireland. *Br. J. Community Nurs.* **2017**, *22*, 138–145. [CrossRef] [PubMed]
18. Derr, R.L.; Sivanandy, M.S.; Bronich-Hall, L.; Rodriguez, A. Insulin-related knowledge among health care professionals in inter-nal medicine. *Diabetes Spectr.* **2007**, *20*, 177–185. [CrossRef]

MDPI
St. Alban-Anlage 66
4052 Basel
Switzerland
Tel. +41 61 683 77 34
Fax +41 61 302 89 18
www.mdpi.com

Diabetology Editorial Office
E-mail: diabetology@mdpi.com
www.mdpi.com/journal/diabetology

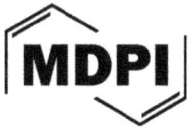

www.ingramcontent.com/pod-product-compliance
Lightning Source LLC
LaVergne TN
LVHW070617100526
838202LV00012B/664